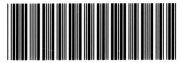

369 0240352

KU-276-303

Medical Radiology

Diagnostic Imaging

For further volumes:
http://www.springer.com/series/4354

Giuseppe Guglielmi

Editor

Osteoporosis and Bone Densitometry Measurements

Foreword by
Maximilian F. Reiser

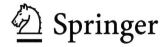 Springer

Editor
Giuseppe Guglielmi
Department of Radiology
University of Foggia
Foggia
Italy

ISSN 0942-5373
ISBN 978-3-642-27883-9   ISBN 978-3-642-27884-6   (eBook)
DOI 10.1007/978-3-642-27884-6
Springer Heidelberg New York Dordrecht London

Library of Congress Control Number: 2013932464

Printed on acid-free paper

Springer is part of Springer Science+Business Media (www.springer.com)

Foreword

Osteoporosis is a disease which is associated with an extraordinary burden for the healthcare systems. As pointed out in this book, the costs for hip fractures in the elderly are already comparable to those of myocardial infarction. Mortality following hip fractures is similar to that of breast cancer. Vertebral, wrist, and humeral fractures due to osteoporosis are also major healthcare issues which greatly reduce the quality of life of the affected patients.

Due to the demographic developments in the near future with an increasing population of elderly persons, osteoporotic fractures will considerably increase. The methods and techniques to assess osteoporosis and to characterize conditions with compromised bone strength that increase fracture risk, have expanded over the past decades. Innovative treatment options allowing for a personalized selection of drugs have been introduced or are under investigation.

Professor Giuseppe Guglielmi and other scientists of international renown contributed most informative chapters pertinent to relevant aspects of osteoporosis. Various methods to diagnose osteoporosis and fracture risk, such as radiography, FRAX, DEXA, axial and peripheral QCT, quantitative ultrasound, and high resolution imaging are dealt with. Moreover, most informative and up-to-date information is provided concerning epidemiology and therapy of osteoporosis as well as complications and important differential diagnoses.

We are confident that this book will be of great value for all disciplines involved in the diagnosis and treatment of osteoporosis—a disease which may become an even more menacing challenge world wide. The series editors of "Medical Radiology—Diagnostic Imaging" would like to express their sincere gratitude to Prof. Guglielmi and authors of "Osteoporosis and Bone Densitometry Measurements" for this invaluable book.

Munich, January 2013   Maximilian F. Reiser

Contents

Contributors

J. E. Adams Manchester Academic Health Science Centre and Radiology Department, Manchester Royal Infirmary, Central Manchester Universities NHS Foundation Trust, Oxford Road, Manchester M13 9WL, UK

Jan S. Bauer Department of Radiology, Technische Universität München, Ismaninger Str. 22, 81675 Munich, Germany

Maria Luisa Brandi Unit of Bone and Mineral Metabolism, Department of Internal Medicine, University of Florence, Medical School, Viale Pieraccini 6, 50139 Florence, Italy

J. Damilakis Department of Medical Physics, University of Crete, P.O. Box 2208, 71003 Heraklion, Crete, Greece

Anastasia N. Fotiadou Hinchingbrooke Hospital NHS Trust, Hinchingbrooke Park, Huntingdon, Cambridgeshire, PE29 6NT, UK

Harry K. Genant Department of Radiology, University of California San Francisco, San Francisco, CA 94143-0628, USA

James F. Griffith Department of Imaging and Interventional Radiology, The Chinese University of Hong Kong, Shatin, Hong Kong, People's Republic of China; Department of Radiology, Boston University, 820, Harrison Avenue, FGH building, 3rd floor, Boston, MA 02118, USA

Ali Guermazi Department of Radiology, Boston University, 820, Harrison Avenue, FGH building, 3rd floor, Boston, MA 02118, USA; Department of Radiology, Quantitative Imaging Center, Musculoskeletal Imaging, Boston University School of Medicine, 820 Harrison Avenue, Boston, MA 02118, USA

Giuseppe Guglielmi Department of Radiology, University of Foggia, Viale Luigi Pinto 1, 71100 Foggia, Italy; Department of Radiology, Scientific Institute "Casa Sollievo della Sofferenza" Hospital, Viale Cappuccini 1, 71013 San Giovanni Rotondo, Foggia, Italy

Lotfi Hacein-Bey Interventional Neuroradiology and Neuroradiology, Radiological Associates of Sacramento Medical Group, Inc, 1500 Expo Parkway, Sacramento, CA 95815, USA

Daichi Hayashi Department of Radiology, Boston University, 820, Harrison Avenue, FGH building, 3rd floor, Boston, MA 02118, USA

Mohamed Jarraya Department of Radiology, Boston University, 820, Harrison Avenue, FGH building, 3rd floor, Boston, MA 02118, USA

Christian R. Krestan Department of Radiology, Vienna General Hospital, Medical University of Vienna, Waehringerstr. 18-20, 1090 Vienna, Austria

Leon Lenchik Department of Radiology, Wake Forest University School of Medicine, Winston-Salem, NC, USA

Thomas M. Link Department of Radiology and Biomedical Imaging, University of California San Francisco, 400 Parnassus Ave, A367, 0628, San Francisco, CA 94143, USA

Salvatore Minisola Department of Internal Medicine and Medical Disciplines, University of Rome "Sapienza", Viale del Policlinico 155, 00161 Rome, Italy

Michelangelo Nasuto Department of Radiology, University of Foggia, Viale Luigi Pinto 1, 71100 Foggia, Italy

Stefan Nemec Department of Radiology, Vienna General Hospital, Medical University of Vienna, Waehringerstr. 18-20, 1090 Vienna, Austria

Ursula Nemec Department of Radiology, Vienna General Hospital, Medical University of Vienna, Waehringerstr. 18-20, 1090 Vienna, Austria

Alexander M. Norbash Department of Radiology, Boston University Medical Center, 820, Harrison Avenue, Boston, MA 02118, USA

Janina M. Patsch Department of Radiology and Biomedical Imaging, University of California, San Francisco, 185 Berry Street, Suite 350, San Francisco, CA 94107, USA

Wilfred C. G. Peh Department of Diagnostic Radiology, Khoo Teck Puat Hospital Alexandra Health, 90 Yishun Central, Singapore 768228, Republic of Singapore

Prisco Piscitelli Department of Internal Medicine, Unit of Bone and Mineral Metabolism, University of Florence, Medical School, Viale Pieraccini 6, 50139 Florence, Italy

S. M. Ploof Department of Radiology, Wake Forest University School of Medicine, Winston-Salem, NC, USA

Elisabetta Romagnoli Department of Internal Medicine and Medical Disciplines, University of Rome "Sapienza", Viale del Policlinico 155, 00161 Rome, Italy

G. Solomou Department of Medical Physics, University Hospital of Heraklion, P.O. Box 1352, 71110 Heraklion, Crete, Greece

Sivasubramanian Srinivasan Department of Diagnostic Radiology, Khoo Teck Puat Hospital Alexandra Health, 90 Yishun Central, Singapore 768228, Republic of Singapore

S. Wuertzer Department of Radiology, Wake Forest University School of Medicine, Winston-Salem, NC, USA

Epidemiology of Osteoporosis and Fragility Fractures

Maria Luisa Brandi and Prisco Piscitelli

Contents

Abstract

According to the latest definition of osteoporosis, both bone mineral density (BMD) and bone quality are important in determining skeletal fragility fractures. Actually, a large proportion of fractures occur in people with BMD values indicating osteopenia or normal status. However, for epidemiological purpose, the prevalence of osteoporosis continues to be assessed on the basis of bone demineralization (2.5 Standard Deviations below the young adult mean values). Osteoporosis should not be regarded as a condition affecting exclusively women, as 20–25 % of hip fragility fractures occur in men, with a higher post-fracture mortality rate if compared to that recorded for females. All osteoporotic fractures should be considered as the first signal of an evolving diseases: fractures occurring at vertebra, forearm, humerus, ribs, feet, and hip are always associated with a higher risk of subsequent fragility fractures, and mortality (which is dramatically increased after hip fractures, up to 25 % at 1 year). A total of 20 % of people living in Western countries are thought to be affected by osteoporosis, with 4 million new fragility fractures occurring in Europe every year (including more than 800,000 hip fractures). Total direct costs of osteoporosis and related fractures are estimated to exceed 25 billion Euros in Europe and 18 billion Dollars in the United States. Medical expenditures are expected to double by the year 2050 based on the expected demographic projections. However, osteoporotic fractures represent even now an increasing problem in Asia and South America, with China, India, and Brazil accounting for 1 million of hip fractures. In this perspective, the World Health Organization (WHO) considers osteoporosis to be second to cardiovascular diseases as a critical health problem worldwide.

M. L. Brandi (✉) · P. Piscitelli
Department of Internal Medicine,
Unit of Bone and Mineral Metabolism,
University of Florence, Medical School,
Viale Pieraccini 6, 50139 Florence, Italy
e-mail: m.brandi@dmi.unifi.it

G. Guglielmi (ed.), *Osteoporosis and Bone Densitometry Measurements*, Medical Radiology. Diagnostic Imaging,
DOI: 10.1007/174_2012_747, © Springer-Verlag Berlin Heidelberg 2013

1   Osteoporosis as a Disease

Osteoporosis has been fairly recognized as a "disease" only in recent years (between 1980s and 1990s), along with the availability of the results from the first large clinical trials on drugs effective for fragility fracture prevention. The definition of osteoporosis has been updated in 2001 because clinical practice highlighted the relevance of other risk factors (i.e. bone quality and micro-architecture) in addition to low bone mineral density (at least 2.5 Standard Deviations below the young adult mean values), as measured by DXA (Dual-energy X-rays Absorptiometry). Therefore, osteoporosis is now considered as a "skeletal disorder characterized by compromised bone strength that increases the risk of fracture". By referring to "bone strength", the new definition includes information concerning both bone density (expressed as grams of mineral per area or volume) and quality (which integrates properties attributable to micro-architecture, turnover, micro-damage accumulation and mineralization status) (NIH Consensus Development Panel on Osteoporosis 2001). The World Health Organization (WHO) considers osteoporosis to be second only to cardiovascular diseases as a critical health problem worldwide (Kanis et al. 2008). Increased life expectancy is associated with a greater frailty of elderly people and a higher prevalence of chronic and degenerative diseases. About 20 % of all post-menopausal women living in western countries would met current WHO criteria for the diagnosis of osteoporosis. In this frame, osteoporosis and its complications—especially hip fractures—represent a challenge for health professionals and decision makers in the twenty first century.

2   The Burden of Osteoporotic Fractures

Data available for those countries characterized by higher proportion of elderly people on the general population have shown that incidence and costs of hip fractures in the elderly are already comparable to those of acute myocardial infarction in the whole adult population (Piscitelli et al. 2007). In white women, the lifetime risk of developing hip fracture is 1 in 6, compared with a 1 in 9 risk of being diagnosed with breast cancer (Gullberg et al. 2007). Furthermore, the current mortality following hip fractures is similar to that observed for breast cancer, with a 5 % acute mortality rate and a 15–25 % 1 year-mortality (Keene et al. 1993). Hip fractures in the elderly are clearly associated with osteoporosis and require a longer period of hospitalization than all other pathologies, with the only exception of psychiatric diseases (Papaioannou et al. 2001). Once hip fracture has occurred, the ability to walk is completely lost

in 20 % of cases, and only 30–40 % of patients recover a degree of autonomy comparable to the period before the fracture (Hagsten et al. 2006; Di Monaco et al. 2006; Zimmermann et al. 2006; Latham 2006). Vertebral fractures or deformities are the most common osteoporotic fractures (Cummings et al. 2002). These fractures usually cause back pain, loss of height, deformity, immobility, and even pulmonary dysfunction, thus resulting in a significant impact on activities of daily living (ADLs); their impact on quality of life can be relevant also in terms of reduced self-esteem (distorted body image) and depression. According to the European Vertebral Osteoporosis Study (EVOS), in about 12 % of both men and women aged 50–80 years old it is possible to detect vertebral deformities, with their prevalence increasing with age in both sexes (O'Neill et al. 1996). Vertebral deformities, even if asymptomatic, are associated with adverse outcomes including back pain, physical impairment (Ettinger et al. 1992; Nevitt et al. 1998), a higher risk of subsequent osteoporotic fractures (Hasserius et al. 2003; Lindsay et al. 2001; Pongchaiyakul et al. 2005) and an increased risk of mortality (Lindsay et al. 2001; Ismail et al. 1998). However, two-thirds of vertebral fractures do not come to clinical attention (Fechtenbaum et al. 2005), and it is very difficult to assess their incidence among general population. Wrist or forearm fractures represent the most common breakage among peri-menopausal women (typically between 40 and 50 years old), with their incidence rising quickly after the menopause, probably as a consequence of a hormone-related fast bone loss process, but reaching a plateau after the age of 65 (Cummings et al. 2002). Wrist fractures are also frequent in men aged <70, but the age-adjusted female-to male ratio remains four to one (Cummings et al. 2002). Wrist fractures increase almost two folds the risk of subsequent hip or vertebral fractures, but also the risk of new forearm breakage and other skeletal fractures is increased by 3.3 times and 2.4 respectively (Klotzbuecher et al. 2000). Humeral fractures represent the third most common fracture in people aged >65 years old and have been associated to a higher risk of subsequent hip fractures (Clinton 2009). Actually, a proximal humeral fracture increases more than five times the risk of hip fracture at 1 year (Clinton 2009). Incidence rates estimated for fractures of the proximal humerus and other skeletal sites increase with age and seem to be more frequent in women with poor neuromuscular function but also in ageing men, with 75 % of these fractures being caused by moderate or low energy trauma (Cummings et al. 2002; Kelsey et al. 1992. Even fractures occurring at foot/ankle or ribs, have been found to double the risk of subsequent hip, vertebral, forearm or other skeletal fractures (Klotzbuecher et al. 2000), thus confirming that all osteoporotic fractures should be considered as the first signal of an evolving diseases. A 10 % loss of bone mass at vertebral sites is associated

Country	Hip fractures (hospitalizations per year)	Other fractures (hospitalizations per year)	Osteoporosis prevalence (if data available)	Expenditures due to hip fractures (million Euros)
Austria	12,000	–	–	156
Belgium	13,000	–	–	160
Denmark	9,600	–	41 % of women >50 18 % of men >50	48
Finland	7,700	–	–	150
France	72,000	46,000	–	600
Germany	135,000	–	6.5 million women and 1.3 million men	1,400
Greece	13,500	–	–	44
Ireland	3,000	–	–	8
Italy	80,000	60,000	4 million women and 800,000 men	1,000
Netherlands	15,000	–	–	180
Portugal	8,500	–	–	51
Spain	31,000	–	2 million women >50 (26 % of people >50)	220
Sweden	17,000	–	15 % of women >50 8 % of men >50	300
Switzerland	16,000	8,000	–	145
UK (Britain)	86,000	–	–	850
USA	270,000	–	54 % of women >50[a] 30 % of men >50[a] (12 million people)	2,900
Canada	30,000	–	25 % of women >50 12 % of men >50	300
Argentina	34,000	–	25 % of women >50	140
Brazil	121,000	–	10 million women >50	1,400
Mexico	–	–	25 % of women >50	120
Australia	20,000	–	27 % of women >60 11 % of men >60	180
Japan	153,000	–		1,120
India	300,000	–	36 million people	–
China	687,000	–	50 % of women >50 22.5 % of men >50 (70 million people)	1,200

[a] US prevalence data refers to Caucasian people; In the US general population, 12 million people >50 years old are expected to have osteoporosis

with a two-fold higher risk of developing vertebral fractures, and similarly, a 10 % loss of bone mass at the hip can double the risk of future hip fracture (Klotzbuecher et al. 2000). According to the International Osteoporosis Foundation (IOF) statistics, one in three women over 50 will experience osteoporotic fractures, as will one man out five (International Osteoporosis Foundation 2012). Osteoporosis is thought to affect over 75 million people in western countries (Europe, USA and Japan), with an estimated incidence of 10 million new fragility fractures per year worldwide (1.6 million occurring at the hip in people >65 years old, 1.7 million at the forearm and 1.4 million classified as clinical vertebral fractures) (Johnell and Kanis 2006). About 50 % of all these fractures are thought to occur in the Western Pacific region and Southeast Asia, with the other 50 % affecting European and American people (no specific data are available for Africa) (Johnell and Kanis 2006). The combined lifetime risk for hip, forearm and vertebral fractures coming to clinical attention is around 40 %, equivalent to the risk of developing cardiovascular diseases (Kanis 2002). Data are particularly impressive for hip fractures, as they are thought to increase by 310 % in men and 240 % in women before 2050 (Cummings et al. 2002). Since now, in European countries, osteoporosis-related disability following fragility fractures is greater than that caused by all cancers (with the exception of lung cancer) and it is comparable to that associated with major chronic non-communicable diseases, such as rheumatoid arthritis, asthma and hypertension (Johnell and Kanis 2006). Osteoporosis should not be regarded as a condition affecting exclusively women, as 20–25 % of hip fragility fractures occur in men, with a higher post-fracture mortality rate if compared to that recorded for females (Cummings et al. 2002). It has been estimated that the lifetime risk of experiencing an osteoporotic fracture in men over the age of 50 is about 30 %, similar to the lifetime risk of developing prostate cancer (Melton et al. 1992). IOF key statistics for Europe lead to an estimation of 4 million new osteoporotic fractures per year (8 per minute or 1 every 8 s), with about 800,000 of these being hip fractures affecting 179,000 men and 611,000 women (International Osteoporosis Foundation 2012; Johnell and Kanis 2006). Total direct costs are estimated to exceed 25 billion Euros and are expected at least to double by the year 2050 (based on the expected demographic projections for Europe) (International Osteoporosis Foundation 2012). In the following table, we have resumed all the main available epidemiological information for different countries in the world concerning the prevalence of osteoporosis, the number of hospital admissions per year due to fractures occurring at hip and other skeletal sites, and estimated expenditures related to osteoporotic fractures (International Osteoporosis Foundation 2012). It must be pointed out that while hip fractures are almost always hospitalized, hospital admissions due to other fractures (i.e. hospitalizations following wrist, forearm, leg, feet, and clinical vertebral fractures) represent only a proportion of the fractures occurring in the general population. Similarly, to the costs sustained at national level for hip fractures should be added also expenditures due to other osteoporotic fractures (those resulting in hospital admissions and surgery, and those requiring more conservative or home-based treatments). It is important to underline the increasing burden of osteoporosis and major fragility fractures—especially hip fractures—in China, India and Latin America.

References

Clinton J (2009) Proximal humeral fracture as a risk factor for subsequent hip fractures. J Bone Joint Surg (Am) 91:503–511

Cummings SR et al (2002) Epidemiology and outcomes of osteoporotic fractures. Lancet 359:1761–1767

Di Monaco M et al (2006) Muscle mass and functional recovery in women with hip fracture. Am J Phys Med Rehabil 85(3):209–215

Ettinger B et al (1992) Contribution of vertebral deformities to chronic back pain and disability. The Study of Osteoporotic Fractures Research Group. J Bone Min Res 7:449–456

Fechtenbaum J et al (2005) Reporting of vertebral fractures on spine X-rays. Osteoporosis Int 16:1823e6

Gullberg B et al (2007) World-wide projections for hip fracture. Osteoporos Int 7:407

Hagsten B et al (2006) Health-related quality of life and selfreported ability concerning ADL and IADL after hip fracture: a randomized trial. Acta Orthop 77(1):114–119

Hasserius R et al (2003) Prevalent vertebral deformities predict increased mortality and increased fracture rate in both men and women: a 10-year population-based study of 598 individuals from the Swedish cohort in the European Vertebral Osteoporosis Study. Osteoporos Int 14:61–68

International Osteoporosis Foundation (2012) Facts and Statistics about osteoporosis and its impact. http://testsite.iofbonehealth.org/docs/facts-and-statistics.html. Accessed 29 July 2012

Ismail AA et al (1998) Mortality associated with vertebral deformity in men and women: results from the European Prospective Osteoporosis Study (EPOS). Osteoporos Int 8:291–297

Johnell O, Kanis JA (2006) An estimate of the worldwide prevalence and disability associated with osteoporotic fractures. Osteoporos Int 17:1726

Kanis JA (2002) Diagnosis of osteoporosis and assessment of fracture risk. Lancet 359:1929

Kanis JA et al (2008) European guidance for the diagnosis and management of osteoporosis in postmenopausal women. Osteoporos Int 19(4):399–428

Keene GS et al (1993) Mortality and morbidity after hip fractures. BMJ 307:1248–1250

Kelsey JL et al (1992) Risk factors for fractures of the distal forearm and proximal humerus. Am J Epidemiol 135:477–489

Klotzbuecher et al (2000) Patients with prior fractures have an increased risk of future fractures: a summary of the literature and statistical synthesis. J Bone Miner Res 15:721–727

Latham NK (2006) Pattern of functional change during rehabilitation of patients with hip fracture. Arch Phys Med Rehabil 87(1):111–116

Lindsay R et al (2001) Risk of new vertebral fracture in the year following a fracture. JAMA 285:320–323

Melton LJ, III, Chrischilles EA, Cooper C et al (1992) Perspective: how many women have osteoporosis? J Bone Miner Res 7:1005

Nevitt MC et al (1998) The association of radiographically detected vertebral fractures with back pain and function: a prospective study. Ann Intern Med 128:793–800

NIH Consensus Development Panel on Osteoporosis (2001) Osteoporosis prevention, diagnosis, and therapy. JAMA 285(6):785–795

O'Neill TW et al (1996) The prevalence of vertebral deformity in European men and women: the European Vertebral Osteoporosis Study. J Bone Miner Res 11:1010–1018

Papaioannou A, Adachi JD, Parkinson W et al (2001) Lengthy hospitalization associated with vertebral fractures despite control for comorbid conditions. Osteoporos Int 12:870–874

Piscitelli P, Guida G, Iolascon G et al (2007) Incidence and costs of hip fractures versus acute myocardial infarction in the Italian population: a 4 years survey. Osteoporos Int 18:211–219

Pongchaiyakul C et al (2005) Asymptomatic vertebral deformity as a major risk factor for subsequent fractures and mortality: a long-term prospective study. J Bone Min Res 20:1349–1355

Zimmermann S et al (2006) The lower extremity gain scale: a performance-based measure to assess recovery after hip fracture. Arch Phys Med Rehabil 87(3):430–436

Therapy of Osteoporosis

Salvatore Minisola and Elisabetta Romagnoli

Contents

Abstract

The goal of any osteoporosis therapy is the prevention of both vertebral and nonvertebral fractures, which in principle can be achieved by inhibiting bone resorption and/or by stimulating bone formation. There are currently several osteoporosis treatment options that may be suitable for various patient populations, including oral and IV bisphosphonates, SERMs, calcitonin, teriparatide, strontium ranelate, and denosumab. The choice of osteoporosis therapy should be individualized based on consideration of the efficacy, safety, cost, convenience (i.e., dosing regimen and delivery), and other non-osteoporosis-related benefits associated with each agent. Given the limitations of current antiosteoporosis drugs, a search for new therapeutics has focused in the last few years on also identifying novel antiresorptives that prevent the decrease in activation frequency and bone formation and on bone anabolics that increase bone formation directly without affecting bone resorption. It will be important to incorporate new and emerging agents into this individualized treatment paradigm to optimize clinical outcomes in patients with osteoporosis.

1 Introduction

Osteoporosis is a systemic skeletal disease characterized by an unbalanced and/or uncoupled bone-remodeling activity leading to bone loss, microarchitectural deterioration of bone, and ultimately fractures at typical sites such as the lumbar spine, the femoral neck, and the distal radius. These fractures are often associated with an increase in morbidity, disability, and mortality, particularly in the elderly. Because of its widespread nature, with a 50 % fracture risk in all women after the age of 50 years and a 25 % risk in men, osteoporosis is a global public health concern and a great socioeconomic burden (Cauley et al. 2000; MacLean et al. 2008; Bolland et al. 2010; Harvey et al. 2010).

S. Minisola (✉) · E. Romagnoli
Department of Internal Medicine and Medical Disciplines,
University of Rome "Sapienza", Viale del Policlinico 155,
00161 Rome, Italy
e-mail: salvatore.minisola@fastwebnet.it

G. Guglielmi (ed.), *Osteoporosis and Bone Densitometry Measurements*, Medical Radiology. Diagnostic Imaging,
DOI: 10.1007/174_2012_651, © Springer-Verlag Berlin Heidelberg 2013

The goal of any osteoporosis therapy is the prevention of both vertebral and nonvertebral fractures, which in principle can be achieved by inhibiting bone resorption and/or by stimulating bone formation. Effective osteoporosis treatment can significantly reduce vertebral and nonvertebral fractures rate and mortality (MacLean et al. 2008; Bolland et al. 2010). On the contrary, untreated osteoporosis was associated with significant increase in hospitalization and costs for medical care (Lindsay et al. 2001; Huybrechts et al. 2006). However, despite the increasing burden of osteoporosis on a global scale, a vast number of individuals at high risk of fracture remain undiagnosed or untreated.

The World Health Organization (WHO)-defined bone mineral density (BMD) T-score of ≤ 2.5 standard deviation is frequently used as both a diagnostic and intervention threshold for osteoporosis (McCloskey 2010). However, the majority of osteoporotic fractures has been shown to occur in individuals with BMD values above the osteoporosis threshold, typically in the osteopenic range (T-score of less than -1 and greater than -2.5) (Siris et al. 2001). The WHO has developed the Fracture Risk Assessment Tool (FRAX®) (Kanis et al. 2009), which calculates the 10-year probability of a major osteoporotic fracture. Risk factors for osteoporotic fracture, according to the FRAX® algorithm, include prior fragility fracture, parental history of hip fracture, current tobacco smoking, use of oral glucocorticoids, rheumatoid arthritis, other causes of secondary osteoporosis, and alcohol consumption of three or more units daily (Kanis et al. 2008). Guidelines originally published in 2008 and updated in 2010 by the National Osteoporosis Foundation (NOF) recommend osteoporosis treatment in postmenopausal women or men aged 50 years and older with a T-score of -2.5 or lower at the femoral neck, hip, or spine or with a prior hip or spine fracture; treatment is also indicated for patients with low bone mass (T-score between -1.0 and -2.5) and a 10-year probability of hip fracture of ≥ 3 % or a 10-year probability of major osteoporosis-related fracture of ≥ 20 %, as determined by FRAX® (National Osteoporosis Foundation 2010).

The choice of osteoporosis therapy should be individualized based on consideration of the efficacy, safety, cost, convenience (i.e., dosing regimen and delivery), and other non-osteoporosis-related benefits associated with each agent (Laroche 2008); Silverman and Christiansen 2012). Daily supplementation with calcium and vitamin D is recommended as a baseline therapy as part of most pharmacologic regimens (National Osteoporosis Foundation 2010). For some women, lifestyle changes alone, including increased calcium and vitamin D intake, exercise, and fall prevention, may be sufficient to reduce the risk of osteoporosis.

Pharmacological treatments for osteoporosis can be divided into two categories: antiresorptive agents and anabolic agents. Antiresorptive drugs suppress bone resorption and are the most commonly agents used for treatment of osteoporosis. Anabolic agents rather stimulate bone formation, thus increasing bone mass and represent a more recent therapeutic approach for osteoporosis treatment.

Given the limitations of current antiosteoporosis drugs, a search for new therapeutics has focused in the last few years on also identifying novel antiresorptives that prevent the decrease in activation frequency and bone formation and on bone anabolics that increase bone formation directly without affecting bone resorption. This chapter summarizes the current status of pharmacological treatment of postmenopausal osteoporosis and the major evidences concerning old and new drugs.

2 Antiresorptive Drugs

2.1 Estrogens

Estrogens represent the oldest antiresorptive therapy recognized to be effective for the prevention of early postmenopausal bone loss and fracture (Riggs et al. 2002; Rossouw et al. 2002; Khosla 2010). However, the use of these agents was largely discouraged by the well-known increased risk of breast and endometrial cancer, cardiovascular disease, and dementia (Riggs et al. 2002; Rossouw et al. 2002). Physiologically, estrogens play a major role in the acquisition of bone mass during growth and pregnancy and have important effects on extraskeletal calcium homeostasis (Heshmati et al. 2002; Riggs et al. 2002). Indeed, estrogens stimulate osteoclast apoptosis and suppress osteoblast and osteocyte apoptosis (Riggs et al. 2002) Estrogen deficiency is also associated with an increased lifespan of osteoclasts and a reduction in osteoblasts lifespan, as well as with a raise in proresorptive cytokines, that lead to a significant bone loss and enhanced mobilization of calcium from the skeleton (Khosla 2010). Some evidences suggested that even the low serum estrogen levels in late postmenopausal women could have beneficial effects on bone (Heshmati et al. 2002). However, large-scale studies on fractures preventions and safety profile associated with estrogen low-dose treatment are still lacking (Khosla 2010).

Current clinical recommendations state that hormone replacement therapy should be used for treatment of menopausal symptoms for the shortest period of time and as osteoporosis therapy after consideration of all other treatments and of all patients' risks and benefits (Rossouw et al. 2002).

2.2 SERMS

Selective estrogen receptor modulators (SERMS) have been developed in order to provide the beneficial effects of estrogens on bone without adverse effects on other tissues. Indeed, SERMS act on estrogens receptor with a tissue-specific mechanism, thus acting as estrogen antagonist on brain and breast and as agonist on bone (Khosla 2010). The only SERMS currently utilized for the treatment of postmenopausal osteoporosis are raloxifene and bazedoxifene.

2.2.1 Raloxifene

Raloxifene is approved for treatment of osteoporosis at the oral dose of 60 mg once-daily. A meta-analysis of seven randomized, double-bind, placebo-controlled trials demonstrated a reduced vertebral fractures risk in postmenopausal women with osteoporosis, but no efficacy was reported for nonvertebral and hip fractures (Rossouw et al. 2002; Seeman et al. 2006). A reduced risk of developing breast cancer was also reported with raloxifene (Khosla 2010). However, raloxifene can increase the risk of venous thromboembolic disease, fatal stroke, and menopausal symptoms (Rossouw et al. 2002; Khosla 2010).

2.2.2 Bazedoxifene

Bazedoxifene is a novel SERM that was recently approved in the European Union for the treatment of osteoporosis in postmenopausal women at high risk of fracture. In a 3-year phase 3 study, bazedoxifene 20 and 40 mg/day significantly reduced the risk of new vertebral fracture by 42 and 37 % relative to placebo, respectively, in postmenopausal women with osteoporosis (Silverman et al. 2008). The incidence of nonvertebral fractures was not significantly different among bazedoxifene, raloxifene, and placebo groups. The results were confirmed in a 2-year extension of the 3-year treatment study that evaluated the longer term efficacy and safety of bazedoxifene in women with postmenopausal osteoporosis (Silverman et al. 2012).

2.3 Bisphosphonates

The introduction of bisphosphonates in clinical practice almost two decades ago was a major advance in the management of postmenopausal osteoporosis. Because of their antifracture efficacy and generally good tolerability, bisphosphonates rapidly became and still remain the mainstay of therapy for postmenopausal osteoporosis (Eastell et al. 2011).

Bisphosphonates are effective in reducing bone turnover, increasing BMD and reducing fracture risk in postmenopausal women with osteoporosis. Their efficacy is based on their ability to restore the rate of bone turnover to premenopausal levels, thereby preventing further deterioration of bone quality in patients with accelerated bone loss. The licensed bisphosphonates exhibit some differences in potency and speed of onset and offset of action. These differences

mean that different agents may be more advantageous in different situations.

These drugs are derivatives of inorganic pyrophosphate and bind to hydroxyapatite crystals in the skeleton (Eastell et al. 2011). Thus, they have a long half-life in the skeleton and are preferentially incorporated and accumulated at sites of accelerated bone turnover, where they act as inhibitors of osteoclast-mediated bone resorption (Favus 2010). Second- and third-generation bisphosphonates have nitrogen-containing side chains and are the agents actually most commonly used for osteoporosis treatment. In Europe the bisphosphonates approved for the treatment and prevention of osteoporosis are: alendronate, risedronate, and ibandronate, given by os, and intravenous ibandronate and zoledronic acid (Russell 2011).

2.3.1 Alendronate

Alendronate is an aminobisphosphonate used for the treatment of postmenopausal osteoporosis nowadays almost exclusively at 70 mg once-weekly oral regimen. The Fracture Intervention Trial (FIT) showed a significant reduction of vertebral fractures in patients with ≥1 vertebral fracture at baseline receiving alendronate for 3 years, and among patients without vertebral fractures at baseline after 4 years of alendronate (Black et al. 1996; Cummings et al. 1998; Bilezikian 2009). A meta-analysis of the combined nonvertebral fractures data from five prospective, randomized, placebo-controlled trials of at least 2 years' duration, found that alendronate significantly reduced the risk of nonvertebral fractures in postmenopausal women with osteoporosis (Karpf et al. 1997). The Fracture Intervention Trial Long-term Extension (FLEX) study evaluated the effects of continuation or discontinuation of alendronate for an additional 5 years (after the first 5 years of therapy) and showed a reduced risk for clinical vertebral fractures, but not for nonvertebral and morphometric vertebral fractures in women receiving alendronate (Black et al. 2006).

2.3.2 Risedronate

Risedronate is a third generation bisphosphonate used for the treatment of osteoporosis nowadays almost exclusively as 35-mg weekly and 75-mg for 2 consecutive days to the month oral dose. VERT-NA and VERT-MN trials showed that risedronate significantly reduced vertebral and nonvertebral fractures and increased BMD at both lumbar spine and femoral neck after 3 years of therapy, compared to placebo, in women with previous vertebral fractures (Harris et al. 1999; Bilezikian 2009). VERT-MN Extension Trial confirmed these results at 5 years (Harris et al. 1999; Sorensen et al. 2003). The Hip Intervention Program trial reported a reduction in the risk of hip fracture in elderly women with confirmed osteoporosis but not in elderly women with risk factors for osteoporosis other than low BMD after 3 years of risedronate (McClung et al. 2001).

2.3.3 Ibandronate

Ibandronate is a potent nitrogen-containing bisphosphonate administered intermittently at the oral dose of 150 mg once-monthly and as intravenous injections of 3 mg every 3 months. The BONE study reported a reduction in new morphometric and clinical vertebral fractures, but not nonvertebral fractures, in women with postmenopausal osteoporosis treated with oral ibandronate (Chesnut et al. 2004). Moreover, subsequent studies showed that the 150 mg once-monthly oral dose and intravenous 3 mg, administered every 3 months, are more efficacious than the daily oral regimen of 2.5 mg (Reginster et al. 2006; Eisman et al. 2008).

2.3.4 Zoledronic Acid

Zoledronic acid represents the most potent amin-obisphosphonate and is approved for the treatment of osteoporosis as a single 15-min infusion at the dosage of 5 mg every 12 months. The HORIZON Pivotal Fracture Trial reported a significant decrease in morphometric and clinical vertebral fractures, hip fractures, nonvertebral fractures, and clinical fractures among postmenopausal women 65–89 years of age treated with once-yearly zoledronic acid infusions over 3 years, compared to placebo (Black et al. 2007). To assess the effect of zoledronate beyond 3 years, an extension study of the HORIZON-PFT in which women on zoledronate for 3 years were randomly assigned to zoledronate or placebo for 3 more years was conducted. Small differences in bone density and markers in those who continued versus those who stopped treatment suggest residual effects, and therefore, after 3 years of annual zoledronate, many patients may discontinue therapy up to 3 years. However, vertebral fracture reductions suggest that those at high fracture risk, particularly vertebral fracture, may benefit by continued treatment (Black et al. 2012).

2.3.5 Safety

Upper gastrointestinal adverse effects represent the most common cause of patients' intolerance and discontinuation of oral bisphosphonates and include nausea, dyspepsia, abdominal pain, gastritis, and other non-specific symptoms. Accordingly, in clinical practice, patients should take these drugs fasting with a full glass of water and maintain an upright posture for at least 30 min after ingestion. Indeed, suboptimal administration of medication is considered the main cause of the erosive oral bisphosphonates-associated esophagitis (Kennel and Drake 2009).

A transient acute phase reaction has been associated with IV bisphosphonates injection, with the higher incidence after the first administration. A flu-like syndrome is the most common clinical presentation, with fever, myalgias, and arthralgias that resolves within 24–72 h and could be ameliorated by anti-inflammatory drugs (Kennel and Drake 2009).

Transient hypocalcemia is a well-recognized effect of IV bisphosphonates injection, particularly in patients with hypoparathyroidism, renal failure, hypovitaminosis D, or in the elderly. Thus, a correct supplementation with calcium and vitamin D in patients which would receive IV bisphosphonates is strongly recommended (Kennel and Drake 2009).

Bisphosphonate-associated osteonecrosis of the jaw is defined as an area of exposed bone in the maxillofacial region that did not heal within 8 weeks in a patient exposed to a bisphosphonate and had not had radiation therapy to the craniofacial region (Khosla et al. 2007). The incidence is relatively low in patients receiving oral bisphosphonates for osteoporosis and considerably higher in patients with malignancy receiving high doses of intravenous bisphosphonates (Khosla et al. 2007). However, a careful oral examination for active or anticipated dental issues and a good oral hygiene are highly recommended (Khosla et al. 2007). Safety concerns associated with the long-term use of bisphosphonates include atypical fractures, such as low-impact subtrochanteric stress fractures or completed fractures of the femur. It has been suggested that in some patients, prolonged administration of bisphosphonates may lead to over-suppression of bone turnover, which no longer permits remodeling to repair microdamage and thereby reduces bone strength. However, the absolute risk of atypical fracture associated with bisphosphonates for the individual patient with a high risk of osteoporotic fractures is small compared with the beneficial effects of the drug (Shane et al. 2010).

Bisphosphonates should not be used in patients with active gastrointestinal symptoms, delayed esophageal emptying, or other esophageal pathology and creatinine clearance less than 30–35 ml/min. However, some post hoc analysis of trials with risedronate reported no difference in the incidence of adverse events in the treatment group regardless of renal function, compared to placebo (Watts and Diab 2010).

2.4 Denosumab

Denosumab is a fully human monoclonal antibody that specifically binds to the receptor activator of nuclear factor-kB ligand (RANKL), thus blocking its interaction with its receptor, RANK, on osteoclasts. This system is essential for the formation, function, and survival of osteoclasts (McClung et al. 2006; Cummings et al. 2009). Hence, denosumab acts as an inhibitor of osteoclasts-mediated bone resorption. The FREEDOM trial reported a reduction in vertebral and nonvertebral fractures, compared to placebo, in postmenopausal women with osteoporosis treated with 60 mg of denosumab every 6 months for 36 months. Moreover, an increase in BMD at both lumbar spine and hip was reported; the drug is also associated with an increase in forearm BMD, suggesting a unique effect on cortical bone (Cummings et al. 2009). The pivotal trial also showed significant reductions in markers of bone turnover, C-telopeptide, and intact serum procollagen type I N-terminal propeptide, over 3 years (Cummings et al. 2009). Reductions in bone turnover were sustained over 4 and 6 years in open-label study extensions (Miller et al. 2011; Papapoulos et al. 2012).

The drug does not require renal clearance, and may be given to patients with renal impairment without dose adjustment, though with careful calcium supplementation because these patients are at higher risk of worsening hypocalcemia. There is some concern that treatment with denosumab may cause significant suppression of bone remodeling, the long-term effects of which are unknown. Adverse effects reported were: eczema, flatulence, cellulitis (including erysipelas), urinary tract and upper respiratory tract infection, constipation, arthralgia (McClung et al. 2006; Cummings et al. 2009).

Denosumab has been approved in Europe for the treatment of postmenopausal osteoporosis as a 60 mg subcutaneous injection every 6 months.

3 Anabolic Drugs

Anabolic drugs stimulate processes and mechanisms associated with bone formation, which is ultimately improved, leading to an increase in bone mass. Moreover, these agents affect a number of skeletal properties besides bone density, such as bone sizes and microarchitecture. The only anabolic therapy currently approved for osteoporosis treatment is the recombinant human parathyroid hormone (PTH).

3.1 Parathyroid Hormone (PTH)

Unlike chronic and continuous secretion of PTH that has a catabolic action on bone, the intermittent administration of low doses of PTH has potent anabolic effects on the skeleton. Indeed, PTH produces a prominent increment of BMD at both lumbar spine and femur and significantly decreases the incidence of vertebral and nonvertebral fractures, by stimulating bone formation and subsequently stimulates both bone formation and resorption (Neer et al. 2001; Canalis et al. 2007). Moreover, positive effects on bone connectivity, bone microarchitecture, and biomechanical properties of bone have been reported (Canalis et al. 2007). Two bioactive forms of PTH are currently available in Europe for osteoporosis treatment: teriparatide, the 1–34 fragments of PTH, and PTH (1–84), the intact human

recombinant molecule. Both the forms are administrated as a daily subcutaneous injection over a period of 24 months.

PTH is indicated in women and men at high risk of osteoporosis-related fractures, including those with vertebral or other osteoporosis-related fractures with BMD in the osteoporosis range, or very low BMD even in the absence of fractures (T-score < −3) and including individuals who have had an incident fracture or a bone loss during therapy with bisphosphonates agents (Canalis et al. 2007; National Osteoporosis Foundation 2010). PTH is also approved for men and women with glucocorticoid-induced osteoporosis at high fracture's risk and in men with hypogonadal osteoporosis (Canalis et al. 2007).

Despite all efforts made with PTH, the limited effect on nonvertebral fractures, the costs, the inconvenient route of administration, the activation of bone resorption, and the loss of efficacy with time suggest that PTH, although the best anabolic option today, will ultimately only partially meet the medical needs. Reducing the impact of some of these limitations constitutes the basis for current attempts to develop small molecules affecting the secretion of endogenous PTH and to use different routes of PTH administration (Roland Baron and Hesse 2012).

3.1.1 Teriparatide [PTH(1–34)]

Teriparatide has been approved for the treatment of osteoporosis at the dose of 20 µg once daily. It has been demonstrated effective in reducing the risk of vertebral and nonvertebral fractures and increasing vertebral, femoral, and total-body BMD, compared to placebo (Neer et al. 2001). In clinical trials, the safety and efficacy of teriparatide therapy has not been demonstrated beyond 2 years of treatment (Canalis et al. 2007). As a consequence, the recommended duration of teriparatide treatment in Europe is 24 months.

3.1.2 Parathyroid Hormone [PTH(1–84)]

Parathyroid hormone is approved in some countries of Europe as 100 µg-daily dose. It was found effective in reducing the risk of new or worsened vertebral fractures in postmenopausal women with osteoporosis and increasing BMD at both vertebral and femoral sites compared to placebo (Greenspan et al. 2007). As for teriparatide, in Europe the recommended duration of PTH (1–84) therapy is 24 months.

3.1.3 Safety

Adverse effects of PTH therapy include mild hypercalcemia, hypercalciuria, a possible rise in serum uric acid concentration, dizziness, nausea, vomiting, headache, and leg cramps (Neer et al. 2001; Canalis et al. 2007; Greenspan et al. 2007; Roland Baron and Hesse 2012). In clinical practice, serum calcium and 24-h urinary calcium excretion is usually checked 1 month after initiating PTH therapy. However, hypercalcemia and hypercalciuria are generally reversed by reducing calcium or vitamin D supplementation and eventually by a dose reduction of PTH to every-other day administration.

PTH is contraindicated in patients with Paget's disease of bone, skeletal metastases, skeletal malignant conditions, history of bone irradiation, unexplained elevations in alkaline phosphatase, myeloma, hyperparathyroidism, hypercalcemia, and end-stage renal failure.

3.1.4 PTH and Antiresorptive Sequential Therapy

Some studies demonstrated a rapid and progressive decline in BMD throughout the period following PTH therapy, particularly during the first 6 months (Bilezikian 2008). Therefore, it is common practice to follow PTH treatment with an antiresorptive agent, usually a bisphosphonate, in order to both exploit its own benefits and maintain densitometric gains achieved with PTH (Canalis et al. 2007; Bilezikian 2008; National Osteoporosis Foundation 2010).

4 Strontium Ranelate

Strontium ranelate is made up of an organic anion (ranelate) and two stable strontium cations and is incorporated into the crystal structure of bone (Marie 2006). In vitro models reported anabolic and antiresorptive actions of strontium ranelate that could both reduce osteoclast-mediated resorption and increase osteoblastic differentiation (Hamdy 2009). Strontium ranelate was found to reduce incidence of new vertebral and nonvertebral fractures in postmenopausal women with osteoporosis in two randomized, placebo controlled trials of 3 years' duration (Meunier et al. 2004; Reginster et al. 2005). The reduction of hip fractures was shown only among a high risk group of patients (Reginster et al. 2005). Strontium ranelate is currently approved in Europe for treatment of postmenopausal osteoporosis at the oral dose of 2 g once daily. Adverse effects include: nausea, diarrhea, headache, dermatitis and eczema, venous-thrombosis embolism event (Meunier et al. 2004; Reginster et al. 2005). Moreover, a few cases of drug rash with eosinophilia and systemic symptoms syndrome were reported. The mechanism associated with this potentially fatal adverse effect is not understood. Anyway, therapy with strontium ranelate should be finally discontinued in case of skin rash.

5 Calcium and Vitamin D

An adequate daily calcium and vitamin D intake is a safe and inexpensive treatment to prevent osteoporosis-related bone loss and fracture and is of utmost importance for any therapeutic intervention. Indeed, calcium and vitamin D supplementation has been demonstrated as effective in reducing risk of fracture and bone loss at both hip and spine on an average of 3–5 years' treatment duration, compared to placebo (Tang et al. 2007).

Furthermore, hypovitaminosis D is a widespread condition with important health consequences such as bone loss, proximal muscle weakness, increase in body sway, falls, and fractures (Lips 2001; Holick 2007; Holick and Chen 2008). Finally, calcium and vitamin D depletion was associated with a reduced response to antiresorptive agents in terms of both BMD changes and anti-fracture efficacy (Nieves et al. 1998; Adami et al. 2009). By the way, a daily calcium intake of at least 1,000 mg/day in men and women younger than 50 years and of 1,200 mg/day for those 50 years and older is strongly recommended (National Osteoporosis Foundation 2010). Moreover, a daily intake of at least 800–1,000 IU of vitamin D is currently recommended as both food fortification and oral supplementation (National Osteoporosis Foundation 2010) and two inactive forms of vitamin D are currently available for oral supplementation: cholecalciferol and ergocalciferol. However, definite clinical recommendations concerning the optimal dose and dose intervals of vitamin D administration needed to achieve and maintain the target vitamin D serum level are still lacking. Accordingly, in clinical practice, an adequate vitamin D serum concentration could be ensured with both daily and intermittent supplementation of high dose of vitamin D. Recent data from our group showed in fact that a single large dose of vitamin D is effective in rapidly and safely enhancing serum vitamin D concentration and that cholecalciferol has a greater potency than ergocalciferol in enhancing serum vitamin D concentration (Romagnoli et al. 2008; Cipriani et al. 2010).

6 Future Directions

6.1 Cathepsin K Inhibitors

Cathepsin K is a serine protease released by activated osteoclasts into the bone resorption compartment beneath osteoclasts during bone remodeling. This protease helps degrade type 1 collagen and other proteins embedded within bone matrix during bone resorption (Costa et al. 2011). Several phase 2 trials with cathepsin K inhibitors such as odanacatib (MK-0822) (Bone et al. 2010) have been completed, demonstrating mild to moderate antiresorptive effect. However, this compound seems to stimulate bone formation on periosteal surfaces while at the same time inhibiting bone resorption on trabecular surfaces. Side effects reported with early cathepsin K inhibitors included morphea.

6.2 Modulating the Canonical Wnt-Signaling Pathway

Although activation of the Wnt signaling pathway is a very promising approach for the development of bone anabolic drugs, safety concerns exist, in particular regarding possible oncogenic effects and uncontrolled formation of bone. However, it is important to mitigate these potential concerns with the fact that therapeutic intervention will not eliminate entirely the endogenous inhibitor and will occur only over a limited period of time.

6.2.1 Sclerostin Antibody

Sclerostin is a secreted cysteine-knot glycoprotein produced by the *SOST* gene almost exclusively in osteocytes (Baron and Rawadi 2007). Osteocytes form new bone at sites of increased mechanical strain. New bone formation caused by mechanical strain is normally stimulated by LRP 5/6 signaling through the canonical Wnt pathway (Li et al. 2005). Sclerostin normally inhibits new bone formation by inhibiting stimulatory interactions of Wnt proteins with the LRP-5/6 receptor on the plasma membrane of osteoblasts and osteoblast precursors on bone surfaces, thereby decreasing Wnt signaling through the canonical β-catenin pathway, and leading to decreased osteoblast recruitment and activation (Robling et al. 2008). LRP-5/6 signaling is normally inhibited by dickkopf/homolog 1 (Dkk1), secreted frizzled-related protein, or both.

A monoclonal antibody to sclerostin has been shown to inhibit sclerostin activity, thereby upregulating osteoblast Wnt signaling through the canonical β-catenin pathway and stimulating osteoblast recruitment and activity (van Bezooijen et al. 2005). Recently, the first human phase I randomized, double-blind, placebo-controlled clinical trial testing ascending single doses of AMG785, a humanized monoclonal sclerostin antibody, in healthy men and postmenopausal women was reported (Padhi et al. 2011). Bone formation markers increased within 1 month after a single sc dose of 10 mg/kg AMG 785 and markers of bone resorption decreased. Likewise, the gain in BMD at the lumbar spine and total hip was comparable or even greater than with rhPTH (Padhi et al. 2011). Injection site reactions were the most frequently reported adverse events. These studies point to the promising future of sclerostin antibodies for the treatment of low bone mass diseases.

6.2.2 Dkk1 Antagonists

Dkk1 is also an endogenous inhibitor of Wnt signaling. Although sclerostin antibodies are probably the preferred and most advanced therapeutic option for osteoporosis, antibodies to Dkk1 are also being developed. If proven safe and efficacious, these antibodies could also find their way to a more general indication in low bone mass diseases, although the possibility that Dkk1 is less restricted to the bone microenvironment than sclerostin may raise more concerns about off-target effects.

7 Conclusions

Currently approved osteoporosis therapies have been demonstrated as effective in lowering fracture risk. However, at the present, we have no comparative study able to give an overall scientific guide in the choice of a drug rather than another (Reid et al. 2009), except in small trials carried out in patients taking glucocorticoids (Reid et al. 2009; Saag et al. 2009). Hence, the choice of osteoporosis therapy should be individualized for each patient, taking into consideration the efficacy, safety, cost, convenience, and other non-osteoporosis-related benefits of each potential drug in relation to the patient's needs (Qaseem et al. 2008). Treatment's discontinuation represents the great challenge for the management of osteoporosis, resulting in increased fracture risk, hospitalization, and health care costs (Kothawala et al. 2007; Siris et al. 2009). Physicians' and patients' awareness about the need to use osteoporosis medication is therefore of utmost importance as well as strategies to improve adherence to treatment. Several clinical trials for osteoporosis treatment are ongoing, testing new antiresorptives, different forms of rhPTH, or agents that activate Wnt signaling. In many of these trials, combinations and sequences of these agents with various antiresorptives are also being tested. The next few years will therefore be very exciting for osteoporosis treatment.

References

Adami S, Giannini S, Bianchi G, Sinigaglia L, Di Munno O, Fiore CE, Minisola S, Rossini M (2009) Vitamin D status and response to treatment in post-menopausal osteoporosis. Osteoporos Int 20:239–244

Baron R, Rawadi G (2007) Targeting the Wnt/beta-catenin pathway to regulate bone formation in the adult skeleton. Endocrinology 148:2635–2643

Bilezikian JP (2008) Combination anabolic and antiresorptive therapy for osteoporosis: opening the anabolic window. Curr Osteoporos Rep 6:24–30

Bilezikian JP (2009) Efficacy of bisphosphonates in reducing fracture risk in postmenopausal osteoporosis. Am J Med 122:S14–S21

Black DM, Cummings SR, Karpf DB, Cauley JA, Thompson DE, Nevitt MC, Bauer DC, Genant HK, Haskell WL, Marcus R, Ott SM, Torner JC, Quandt SA, Reiss TF, Ensrud KE, Fracture Intervention Trial Research Group (1996) Randomised trial of effect of alendronate on risk of fracture in women with existing vertebral fractures. Lancet 348:1535–1541

Black DM, Schwartz AV, Ensrud KE, Cauley JA, Levis S, Quandt SA, Satterfield S, Wallace RB, Bauer DC, Palermo L, Wehren LE, Lombardi A, Santora AC, Cummings SR, FLEX Research Group (2006) Effects of continuing or stopping alendronate after 5 years of treatment. The fracture intervention trial long-term extension (FLEX): a randomized trial. JAMA 296:2927–2938

Black DM, Delmas PD, Eastell R, Reid IR, Boonen S, Cauley JA, Cosman F, Lakatos P, Leung PC, Man Z, Mautalen C, Mesenbrink P, Hu H, Caminis J, Tong K, Rosario-Jansen T, Krasnow J, Hue TF, Sellmeyer D, Eriksen EF, Cummings SR, HORIZON Pivotal Fracture Trial (2007) Once-yearly zoledronic acid for treatment of postmenopausal osteoporosis. N Engl J Med 356:1809–1822

Black DM, Reid IR, Boonen S, Bucci-Rechtweg C, Cauley JA, Cosman C, Cummings SR, Hue TF, Lippuner K, Lakatos P, Leung PC, Man Z, Martinez RLM, Tan M, Ruzycky ME, Su G, Eastell R (2012) The effect of 3 versus 6 years of zoledronic acid treatment of osteoporosis: a randomized extension to the HORIZON-pivotal fracture trial (PFT). J Bone Miner Res 27:243–254

Bolland MJ, Grey AB, Gamble GD, Reid IR (2010) Effect of osteoporosis treatment on mortality: a meta-analysis. J Clin Endocrinol Metab 95:1174–1181

Bone HG, McClung MR, Roux C, Recker RR, Eisman JA, Verbruggen N, Hustad CM, Da Silva C, Santora AC, Ince BA (2010) Odanacatib, a cathepsin-K inhibitor for osteoporosis: a two-year study in postmenopausal women with low bone density. J Bone Miner Res 25:937–947

Canalis E, Giustina A, Bilezikian JP (2007) Mechanisms of anabolic therapies for osteoporosis. N Engl J Med 357:905–916

Cauley JA, Thompson DE, Ensrud KC, Scott JC, Black D (2000) Risk of mortality following clinical fractures. Osteoporos Int 11:556–561

Chesnut CH III, Skag A, Christiansen C, Recker R, Stakkestad JA, Hoiseth A, Felsenberg D, Huss H, Gilbride J, Schimmer RC, Delmas PD, Oral Ibandronate Osteoporosis Vertebral Fracture Trial In North America And Europe (BONE) (2004) Effects of oral ibandronate administered daily or intermittently on fracture risk in postmenopausal osteoporosis. J Bone Miner Res 19:1241–1249

Cipriani C, Romagnoli E, Scillitani A, Chiodini I, Clerico R, Carnevale V, Mascia ML, Battista C, Viti R, Pileri M, Eller-Vainicher C, Minisola S (2010) Effect of a single oral dose of 600,000 IU of cholecalciferol on serum calciotropic hormones in young subjects with vitamin D deficiency: a prospective intervention study. J Clin Endocrinol Metab 95:4771–4777

Costa AG, Cusano NE, Silva BC, Cremers S, Bilezikian JP (2011) Cathepsin K: its skeletal actions and role as a therapeutic target in osteoporosis. Nat Rev Rheumatol 7:447–456

Cummings SR, Black DM, Thompson DE, Applegate WB, Barrett-Connor E, Musliner TA, Palermo L, Prineas R, Rubin SM, Scott JC, Vogt T, Wallace R, Yates AJ, LaCroix AZ (1998) Effect of alendronate on risk of fracture in women with low bone density but without vertebral fractures. Results from the Fracture Intervention Trial. JAMA 280:2077–2082

Cummings SR, San Martin J, McClung MR, Siris ES, Eastell R, Reid IR, Delmas P, Zoog HB, Austin M, Wang A, Kutilek S, Adami S, Zanchetta J, Libanati C, Siddhanti S, Christiansen C, FREEDOM trial (2009) Denosumab for prevention of fractures in postmenopausal women with osteoporosis. N Engl J Med 361:756–765

Eastell R, Walsh JS, Watts NB, Siris E (2011) Bisphosphonates for postmenopausal osteoporosis. Bone 49:82–88

Eisman JA, Civitelli R, Adami S, Czerwinski E, Recknor C, Prince R, Reginster JY, Zaidi M, Felsenberg D, Hughes C, Mairon N, Masanauskaite D, Reid DM, Delmas PD, Recker RR (2008) Efficacy and tolerability of intravenous ibandronate injections in postmenopausal osteoporosis: 2-year results from the DIVA study. J Rheumatol 35:488–497

Favus MJ (2010) Bisphosphonates for osteoporosis. N Engl J Med 363:2027–2035

Greenspan SL, Bone HG, Ettinger MP, Hanley DA, Lindsay R, Zanchetta JR, Blosch CM, Mathisen AL, Morris SA, Marriott TB, Treatment of Osteoporosis with Parathyroid Hormone Study Group (2007) Effect of recombinant human parathyroid hormone (1-84) on vertebral fracture and bone mineral density in postmenopausal women with osteoporosis: a randomized trial. Ann Intern Med 146:326–339

Hamdy NA (2009) Strontium ranelate improves bone microarchitecture in osteoporosis. Rheumatology (Oxford) 48(Suppl 4):iv9–iv13

Harris ST, Watts NB, Genant HK, McKeever CD, Hangartner T, Keller M, Chesnut CH 3rd, Brown J, Eriksen EF, Hoseyni MS, Axelrod DW, Miller PD (1999) Effects of risedronate treatment on vertebral and nonvertebral fractures in women with postmenopausal osteoporosis. A randomized controlled trial. JAMA 282:1344–1352

Harvey N, Dennison E, Cooper C (2010) Osteoporosis: impact on health and economics. Nat Rev Rheumatol 6:99–105

Heshmati HM, Khosla S, Robins SP, O'Fallon WM, Melton LJ 3rd, Riggs BL (2002) Role of low levels of endogenous estrogen in regulation of bone resorption in late postmenopausal women. J Bone Miner Res 17:172–178

Holick MF (2007) Vitamin D deficiency. N Engl J Med 357:266–281

Holick MF, Chen TC (2008) Vitamin D deficiency: a worldwide problem with health consequences. Am J Clin Nutr 87:1080S–1086S

Huybrechts KF, Ishak KJ, Caro JJ (2006) Assessment of compliance with osteoporosis treatment and its consequences in a managed care population. Bone 38:922–928

Kanis JA, Burlet N, Cooper C, Delmas PD, Reginster JY, Borgstrom F, Rizzoli R (2008) European guidance for the diagnosis and management of osteoporosis in postmenopausal women. Osteoporos Int 19:399–428

Kanis JA, Oden A, Johansson H, Borgstrom F, Strom O, McCloskey E (2009) FRAX® and its applications to clinical practice. Bone 44:734–743

Karpf DB, Shapiro DR, Seeman E, Ensrud KE, Johnston CC Jr, Adami S, Harris ST, Santora AC II, Hirsch LJ, Oppenheimer L, Thompson D (1997) Prevention of nonvertebral fractures by alendronate: a meta-analysis. JAMA 277:1159–1164

Kennel KA, Drake MT (2009) Adverse effects of bisphosphonates: implications for osteoporosis management. Mayo Clin Proc 84:632–637

Khosla S (2010) Update on estrogens and the skeleton. J Clin Endocrinol Metab 95:3569–3577

Khosla S, Burr D, Cauley J, Dempster DW, Ebeling PR, Felsenberg D, Gagel RF, Gilsanz V, Guise T, Koka S, McCauley LK, McGowan J, McKee MD, Mohla S, Pendrys DG, Raisz LG, Ruggiero SL, Shafer DM, Shum L, Silverman SL, Van Poznak CH, Watts N, Woo SB, Shane E (2007) Bisphosphonate associated osteonecrosis of the jaw: report of a task force of the American Society for Bone and Mineral Research. J Bone Miner Res 22:1479–1491

Kothawala P, Badamgarav E, Ryu S, Miller RM, Halbert RJ (2007) Systematic review and meta-analysis of real-world adherence to drug therapy for osteoporosis. Mayo Clin Proc 82:1493–1501

Laroche M (2008) Treatment of osteoporosis: all the questions we still cannot answer. Am J Med 121:744–747

Li X, Zhang Y, Kang H et al (2005) Sclerostin binds to LRP5/6 and antagonizes canonical Wnt signaling. J Biol Chem 280:19883–19887

Lindsay R, Silverman SL, Cooper C, Hanley DA, Barton I, Broy SB, Licata A, Benhamou L, Geusens P, Flowers K, Stracke H, Seeman E (2001) Risk of new vertebral fracture in the year following a fracture. JAMA 285:320–323

Lips P (2001) Vitamin D deficiency and secondary hyperparathyroidism in the elderly: consequences for bone loss and fractures and therapeutic implications. Endocr Rev 22:477–501

MacLean C, Newberry S, Maglione M, McMahon M, Ranganath V, Suttorp M, Mojica W, Timmer M, Alexander A, McNamara M, Desai SB, Zhou A, Chen S, Carter J, Tringale C, Valentine D, Johnsen B, Grossman J (2008) Systematic review: comparative effectiveness of treatments to prevent fractures in men and women with low bone density or osteoporosis. Ann Intern Med 148:197–213

Marie PJ (2006) Strontium ranelate: a dual mode of action rebalancing bone turnover in favour of bone formation. Curr Opin Rheumatol 18(Suppl 1):S11–S15

McCloskey E (2010) FRAX: identifying people at high risk of fracture. International Osteoporosis Foundation. http://www.iofbonehealth.org/download/osteofound/filemanager/publications/pdf/FRAX-report-09.pdf. Accessed 12 Jan 2011

McClung MR, Geusens P, Miller PD, Zippel H, Bensen WG, Roux C, Adami S, Fogelman I, Diamond T, Eastell R, Meunier PJ, Wasnich RD, Greenwald M, Kaufman JM, Chesnut CH, Reginster JY (2001) Effect of risedronate on the risk of hip fracture in elderly women. N Engl J Med 344:333–340

McClung MR, Lewiecki EM, Cohen SB, Bolognese MA, Woodson GC, Moffett AH, Peacock M, Miller PD, Lederman SN, Chesnut CH, Lain D, Kivitz AJ, Holloway DL, Zhang C, Peterson MC, Bekker PJ (2006) Denosumab in postmenopausal women with low bone mineral density. N Engl J Med 354:821–831

Meunier PJ, Roux C, Seeman E, Ortolani S, Badurski JE, Spector TD, Cannata J, Balogh A, Lemmel EM, Pors-Nielsen S, Rizzoli R, Genant HK, Reginster JY (2004) The effects of strontium ranelate on the risk of vertebral fracture in women with postmenopausal osteoporosis. N Engl J Med 350:459–468

Miller PD, Wagman RB, Peacock M, Lewiecki EM, Bolognese MA, Weinstein RL, Ding B, San Martin J, McClung MR (2011) Effect of denosumab on bone mineral density and biochemical markers of bone turnover: six-year results of a phase 2 clinical trial. J Clin Endocrinol Metab 96:394–402

National Osteoporosis Foundation (2010) Clinician's guide to prevention and treatment of osteoporosis. http://www.nof.org/sites/default/files/pdfs/NOF_ClinicianGuide2009_v7.pdf. Accessed 23 July 2010

Neer RM, Arnaud CD, Zanchetta JR, Prince R, Gaich GA, Reginster JY, Hodsman AB, Eriksen EF, Ish-Shalom S, Genant HK, Wang O, Mitlak BH (2001) Effect of parathyroid hormone (1-34) on fractures and bone mineral density in postmenopausal women with osteoporosis. N Engl J Med 344:1434–1441

Nieves JW, Komar L, Cosman F, Lindsay R (1998) Calcium potentiates the effect of estrogen and calcitonin on bone mass: review and analysis. Am J Clin Nutr 67:18–24

Padhi D, Jang G, Stouch B, Fang L, Posvar E (2011) Single-dose, placebo-controlled, randomized study of AMG 785, a sclerostin monoclonal antibody. J Bone Miner Res 26:19–26

Papapoulos S, Chapurlat R, Libanati C, Brandi ML, Brown JP, Czerwiski E, Krieg M-A, Man Z, Mellström D, Radominski SC, Reginster JY, Resch H, Román JA, Roux C, Vittinghoff E, Austin M, Daizadeh N, Bradley MN, Grauer A, Cummings SR, Bone HG (2012) Five years of denosumab exposure in women with postmenopausal osteoporosis: results from the first two years of the FREEDOM extension. J Bone Miner Res 27:694–701

Qaseem A, Snow V, Shekelle P, Hopkins R Jr, Forciea MA, Owens DK, Clinical Efficacy Assessment Subcommittee of the American College of Physicians (2008) Pharmacologic treatment of low bone density or osteoporosis to prevent fractures: a clinical practice guideline from the American College of Physicians. Ann Intern Med 149:404–415

Reginster JY, Seeman E, De Vernejoul MC, Adami S, Compston J, Phenekos C, Devogelaer JP, Curiel MD, Sawicki A, Goemaere S, Sorensen OH, Felsenberg D, Meunier PJ (2005) Strontium ranelate reduces the risk of nonvertebral fractures in postmenopausal women with osteoporosis: treatment of peripheral osteoporosis (TROPOS) study. J Clin Endocrinol Metab 90:2816–2822

Reginster JY, Adami S, Lakatos P, Greenwald M, Stepan JJ, Silverman SL, Christiansen C, Rowell L, Mairon N, Bonvoisin B, Drezner MK, Emkey R, Felsenberg D, Cooper C, Delmas PD, Miller PD (2006) Efficacy and tolerability of once-monthly oral ibandronate in postmenopausal osteoporosis: 2 year results from the MOBILE study. Ann Rheum Dis 65:654–661

Reid DM, Devogelaer JP, Saag K, Roux C, Lau CS, Reginster JY, Papanastasiou P, Ferreira A, Hartl F, Fashola T, Mesenbrink P, Sambrook PN, HORIZON Investigators (2009) Zoledronic acid and risedronate in the prevention and treatment of glucocorticoid-induced osteoporosis (HORIZON): a multicentre, double-blind, double-dummy, randomised controlled trial. Lancet 373:1253–1263

Riggs BL, Khosla S, Melton LJ 3rd (2002) Sex steroids and the construction and conservation of the adult skeleton. Endocr Rev 23:279–302

Robling AG, Niziolek PJ, Baldridge LA, Condon KW, Allen MR, Alam I, Mantila SM, Gluhak-Heinrich J, Bellido TM, Harris SE, Turner CH (2008) Mechanical stimulation of bone in vivo reduces osteocyte expression of Sost/sclerostin. J Biol Chem 283:5866–5875

Roland Baron R, Hesse E (2012) Update on bone anabolics in osteoporosis treatment: rationale, current status, and perspectives. J Clin Endocrinol Metab 97:311–325

Romagnoli E, Mascia ML, Cipriani C, Fassino V, Mazzei F, D'Erasmo E, Carnevale V, Scillitani A, Minisola S (2008) Short and long-term variations in serum calciotropic hormones after a single very large dose of ergocalciferol (vitamin D2) or cholecalciferol (vitamin D3) in the elderly. J Clin Endocrinol Metab 93:3015–3020

Rossouw JE, Anderson GL, Prentice RL, LaCroix AZ, Kooperberg C, Stefanick ML, Jackson RD, Beresford SA, Howard BV, Johnson KC, Kotchen JM, Ockene J (2002) Writing Group for the Women's Health Initiative Investigator Risks and benefits of estrogen plus progestin in healthy postmenopausal women: principal results from the Women's Health Initiative randomized controlled trial. JAMA 288:321–333

Russell G (2011) Bisphosphonates: the first 40 years. Bone 49:2–19

Saag KG, Zanchetta JR, Devogelaer JP, Adler RA, Eastell R, See K, Krege JH, Krohn K, Warner MR (2009) Effects of teriparatide versus alendronate for treating glucocorticoid-induced osteoporosis: thirty-six-month results of a randomized, double-blind, controlled trial. Arthritis Rheum 60:3346–3355

Seeman E, Crans GG, Diez-Perez A, Pinette KV, Delmas PD (2006) Anti-vertebral fracture efficacy of raloxifene: a meta-analysis. Osteoporos Int 17:313–316

Shane E, Burr D, Ebeling PR, Abrahamsen B, Adler RA, Brown TD, Cheung AM, Cosman F, Curtis JR, Dell R, Dempster D, Einhorn TA, Genant HK, Geusens P, Klaushofer K, Koval K, Lane JM, McKiernan F, McKinney R, Ng A, Nieves J, O'Keefe R, Papapoulos S, Sen HT, van der Meulen MCH, Weinstein RS, Whyte M (2010) Atypical subtrochanteric and diaphyseal femoral fractures: report of a Task Force of the American Society for Bone and Mineral Research. J Bone Miner Res 25:2267–2294

Silverman S, Christiansen C (2012) Individualizing osteoporosis therapy. Osteoporos Int 23:797–809

Silverman SL, Christiansen C, Genant HK, Vukicevic S, Zanchetta JR, de Villiers TJ, Constantine GD, Chines AA (2008) Efficacy of bazedoxifene in reducing new vertebral fracture risk in postmenopausal women with osteoporosis: results from a 3-year, randomized, placebo-, and active controlled clinical trial. J Bone Miner Res 23:1923–1934

Silverman SL, Chines AA, Kendler DL, Kung AWC, Teglbjaerg CS, Felsenberg D, Mairon N, Constantine GD, Adachi JD, The Bazedoxifene Study Group (2012) Sustained efficacy and safety of bazedoxifene in preventing fractures in postmenopausal women with osteoporosis: results of a 5-year, randomized, placebo-controlled study. Osteoporos Int 23:351–363

Siris ES, Miller PD, Barrett-Connor E, Faulkner KG, Wehren LE, Abbott TA, Berger ML, Santora AC, Sherwood LM (2001) Identification and fracture outcomes of undiagnosed low bone mineral density in postmenopausal women: results from the National Osteoporosis Risk Assessment. JAMA 286:2815–2822

Siris ES, Selby PL, Saag KG, Borgström F, Herings RM, Silverman SL (2009) Impact of osteoporosis treatment adherence on fracture rates in North America and Europe. Am J Med 122(Suppl 2):S3–S13

Sorensen OH, Crawford GM, Mulder H, Hosking DJ, Gennari C, Mellstrom D, Pack S, Wenderoth D, Cooper C, Reginster JY (2003) Long-term efficacy of risedronate: a 5-year placebo-controlled clinical experience. Bone 32:120–126

Tang BM, Eslick GD, Nowson C, Smith C, Bensoussan A (2007) Use of calcium or calcium in combination with vitamin D supplementation to prevent fractures and bone loss in people aged 50 years and older: a meta-analysis. Lancet 370:657–666

van Bezooijen RL, Papapoulos SE, Löwik CW (2005) Bone morphogenetic proteins and their antagonists: the sclerostin paradigm. J Endocrinol Invest 28(8 Suppl):15–17

Watts N, Diab DL (2010) Long-term use of bisphosphonates in osteoporosis. J Clin Endocrinol Metab 95:1555–1565

Radiography in Osteoporosis

Sivasubramanian Srinivasan and Wilfred C. G. Peh

Contents

Abstract

The pathological changes of osteoporosis are due to resorption of the cortical and trabecular bone. The main radiographic findings include changes in the trabecular pattern, cortical thinning, and decreased bone density which are more prominent in the axial skeleton. Although the most common cause is primary osteoporosis, one has to be aware of the secondary causes as well. Conventional radiography helps in evaluating the secondary causes of osteoporosis, to confirm or rule out fractures and to diagnose concomitant or predisposing conditions. However, radiographs have certain limitations. Radiography only helps in qualitative assessment and cannot be considered as a tool for quantitative assessment. This chapter aims to review the radio-pathological changes and various causes of osteoporosis.

1 Key points

- Conventional radiography helps in subjective quantification of bone density, microstructural changes in the trabeculae, fractures, and deformities due to osteoporosis.
- Approximately 20–40 % of bone mass has to be lost for a bone to appear osteopenic and various technical factors also affect the appearance of the bone density in the radiographs.
- Primary osteoporosis (post-menopausal or senile osteoporosis) is the most common cause of osteoporosis. Radiographs are useful for visualizing the deformities or fractures of spine, to assess the trabecular pattern of the femoral head, and also in the distal appendicular skeleton. Radiographs are also useful in assessing the response to medications used for the treatment of osteoporosis.
- Secondary osteoporosis may be due to numerous causes and radiographs are often helpful in the differential diagnosis and for follow-up of the particular causative

S. Srinivasan · W. C. G. Peh (✉)
Department of Diagnostic Radiology,
Khoo Teck Puat Hospital Alexandra Health,
90 Yishun Central, Singapore 768228,
Republic of Singapore
e-mail: wilfred.peh@gmail.com

G. Guglielmi (ed.), *Osteoporosis and Bone Densitometry Measurements*, Medical Radiology. Diagnostic Imaging,
DOI: 10.1007/174_2012_728, © Springer-Verlag Berlin Heidelberg 2013

clinical condition such as hyperparathyroidism and steroid-induced osteoporosis.

- Osteoporosis can be regional or occasionally localized to a particular limb in conditions such as reflex sympathetic dystrophy.

2   Introduction

Osteoporosis is the most common metabolic bone disorder and is defined by the World Health Organization (WHO) as "skeletal disease characterized by low bone mass and micro architectural deterioration of bone tissue, with a consequent increase in bone fragility and susceptibility to fracture" (Guglielmi et al. 2011). Although there are various methods such as dual-energy X-ray absorptiometry (DXA) and quantitative computed tomography (q-CT) for quantifying the bone density, conventional radiography helps in subjectively assessing the density of the bone and also in detection of fracture and alterations in the bone resorption in certain conditions such as hyperparathyroidism (Grampp et al. 1996, 1997). It also helps in diagnosis and follow-up of associated fractures. Recently, magnetic resonance (MR) imaging and micro-CT have been used as research tools for assessment of bone microarchitecture. We use the term "osteopenia" to refer to the rarefaction and decreased bone density seen on radiographs.

3   Pathological Changes Occurring in Osteoporosis

The bone remodeling unit consists of osteoblasts which are mononucleate cells forming the connective tissue matrix (osteoid) which later mineralizes to become bone, and osteoclasts which are multinuclear giant cells capable of digesting calcified bone matrix (Nijweide et al. 1986; D'ipolito et al. 1999). Primary osteoporosis or age-related bone loss results from imbalance between the osteoblasts and osteoclasts. Bone can be structurally classified into cortical bone and trabecular bone (Grampp et al. 1997; Guglielmi et al. 2011).

3.1   Cortical Bone

Cortical bone is the dense bone surrounding the marrow space and has an inner surface (endosteal surface) and an outer surface (periosteal surface). The Haversian and Volkmann channels are present within the cortex (intracortical region). The cortical bone is less metabolically active compared to trabecular bone (Bart 2008). The resorption at the endosteal surface is greater relative to bone

deposition, and this process increases with age. Hence, the marrow space appears wider with age (Bart 2008; Jergas 2008) (Fig. 1).

3.2   Trabecular Bone

Trabecular bone comprises the deeper part of the bone and is arranged as a lattice-work of thin sheets of varying thickness, with the interstices containing bone marrow or fat (Eriksen et al. 1994). The trabecular bone is most prominent in the axial skeleton, especially the spine (Bailey et al. 2000), and the distal aspect of the appendicular long bones, particularly the proximal end of femur and the distal end of radius. Trabecular bone has a greater surface area and compared to cortical bone, responds faster to metabolic changes (Grampp et al. 1997). Loss of trabecular bone usually occurs in a typical sequential fashion. Non-weight-bearing trabeculae are lost first. The weight-bearing trabeculae may appear prominent due to the loss of the rest of the trabeculae, and may become stronger and thickened.

Bone mass decreases with age. The loss of bone mass depends upon the rate of bone loss and also the peak bone mass attained in early life. Men have a greater peak bone mass and hence, the incidence of osteoporosis is less. The factors which influence peak bone mass include dietary calcium, sex hormone status, nutrition, physical activity, and genetic factors.

4   Radiography: Technical Considerations

The amount of X-ray absorption increases with the third power of atomic number (Wolbarst 1993), hence the absorption is directly proportional to the amount of calcium. Reduction in the bone mass or reduction in the calcium causes decrease in the absorption of the X-rays, resulting in increased lucency or radiolucency of the bones. Prediction of bone density by radiographs alone is poor when compared to standard densitometry, especially in the early stages (Epstein et al. 1986; Finsen and Anda 1988). Detection of osteopenia is possible only after 20–40 % of bone mass is lost (Grampp et al. 1997).

Many technical factors and patient factors (Heuck and Schmidt 1960; Jergas 2008) also interfere with the appearance of the bone quality on radiographs (Table 1). Hence, radiographs can assess gross morphology, presence of increased translucency, cortical changes, changes in the trabeculae and fractures, but cannot accurately quantify the degree of osteoporosis. The interobserver variability of assessing the density and detection of osteopenia is significant (Epstein et al. 1986; Williamson et al. 1990). Recently, digital radiography has increasingly been used to

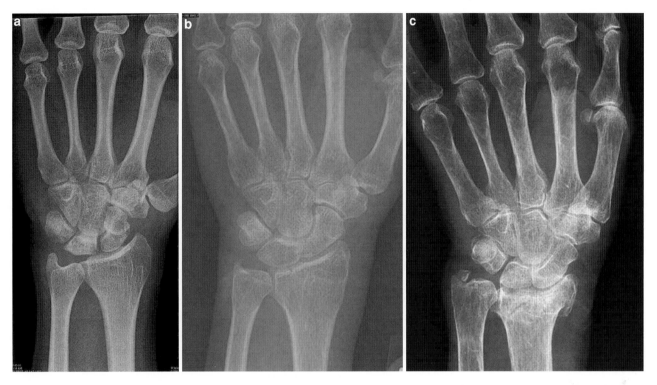

Fig. 1 Bony cortical changes with age. **a** Frontal hand radiograph of a 18-year-old woman shows normal cortical thickness in all the bones. **b** Frontal hand radiograph of a 40-year-old woman shows mild medullary widening due to endosteal resorption. This is age-related. **c** Frontal hand radiograph of a 101-year-old woman shows significant thinning of the cortex, in addition to the old osteoporotic fractures of the distal radius and ulna

Table 1 Factors affecting the radiographic appearance of the bone (Jergas 2008; Heuck and Schmidt 1960)

Technical factors
Exposure time
X-ray tube—anode, voltage
X-ray beam filtration
Film characteristics—e.g. speed, type of the screen, the emulsion
Patient factors
Density or thickness of the bone
Mineral content
Thickness of the soft tissue
Amount of scatter

evaluate osteoporosis (Hauschild et al. 2009). However, it provides no significant benefit compared to conventional radiographs (Wagner et al. 2005).

5 Classification of Osteoporosis

Osteoporosis can be broadly classified as primary and secondary osteoporosis. There are however various other classification systems.

5.1 Primary Osteoporosis

Primary osteoporosis mainly occurs due to advancing age and decrease in sex hormones (Albright 1947; Riggs and Melton 1983, 1986; Khosla et al. 2011). Primary osteoporosis can be subclassified into post-menopausal (Type I) and age–related or senile (Type II) osteoporosis.

5.1.1 Post-Menopausal (Type I) Osteoporosis

This is mainly due to estrogen deficiency after menopause and results in accelerated loss of trabecular bone, with increase in the risk of fractures, especially in the spine and wrist and to a lesser extent, in the hips. This is followed by a phase of slower bone loss, affecting mainly the cortical bone. This occurs along with decrease in number of osteoblasts and rate of bone formation, all of which contribute to the age-related osteoporosis.

5.1.2 Age-Related or Senile (Type II) Osteoporosis

With advancing age, the rate of bone formation decreases, resulting in proportionate loss of cortical and trabecular bone (Riggs and Melton 1983, 1986). However, women are more prone as men acquire more bone during puberty, and due to abrupt absence of estrogen, women tend to lose more bone. Fractures commonly occur in the hip and proximal aspect of long bones, such as the tibia, humerus, and proximal femur. Elderly patients, especially those residing in nursing homes, have a greater risk due to certain factors, such as cognitive impairment, gait and balance disorders, weakness, decreased acuity of vision and medications. 85 % of elderly older than 85 years have osteoporosis. Hip and non-vertebral fractures are approximately three times more common in this population (Vu et al. 2006).

5.2   Secondary Osteoporosis

Secondary osteoporosis is defined as bone loss that results from specific, well-defined clinical disorders (Fitzpatrick 2002). There are numerous causes of secondary osteoporosis (Anil et al. 2010), which include genetic or storage disorders, endocrine disorders, disorders of the gastrointestinal tract, medication-induced osteopenia/osteoporosis, malignancy and restricted mobility (Table 2). Approximately 20–30 % of post-menopausal women and 50 % of men with osteoporosis have secondary causes of osteoporosis (Fitzpatrick 2002). Finding the exact cause of osteoporosis is necessary for appropriate treatment and prognosis.

5.3   Other Classifications

Osteoporosis can also be classified according to distribution into generalized or regional forms (Anil et al. 2010). The former can be primary or secondary osteoporosis which cause generalized loss of the bones, whereas the latter involves a particular region or bones of one limb. Examples include migratory osteoporosis, transient osteoporosis, Sudeck's reflex sympathetic dystrophy, and osteoporosis secondary to infection and inflammatory arthritis.

Other rare unclassified types of osteoporosis include idiopathic osteoporosis (Bordier et al. 1973; Pacifici et al. 1990), which is a reversible condition seen in middle-aged men that is associated with rapid bone turnover. The exact etiology is unknown, although increased interleukin-1 and pulsatile increase in parathyroid hormone are hypothesized (Harms et al. 1989). A form of idiopathic osteoporosis that can also occur in children, and is known as juvenile idiopathic osteoporosis (Smith 1995), in which compression fractures of the spine and fractures of metaphysis of long bones have been reported.

6   Role of Radiographs in Osteoporosis

The role of imaging in osteoporosis is to achieve an early diagnosis so that appropriate treatment can be initiated early (Keen 2007). Radiography is not the mainstay in the diagnosis of osteoporosis. Although quantification of bone

Table 2 Causes of secondary osteoporosis (Fitzpatrick 2002)

| Hormone-related disorders |
| Hyperparathyroidism |
| Corticosteroid-induced osteoporosis. |
| Rickets/osteomalacia |
| Gonadal insufficiency (primary or secondary) |
| Hyperthyroidism |
| Type 1 diabetes mellitus |
| Gastrointestinal disease |
| Celiac disease/malabsorption syndromes |
| Chronic cholestatic diseases |
| Gastrectomy |
| Inflammatory bowel disease |
| Parenteral nutrition |
| Primary biliary cirrhosis |
| Severe liver disease |
| Marrow-related disorders |
| Hemophilia |
| Leukemia |
| Lymphoma |
| Mastocytosis |
| Multiple myeloma |
| Pernicious anemia |
| Sickle cell anemia |
| Thalassemia |
| Storage disorders |
| Genetic disorders |
| Hypophosphatasia |
| Osteogenesis imperfecta |
| Miscellaneous causes |
| Organ transplantation |
| Heparin-induced osteoporosis |

density is difficult with conventional radiographs, they are often required along with DXA or MR imaging to:
1. Confirm or rule out fractures,
2. Detect concomitant or pre-disposing abnormalities such as osteoarthritis,
3. Aid in the diagnosis of secondary causes such as Cushing's disease or hyperparathyroidism, although the appearance in majority of the conditions remains similar (Anil et al. 2010).

6.1   Main Radiographic Findings

The main radiographic findings of osteoporosis are altered trabecular pattern, cortical thinning, and increased radiolucency.

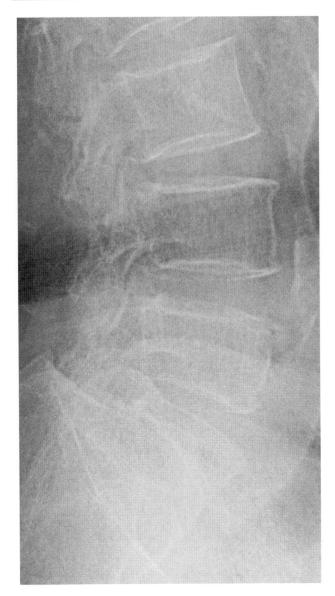

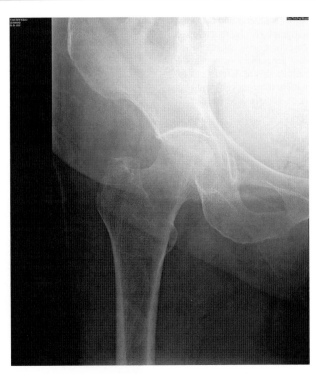

Fig. 3 Frontal radiograph of the right hip shows generalized increased bone radiolucency

Fig. 2 Lateral lumbar spine radiograph of a 60-year-old woman shows prominent vertical trabeculae

Fractures and deformities need to be assessed radiographically, with failure to diagnosis fractures being a problematic area.

6.1.1 Altered Trabecular Pattern

Compared to cortical bone, cancellous bone responds faster to metabolic stimuli. The trabeculae of the cancellous bone are laid down corresponding to the compressive and tensile forces acting on it. The trabeculae can be well appreciated in bones, such as the distal radius, calcaneum, and femoral neck (von Meyer 1867; Benhamou et al. 1994; Link et al. 1999). The trabeculae which are not involved in weight-bearing are lost first. The primary trabeculae or the weight-bearing trabeculae become thickened, possibly due to a compensatory mechanism or to callus from microfractures (Fig. 2). Later in the advanced stage, even the primary weight-bearing trabeculae are lost, resulting in the translucent appearance of bone on radiographs (Vernon-Roberts and Pirie 1973; Geraets et al. 1990).

6.1.2 Cortical Thinning

Involvement of the cortical bone occurs at three sites, namely: endosteal, periosteal, and intracortical (Grampp et al. 1997). In physiological remodeling of bones, the activity affects both the endosteal and periosteal surfaces. However, in involutional osteoporosis, it predominantly involves the endosteal surface, leading to thinning of the cortex. The response of endosteal, periosteal, and cortical resorption differs according to the etiology (Meunier et al. 1972; Genant et al. 1973). For example, in hyperparathyroidism, subperiosteal resorption can be seen in the radiographs as irregularities or erosions in the outer surface of the metacarpals. Intracortical bone resorption can be seen in the inner aspect of the cortex as striations or trabaculations, which are also features of hyperparathyroidism.

6.1.3 Increased Radiolucency

The bone density is directly proportional to the absorption of the X-rays and increases with the third power of atomic number (Wolbarst 1993). In osteoporosis, the decreased mineralization results in reduced absorption with resultant increased lucency of the bone (Fig. 3). There should be approximately 20–40 % bone loss for increased radiolucency to appear on radiographs (Ardran 1951; Harris and Heaney 1969; Epstein et al. 1986; Finsen and Anda 1988).

Fig. 4 **a** Lateral and **b** frontal radiographs of the thoracic spine in a patient with osteoporosis show generalized osteopenia and resultant severe deformities in multiple thoracic vertebral bodies due to compression fractures

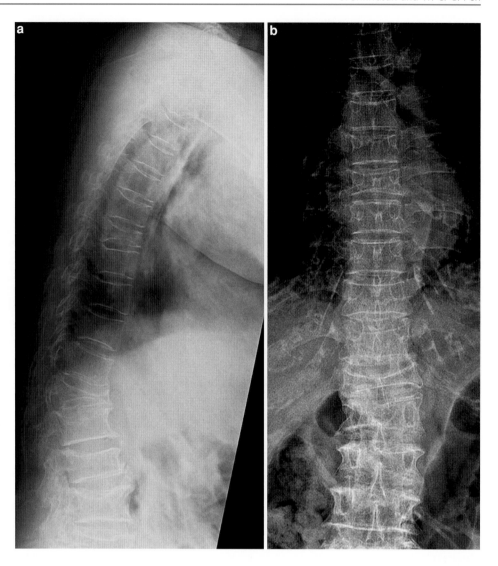

6.1.4 Fractures and Deformities

The common sites of fractures include the spine, hip, and proximal femur (Johnell et al. 2004; Cranney et al. 2007). Fractures can also occur in the proximal humerus, pelvis, clavicle, and scapula.

6.1.5 Failure to Diagnose Fractures

Asymptomatic fractures are often missed on routine radiographs and the false negative rate may be very high, in the range of 29–45 % (Gehlbach et al. 2000; Delmas et al. 2005, Lems 2007). Lems (2007) highlighted three important causes for missing the fractures, especially in the vertebral column:

1. Lack of clinical symptoms, unlike the pelvis or hips, and these occur during routine activities such as walking or climbing stairs,
2. Overlooked on routine radiographs,
3. Presence of more severe pathologies such as malignancy. Improvement of detection of the fractures can be achieved by educating the radiologists to differentiate

fractures from other pathologies which mimic fracture such as degenerative disease, and ankylosing spondylitis. The "Vertebral Fracture Initiative", an educational program from International Osteoporosis Foundation, is one such example to help educate radiologists (Lems 2007).

6.2 Involvement of Specific Regions

6.2.1 Spine

Radiography continues to play an important role in evaluation of osteoporosis of the spine, especially for the assessment of bony outline, including the endplates, alignment, vertebral height, and for fractures. The lateral view of the thoracic and lumbar spine is the most useful projection (Figs. 4 and 5). MR imaging of the spine can be used to detect acute fractures and also differentiate involutional osteoporosis from metastatic disease, if radiographs are equivocal.

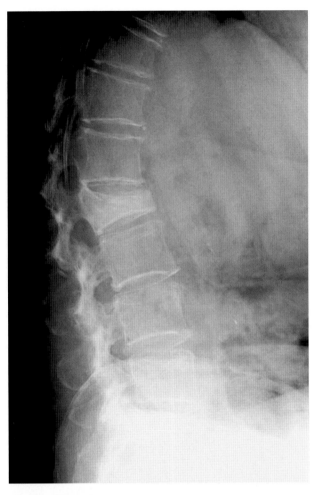

Fig. 5 Lateral radiograph of the lumbar spine shows anterior wedge compression fracture of L2 vertebral body. The apparent sclerosis in the involved vertebral body is due to healing. The rest of the vertebral bodies appear osteopenic

The signs which favor osteoporosis rather than metastasis include (Jung et al. 2003):

1. Hypointense band on T1- and T2-weighted images,
2. Sparing of normal marrow signal intensity of the vertebral body,
3. Retropulsion of the posterior bone fragment,
4. Compression fractures at multiple levels.

6.2.2 Pelvis and Hips

The prominent sites in the pelvis and hips include the iliac blades, femoral neck and greater trochanter, pubis and supraacetabular region. Most visible trabecular changes are present at the proximal end of the femur (Fig. 6). Thinning of the cortex is usually seen at the iliac crests, pubic rami, ischia, and proximal femur (Anil et al. 2010).

Proximal Femur

Trabeculae in the femur can be divided into five groups based on the orientation and function (Fig. 6). The principal

compressive group trabeculae are the uppermost trabeculae and thicker than the rest of the trabeculae. These extend as curved lines from the medial aspect of the metaphysis to the superior aspect of the femoral head. The secondary compressive group arises near the lesser trochanter and curves upwards laterally toward greater trochanter and upper neck in a fan-shaped manner. These are usually thin and sparse. The greater trochanteric group is situated in the greater trochanter in a curvilinear fashion. The principal tensile group arises from below the greater trochanter and extends to the inferior aspect of the femoral head, passing through the femoral neck. Secondary tensile group start below the principal tensile trabeculae and end superiorly along the upper end of femur (just after midline).

Ward's triangle (Singh et al. 1970, 1972, 1973) is an area with loose and thin trabeculae. This triangle becomes prominent in osteoporosis. As osteoporosis worsens, the triangle opens up laterally. Based on this sequence, Singh and coworkers (Singh et al. 1970, 1972) proposed an index which can be used as a scale for assessing the severity of osteoporosis (Fig. 7). The classification ranges from grade VI (normal with visualization of all the trabeculae) to grade I (loss of even the primary compressive trabeculae). Singh et al. later added grade VII in people with dense bones. However, recent studies have indicated poor correlation between Singh's index and bone density assessed by bone mineral densitometry techniques (Hübsch et al. 1992; Koot et al. 1996; Salamat et al. 2010).

Acute Hip Fractures

Fractures of the hip are broadly classified into femoral neck fractures and trochanteric fractures (Greenspan et al. 1994; Mautalen et al. 1996). The femoral neck fractures are intracapsular fractures (Fig. 8) and have a higher risk of avascular necrosis of the femoral head, compared to the extracapsular trochanteric fractures. Open reduction and internal fixation is the preferred treatment for femoral neck fractures. Trochanteric fractures (Fig. 9) are seen in advanced osteoporosis and in the elderly age group. Identification of undisplaced femoral neck fractures may be difficult and may not be diagnosed on the initial radiographs. Only a linear sclerotic band or angulation of trabeculae may be seen, even after careful evaluation. In doubtful cases, MR imaging is helpful and it can detect fractures that are less than 6 hours old (Anil et al. 2010).

Insufficiency Fractures

These can occur in the subchondral region and are often confused with avascular necrosis. The diagnosis is mainly radiological (Rafii et al. 1997; Yamamoto et al. 2000). The presentation is usually acute in elderly women. Subchondral lucency may be seen on radiographs, and are often missed on the initial radiograph. MR imaging is very useful in diagnosing these insufficiency fractures which are typically

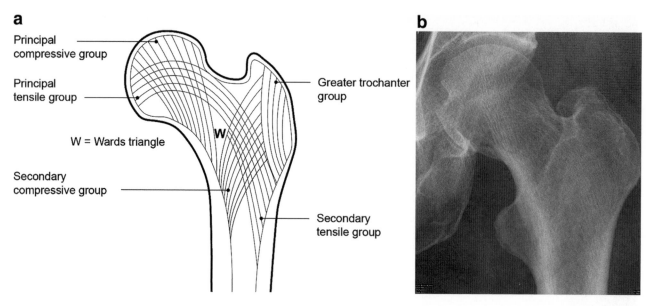

Fig. 6 Trabecular patterns in the proximal femur. **a** *Line diagram* shows the various groups of trabaculae and Ward's triangle. **b** Left hip radiograph of a normal adult shows the various trabacular groups and Ward's triangle

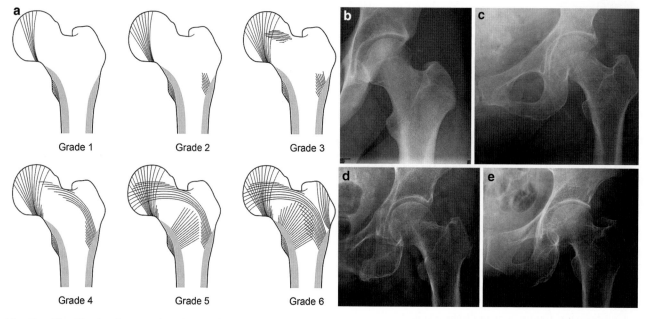

Fig. 7 **a** Classification for assessing the severity of osteoporosis according to the Singh index (Grade 6 to grade 1). **b** Normal trabecular pattern—grade 6. **c** Grade 5. **d** Grade 4. **e** Grade 3

seen as hypointense lines on T1- and T2- weighted images (Fig. 10). Proximal femur fractures should be differentiated from pathological fractures due to metastatic disease, especially when the fracture is located in the subtrochanteric region or in the lesser trochanter (Dijkstra et al. 1997).

Insufficiency fractures due to osteoporosis (Fig. 11) can occur in the sacrum, pubis, and less commonly, in the acetabulum and supraacetabular margins (De Smet and Neff 1985; Peh et al. 1996). The sacral fracture is identified by increased density due to the callus and focal periosteal reaction. MR imaging (Fig. 12) and bone scintigraphy are more sensitive than radiographs for detecting these fractures which may be incidentally seen during routine bone scintigraphy done for screening for metastasis. The pattern of sacral fractures may be H-shaped (described as the Honda sign), I-shaped, or arc-shaped.

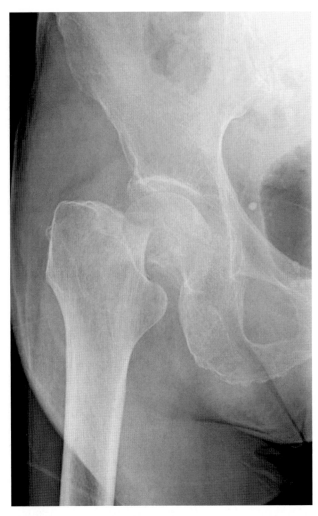

Fig. 8 Right hip radiograph of a 70-year-old woman shows an intracapsular fracture of the femoral neck

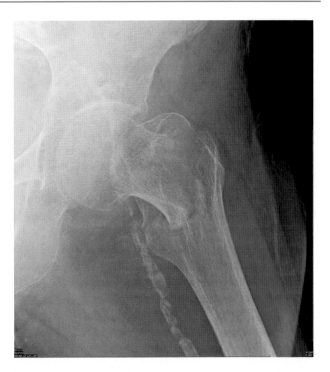

Fig. 9 Left hip radiograph of a 82-year-old woman shows an (extracapsular) intertrochanteric fracture

6.2.3 Appendicular Skeleton

Distal Radius

A fall on outstretched hand may result in a fracture of the distal radius with dorsal angulation, typically known as Colle's fracture (Cooney et al. 1980; O'Neill et al. 2001). It is more common in the left hand, although it depends on the bone mass between the dominant and non-dominant hand and the nature of fall (Fig. 13).

Humerus

Osteoporotic fractures are common in the surgical neck of the humerus (Fig. 14) and usually occur due to falls with direct landing on the shoulder (Palvanen et al. 2000). Clinton et al. (2009) proved that the incidence of humeral fractures increases the risk of hip fracture by more than five times in the first year.

Hand

Radiogrammetric measurements were initially applied to the metacarpal bones, especially the second or third metacarpal. The corticomedullary index is calculated by the combined cortical thickness divided by total bone width (Fig. 15). Another complex calculation exists where the cortical area is calculated. However, some studies have suggested that the correlation between radiogrammetry and other quantitative methods is poor. Recently, digital radiogrammetric techniques have evolved, which have a greater accuracy in quantifying the density compared to conventional radiogrammetry.

Cortical bone loss, measured in the second metacarpal by digital radiogrammetric methods, is similar to bone loss in the distal radius, lumbar spine, and iliac crest. However, correlation was poor with the proximal femur (Ives and Brickley 2005). Computer-aided calculations of cortical thickness, bone width, and bone volume per area have been obtained with digital X-ray radiogrammetry (DXR). DXR is simple, inexpensive, has a low radiation dose, and can be used as a screening tool in high risk patients before referring them for DXA (Pfeil et al. 2011).

Calcaneum

The trabecular pattern of the calcaneum (Fig. 16) is similar to that of the proximal femur and is easily visualized in the radiographs (Diard et al. 2007; Jhamaria et al. 1983). There

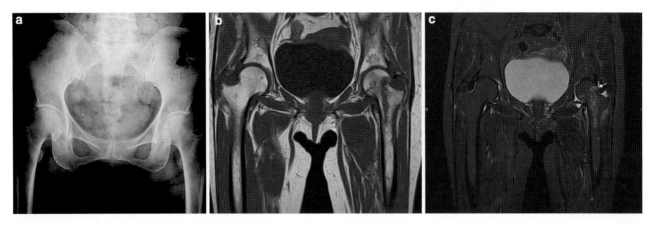

Fig. 10 Insufficiency fracture in the femoral neck. **a** Frontal pelvic radiograph of an elderly woman shows no obvious fracture. **b** Coronal T1-weighted and **c** fat-suppressed T2-weighted MR images show the subcapital linear insufficiency fracture (*arrows*). Adjacent edema is also noted

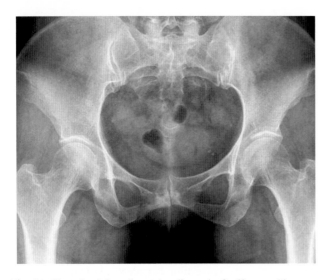

Fig. 11 Frontal pelvic radiograph radiograph of a 60-year-old woman shows an insufficiency fracture of the right inferior pubic ramus

are two sets of compression trabeculae and two sets of tensile trabeculae in the calcaneum (Fig. 16). Jhamaria et al. (1983) classified osteoporosis from grade V (normal) to grade I (severe osteoporosis).

6.3 Secondary Causes of Osteoporosis

6.3.1 Hyperparathyroidism

Hyperparathyroidism can be primary or secondary. Primary hyperparathyroidism is caused by a functioning adenoma of the parathyroid gland. Secondary hyperparathyroidism is usually due to long-standing hypocalcemia, with the most

common cause being chronic renal failure, which stimulates secretion of parathyroid hormone. The diagnosis of primary hyperparathyroidism is usually made by laboratory tests. The radiographs provide useful information regarding the nature of bone involvement and severity. Apart from diffuse osteopenia, the radiographical changes in the bone include subperiosteal, intracortical, endosteal, subchondral, subligamentous/subtendinous, and trabecular bone resorption. The most characteristic feature is subperiosteal bone resorption which is seen usually in the bones of hand and feet. The outer cortex becomes indistinct and scalloping or erosions appear in late stages.

Intracortical tunneling causes a striated appearance in the cortex and endosteal resorption results in thinning of the cortex and widening of the medullary canal. Subchondral resorption occurs beneath the articular cartilage (such as in sacroiliac joint) and results in pseudo-widening of the joint space in the radiographs (Hayes and Conway 1991). Other rare features of primary hyperparathyroidism include development of expansile lytic lesions known as 'brown tumors' and chondrocalcinosis, due to deposition of calcium pyrophosphate dehydrate (CPPD) crystals in the cartilages. In secondary hyperparathyroidism, apart from erosions, sclerosis is common in the axial skeleton, especially in the bone margins due to condensation of the trabeculae. The typical appearance in the vertebral body (Fig. 17) is known as rugger jersey spine and is due to subchondral sclerosis (Resnick 1981).

6.3.2 Steroid-Induced Osteoporosis

The main pathology in endogenous or exogenous glucocorticosteroid-induced osteoporosis is decreased osteoblastic activity and normal osteoclastic activity (Sissons 1956). It is most marked in the spine and ribs. Exuberant callus with marginal trabecular condensation is characteristic

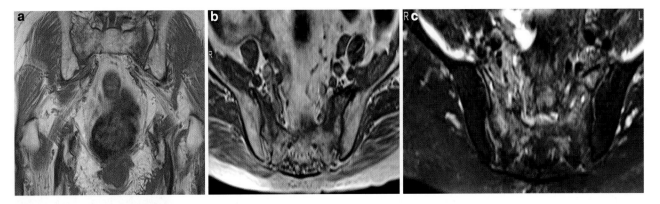

Fig. 12 Insufficiency fracture of the sacrum. **a** Coronal and **b** axial T1-weighted MR images of the sacrum show vertically-orientated hypointense fracture lines involving both sacral ala. **c** Axial fat-suppressed T2-weighted MR image shows prominent hyperintense marrow edema around the fractures

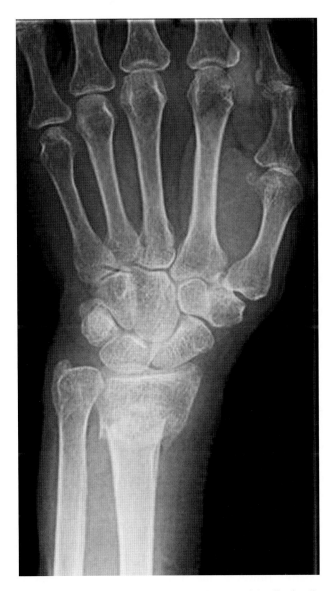

Fig. 13 Frontal wrist radiograph shows a fracture of the distal radius in an osteoporotic patient

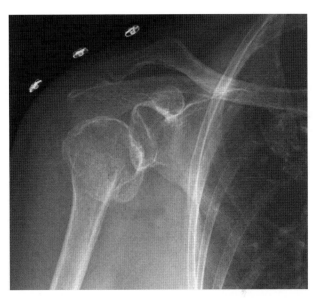

Fig. 14 Frontal shoulder radiograph shows a fracture of the surgical neck of the humerus

finding in steroid-induced osteoporosis. A few recent studies have proven that the bone density is maintained and incidence of fractures are less with prophylactic bisphosphonate therapy (Stoch et al. 2009).

6.3.3 Osteomalacia

In Osteomalacia, even though vitamin D deficiency leads to osteopenia, the pathology is different. There is significant amount of unmineralized osteoid in osteomalacia, in contrast to osteoporosis where there is reduction in the mineralized osteoid. Other than osteopenia, the radiographical findings include pseudofracture or linear lucencies which are seen perpendicular to the long axis of bone. These pseudofractures represent the accumulation of unmineralized osteoid. The common locations include the pelvis,

Fig. 15 Radiogrammetry which was used for quantification for bone density in the past. **a** Diagram shows the cross-section of bone with measurements of the cortical thickness and cortical index. **b** Frontal radiograph shows measurement of the cortical thickness in the second metacarpal

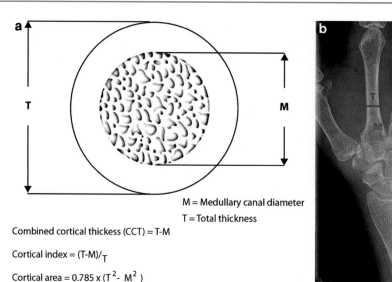

M = Medullary canal diameter

T = Total thickness

Combined cortical thickess (CCT) = T-M

Cortical index = (T-M)/$_T$

Cortical area = 0.785 x (T^2- M^2)

Fig. 16 **a** Calcaneal trabeculae. *Line diagram* shows the various normal groups of trabeculae. **b** Lateral calcaneal radiograph of a 71-year-old woman shows the trabecular pattern. The tensile trabaculae are less prominent

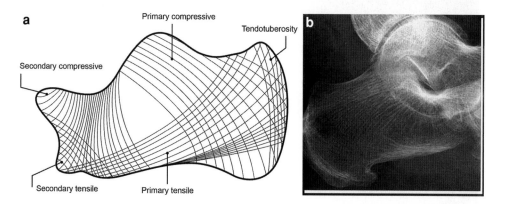

femoral neck, and scapula. These are often symmetrical. The involved bones are prone to develop deformities and fractures (Kienböck 1940; Reginato et al. 1999).

6.3.4 Hyperthyroidism

Thyroid hormone promotes bone resorption and generalized osteopenia is often seen in patients with hyperthyroidism, especially in thyrotoxicosis. Radiographic findings are similar to diffuse osteoporosis, with more cortical involvement and tunnelling (Toh et al. 1985).

6.3.5 Other Important Causes of Secondary Osteoporosis

Other causes include heparin-induced osteoporosis (Nelson-Piercy 1997) and nutrition-related osteoporotic disorders which may be indistinguishable radiographically from involutional osteoporosis. Marrow proliferative disorders such as myeloma may cause diffuse osteopenia and may produce punched-out lytic lesions in the bones. The diagnosis is usually by laboratory investigations.

6.4 Osteoporosis in the Young

6.4.1 Marrow Disorders

Marrow disorders include congenital hemolytic anemias, storage disorders, and leukemias. Blood investigations and further imaging like CT and MR imaging are helpful for the diagnosis and assessing severity of these conditions.

6.4.2 Idiopathic Juvenile Osteoporosis

Idiopathic juvenile osteoporosis (IJO) is a very rare disorder occurring in prepubertal children in the age range of 2–14 years, and is characterized by bone pain, osteopenia, fractures, and deformities (Schippers 1938). Changes are seen in the vertebrae which show diffuse osteopenia and subsequent deformities or compression fractures (Marhaug 1993; Lorenc 2002). In the appendicular skeleton, the fractures are characteristically seen in the metaphyses. This is a self limiting condition which resolves during and after puberty. However, the deformities may sometimes be severe and can be irreversible when the patients grow as

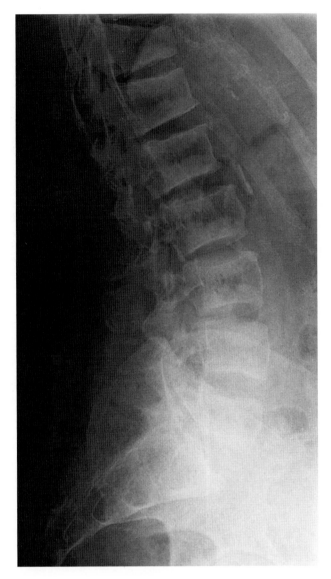

Fig. 17 Lateral thoraco-lumbar radiograph of a 40-year-old woman with secondary hyperparathyroidism. There is osteopenia with marginal sclerosis of multiple vertebral bodies giving the typical rugger-jersey spine appearance

adults. Bisphonates are considered to be effective in preventing these deformities (Melchior et al. 2005).

6.4.3 Rickets

Rickets are due to defect in mineralization of the osteoid. This may either be due to nutrition-related (Vitamin D deficiency) or vitamin D resistant hypophosphatemic rickets which is otherwise known as renal rickets. The classical radiographical changes, apart from osteopenia, include changes in the metaphysis, such as cupping, fraying, and splaying due to weight-bearing and rapid growth (Cheema et al. 2003). The provisional zone of calcification is widened. The changes are usually seen in the distal radial metaphysis, proximal humerus, distal ends of femur and tibia. The metaphyseal

changes are well seen in nutritional rickets which occur in younger children (Swischuk and Hayden 1979).

6.5 Regional or Localized Osteoporosis

6.5.1 Reflex Sympathetic Dystrophy

Reflex sympathetic dystrophy (RSD), otherwise known as complex regional pain syndrome (CPRS), is characterized by intense pain, allodynia (pain caused by touch), vasomotor disturbances, and delayed functional recovery after minor trauma. This condition is thought to be caused by excessive sympathetic stimulation although blockade of sympathetic stimulation has not found to be an effective treatment in several patients (Albazaz et al. 2008). Although the diagnosis is mainly based on clinical findings, bone scintigraphy is often used to confirm the diagnosis of RSD (Lee and Weeks 1995). Focal/regional osteoporosis is seen in around 60 % of patients with RSD, although it may be nonspecific due to disuse secondary to pain (Fig. 18). Soft tissue changes such as swelling or atrophy are also considered nonspecific.

6.5.2 Transient Osteoporosis of Hip

Transient osteoporosis of hip is a self-limiting condition known to occur in late pregnancy, although nearly two-thirds of patients are middle-aged men aged between 40 and 70 years (Kalliakmanis et al. 2006). The patients affected by this condition often present with pain of the hip with limitation of movement. The exact etiology and mechanism are not well understood. Proposed mechanisms include genetic predisposition, intermittent compression of obturator nerve, non-traumatic reflex sympathetic dystrophy, fatty marrow conversion, hormone imbalance, and microfractures (Rocchietti March et al. 2010). The diagnosis is based on the history and radiographic features of osteopenia involving the femoral head and neck. MR imaging usually shows increased signal on T2-weighted images. Bone scintigraphy may show increased uptake in the affected hip during the early stages. The clinical and radiographic findings often disappear after weeks or months. Other similar conditions, such as osteonecrosis, osteomyelitis, inflammatory arthritis, and neoplasm should be ruled out if symptoms persist.

6.5.3 Regional Migratory Osteoporosis

Regional migratory osteoporosis is another self-limiting type of osteoporosis which involves a few weight-bearing joints of the lower limb. This condition is characterized by pain in the affected joint and osteopenia which proceeds from proximal to distal joints in the lower limb. The migration of affected region may be within the same joint (Yamasaki et al. 2003). This condition is considered to be part of the spectrum of transient osteoporosis by some authors (Duncan et al. 1969; Toms et al. 2005).

Fig. 18 **a** Frontal and **b** lateral wrist radiographs of a patient with distal radial fracture who developed reflex sympathetic dystrophy. Diffuse osteopenia and soft tissue swelling are present

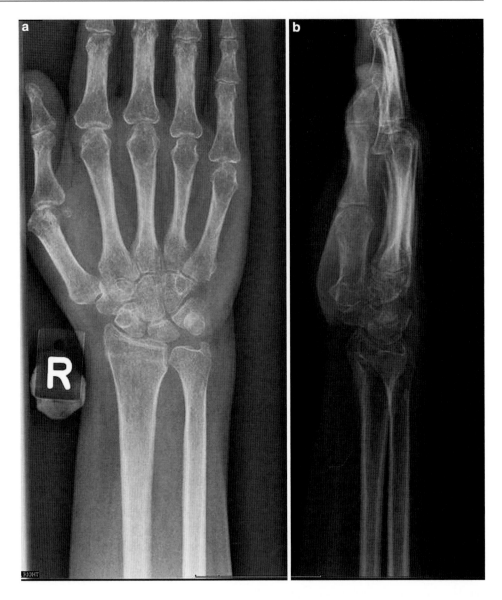

6.5.4 Disuse Osteoporosis

Disuse osteoporosis refers to decrease in bone density, due to reduction in the mechanical stress which results in increased resorption by osteoclast activity and inhibition of osteoblasts (Takata and Yasui 2001). Disuse osteoporosis may be due to muscular paralysis due to neuronal injury (central or peripheral) or due to restriction of movement of limb or part of the body. Radiographic findings include osteopenia, coarsened trabeculae, and thinning of the cortex in the affected bones. The weight-bearing bones are more severely affected than the non-weight bearing ones (Doty and DiCarlo 1995).

7 Conclusion

Radiography is a cheap and widely available modality. Conventional radiography may not be helpful in quantification of the bone density but it is very useful tool in assessing the quality

of bone and for screening of deformities and fractures. Radiography is also helpful in assessing the changes in the pattern of resorption in conditions such as hyperparathyroidism. It can be used in conjunction with other modalities, such as DEXA, MR imaging, and quantitative CT for the differential diagnosis and follow-up evaluation of elderly patients with osteoporosis.

References

Albazaz R, Wong Y, Homer-Vanniasinkam S (2008) Complex regional pain syndrome: a review. Ann Vasc Surg 22(2):297–306

Albright F (1947) Osteoporosis. Ann Intern Med 27(6):861–882

Anil G, Guglielmi G, Peh WCG (2010) Radiology of osteoporosis. Radiol Clin North Am 48(3):497–518

Ardran G (1951) Bone destruction not demonstrable by radiography. Br J Radiol 24(278):107–109

Bailey D, Martin A, McKay H, Whiting S, Mirwald R (2000) Calcium accretion in girls and boys during puberty: a longitudinal analysis. J Bone Miner Res 15(11):2245–2250

Bart (2008) Normal bone anatomy and physiology. Clin J Am Soc Nephrol 3(Suppl):131–139

Benhamou C, Lespessailles E, Jacquet G et al (1994) Fractal organization of trabecular bone images on calcaneus radiographs. J Bone Miner Res 9(12):1909–1918

Bordier PJ, Miravet L, Hioco D (1973) Young adult osteoporosis. Clin Endocrinol Metab 2:277–292

Cheema J, Grissom L, Harcke H (2003) Radiographic characteristics of lower-extremity bowing in children. Radiographics 23(4): 871–880

Clinton J, Franta A, Polissar N et al (2009) Proximal humeral fracture as a risk factor for subsequent hip fractures. J Bone Joint Surg Am 91(3):503–511

Cooney W, Dobyns J, Linscheid R (1980) Complications of Colles' fractures. J Bone Joint Surg Am 62(4):613–619

Cranney A, Jamal S, Tsang J, Josse R, Leslie W (2007) Low bone mineral density and fracture burden in postmenopausal women. Can Med Assoc J 177(6):575–580

Delmas P, van de Langerijt L, Watts N et al (2005) Underdiagnosis of vertebral fractures is a worldwide problem: the IMPACT study. J Bone Miner Res 20(4):557–563

De Smet A, Neff J (1985) Pubic and sacral insufficiency fractures: clinical course and radiologic findings. Am J Roentgenol 145(3): 601–606

Diard F, Hauger O, Moinard M, Brunot S, Marcet B (2007) Pseudo-cysts, lipomas, infarcts and simple cysts of the calcaneus: are there different or related lesions? JBR-BTR 90(5):315–324

Dijkstra P, Oudkerk M, Wiggers T (1997) Prediction of pathological subtrochanteric fractures due to metastatic lesions. Arch Orthop Trauma Surg 116(4):221–224

D'ippolito G, Schiller PC, Ricordi C, Roos BA, Howard GA (1999) Age-related osteogenic potential of mesenchymal stromal stem cells from human vertebral bone marrow. J Bone Miner Res 14(7): 1115–1122

Doty S, DiCarlo E (1995) Pathophysiology of immobilization osteoporosis. Curr Opin Orthop 6(5):45–49

Duncan H, Frame B, Frost H, Arnstein AR (1969) Regional migratory osteoporosis. South Med J 62:41–44

Epstein DM, Dalinka MK, Kaplan FS, Aronchick JM, Marinelli DL, Kundel HL (1986) Observer variation in the detection of osteopenia. Skeletal Radiol 15:347–349

Eriksen EF, Axelrod DW, Melsen F, Obrant K (1994) Bone histomorphometry. Raven Press, New York

Finsen V, Anda S (1988) Accuracy of visually estimated bone mineralization in routine radiographs of the lower extremity. Skeletal Radiol 17:270–275

Fitzpatrick LA (2002) Secondary causes of osteoporosis. Mayo Clin Proc 77:453–468

Gehlbach S, Bigelow C, Heimisdottir M, May S, Walker M, Kirkwood J (2000) Recognition of vertebral fracture in a clinical setting. Osteoporos Int 11(7):577–582

Genant H, Heck L, Lanzl L, Rossmann K, Horst J, Paloyan E (1973) Primary hyperparathyroidism. A comprehensive study of clinical, biochemical and radiographic manifestations. Radiology 109(3):513–524

Geraets W, Van der Stelt P, Netelenbos C, Elders P (1990) A new method for automatic recognition of the radiographic trabecular pattern. J Bone Miner Res 5(3):227–233

Grampp S, Jergas M, Lang P et al (1996) Quantitative CT assessment of the lumbar spine and radius in patients with osteoporosis. Am J Roentgenol 167:133–140

Grampp S, Steiner E, Imhof H (1997) Radiological diagnosis of osteoporosis. Eur Radiol 7(Suppl 2):11–19

Greenspan S, Myers E, Maitland L et al (1994) Trochanteric bone mineral density is associated with type of hip fracture in the elderly. J Bone Miner Res 9(12):1889–1894

Guglielmi G, Muscarella S, Bazzocchi A (2011) Integrated imaging approach to osteoporosis: state-of-the-art review and update. Radiographics 31(5):1343–1364

Harms HM, Kaptaina U, Kulpmann WR et al (1989) Pulse amplitude and frequency modulation of parathyroid hormone in plasma. J Clin Endocrinol Metab 69:843–851

Hauschild O, Ghanem N, Oberst M et al (2009) Evaluation of Singh index for assessment of osteoporosis using digital radiography. Eur J Radiol 71(1):152–158

Harris W, Heaney R (1969) Skeletal renewal and metabolic bone disease. New Engl J Med 280:193–202

Hayes CW, Conway WF (1991) Hyperparathyroidism. Radiol Clin North Am 29:85–96

Heuck F, Schmidt E (1960) Die quantitative Bestimmung des Mineralgehaltes des Knochens aus dem Röntgenbild. Fortschr Röntgenstr 93:523–554

Hübsch P, Kocanda H, Youssefzadeh S et al (1992) Comparison of dual energy X-ray absorptiometry of the proximal femur with morphologic data. Acta Radiol 33:477–481

Ives R, Brickley M (2005) Metacarpal radiogrammetry: a useful indicator of bone loss throughout the skeleton? J Archaeol Sci 32:1552–1559

Jergas M (2008) Radiology of osteoporosis. In: Grampp S (ed) Radiology of osteoporosis. Springer, Berlin, pp 77–103

Jhamaria N, Lal K, Udawat M et al (1983) The trabecular pattern of the calcaneum as an index of osteoporosis. J Bone Joint Surg Br 65(2):195–198

Johnell O, Kanis J, Odén A et al (2004) Fracture risk following an osteoporotic fracture. Osteoporos Int 15(3):175–179

Jung H, Jee W, McCauley T, Ha K, Choi K (2003) Discrimination of metastatic from acute osteoporotic compression spinal fractures with MR imaging. Radiographics 23(1):179–187

Kalliakmanis AG, Pneumaticos S, Plessas S (2006) Transient hip osteoporosis. Orthopedics 29(3):263–264

Keen R (2007) Osteoporosis: strategies for prevention and management. Best practice and research. Clin Rheumatol 21(1):109–122

Khosla S, Melton LJ 3rd, Riggs BL (2011) The unitary model for estrogen deficiency and the pathogenesis of osteoporosis: is a revision needed? J Bone Miner Res 26:441

Kienböck R (1940) Osteomalazie, osteoporose, osteopsathyrose, porotische kyphose. Fortschr Röntgenstr 61:159

Koot VCM, Kesselaer SM, Clevers GJ et al (1996) Evaluation of the Singh index for measuring osteoporosis. J Bone Joint Surg Br 78:831–834

Lee G, Weeks P (1995) The role of bone scintigraphy in diagnosing reflex sympathetic dystrophy. J Hand Surg 20(3):458–463

Lems W (2007) Clinical relevance of vertebral fractures. Ann Rheum Dis 66(1):2–4

Link T, Majumdar S, Grampp S et al (1999) Imaging of trabecular bone structure in osteoporosis. Eur Radiol 9(9):1781–1788

Lorenc R (2002) Idiopathic juvenile osteoporosis. Calcif Tissue Int 70(5):395–397

Marhaug G (1993) Idiopathic juvenile osteoporosis. Scand J Rheumatol 22:45–47

Mautalen C, Vega E, Einhorn T (1996) Are the etiologies of cervical and trochanteric hip fractures different? Bone 18(3 Suppl): 133–137

Melchior R, Zabel B, Spranger J, Schumacher R (2005) Effective parenteral clodronate treatment of a child with severe juvenile idiopathic osteoporosis. Eur J Pediatr 164(1):22–27

Meunier P, S-Bianchi G, Edouard C et al (1972) Bony manifestations of thyrotoxicosis. Orthop Clin North Am 3:745–774

Nelson-Piercy C (1997) Hazards of heparin: allergy, heparin-induced thrombocytopenia and osteoporosis. Baillière's Clin Obstetr Gynaecol 11(3):489–509

Nijweide P, Burger E, Feyen J (1986) Cells of bone: proliferation, differentiation, and hormonal regulation. Physiol Rev 66(4):855–886

O'Neill T, Cooper C, Finn J et al (2001) Incidence of distal forearm fracture in British men and women. Osteoporos Int 12(7):555–558

Pacifici R, Rothstein M, Rifas L et al (1990) Increased monocyteinterleukin-1 activity and decreased vertebral bone density in patients with fasting idiopathic hypercalciuria. J Clin Endocrinol Metab 71:138–145

Palvanen M, Kannus P, Parkkari J et al (2000) The injury mechanisms of osteoporotic upper extremity fractures among older adults: a controlled study of 287 consecutive patients and their 108 controls. Osteoporos Int 11(10):822–831

Peh WCG, Khong PL, Yin YM et al (1996) Imaging of pelvic insufficiency fractures. Radiographics 16:335–348

Pfeil A, Haugeberg G, Hansch A et al (2011) Value of digital X-ray radiogrammetry in the assessment of inflammatory bone loss in rheumatoid arthritis. Arthritis Care Res 63:666–674

Rafii M, Mitnick H, Klug J, Firooznia H (1997) Insufficiency fracture of the femoral head: MR imaging in three patients. Am J Roentgenol 168(1):159–163

Reginato AJ, Falasca GF, Pappu R et al (1999) Musculoskeletal manifestations of osteomalacia: report of 26 cases and literature review. Semin Arthritis Rheum 28:287–304

Resnick D (1981) The "rugger jersey" vertebral body. Arthritis Rheum 24:1191–1194

Riggs BL, Melton LJ III (1983) Evidence for two distinct syndromes of involutional osteoporosis. Am J Med 75(6):899–901

Riggs BL, MeltonLJ III (1986) Involutional osteoporosis. N Engl J Med 314:1676–1686

Rocchietti March M, Tovaglia V, Meo A et al (2010) Transient osteoporosis of the hip. Hip Int 20(3):297–300

Salamat MR, Rostampour N, Zofaghari SJ et al (2010) Comparison of singh index accuracy and dualenergy X-ray absorptiometry bone mineral density measurement for evaluating osteoporosis Iran. J Radiat Res 8(2):123–128

Schippers JC (1938) Over een geval van spontane algemene osteoporose bij een klein meisje. Maandschr Kindergeneeskunde 8:107

Singh M, Nagrath A, Maini P (1970) Changes in trabecular pattern of the upper end of the femur as an index of osteoporosis. J Bone Joint Surg 52(3):457–467

Singh M, Riggs B, Beabout J, Jowsey J (1972) Femoral trabecularpattern index for evaluation of spinal osteoporosis. Ann Intern Med 77(1):63–67

Singh M, Riggs B, Beabout J, Jowsey J (1973) Femoral trabecular pattern index for evaluation of spinal osteoporosis. A detailed methodologic description. Mayo Clin Proc 48(3):184–189

Sissons H (1956) The osteoporosis of Cushing's syndrome. J Bone Joint Surg Br 38(1):418–433

Smith R (1995) Idiopathic juvenile osteoporosis: experience of twenty-one patients. Br J Rheumatol 34(1):68–77

Stoch S, Saag K, Greenwald M et al (2009) Once-weekly oral alendronate 70 mg in patients with glucocorticoid-induced bone loss: a 12-month randomized, placebo-controlled clinical trial. J Rheumatol 36(8):1705–1714

Swischuk L, Hayden C (1979) Rickets: a roentgenographic scheme for diagnosis. Pediatr Radiol 8(4):203–208

Takata S, Yasui N (2001) Disuse osteoporosis. J Med Invest 48(3–4):147–156

Toh SH, Claunch BC, Brown PH (1985) Effect of hyperthyroidism and its treatment on bone mineral content. Arch Intern Med 145:883–886

Toms A, Marshall T, Becker E et al (2005) Regional migratory osteoporosis: a review illustrated by five cases. Clin Radiol 60(4):425–438

Vernon-Roberts B, Pirie C (1973) Healing trabecular microfractures in the bodies of lumbar vertebrae. Ann Rheum Dis 32(5):406–412

von Meyer H (1867) Die architektur der spongiosa (The architecture of the spongiosa) Reichert und Dubois-Reymonds Archiv 34:615–628 (in German)

Vu MQ, Weintraub N, Rubenstein LZ (2006) Falls in the nursing home: are they preventable? J Am Med Dir Assoc 7:S53

Wagner S, Stäbler A, Sittek H et al (2005) Diagnosis of osteoporosis: visual assessment on conventional versus digital radiographs. Osteoporos Int 16(12):1815–1822

Williamson MR, Boyd CM, Williamson SL (1990) Osteoporosis: diagnosis by plain chest film versus dual photon bone densitometry. Skeletal Radiol 19:7–30

Wolbarst AB (1993) Dependence of attenuation on atomic number and photon energy. In: Physics of Radiology. Appleton and Lange, Norwalk, pp 113–121

Yamasaki S, Masuhara K, Miki H et al (2003) Three cases of regional migratory osteoporosis. Arch Orthop Trauma Surg 123(8):439–441

Yamamoto T, Schneider R, Bullough P (2000) Insufficiency subchondral fracture of the femoral head. Am J Surg Pathol 24(3):464–468

Imaging of Insufficiency Fractures

Christian R. Krestan, Ursula Nemec, and Stefan Nemec

Contents

Abstract

This review article focuses on occurrence, imaging, and differential diagnosis of insufficiency fractures. Prevalence and the most common sites of insufficiency fractures and their clinical implications are discussed. Insufficiency fractures are due to normal stress exerted on weakened bone. Most commonly, postmenopausal osteoporosis is the cause for insufficiency fractures. Additional conditions affecting bone turnover include osteomalacia, chronic renal failure, and high dose corticosteroid therapy. It is a challenge for the radiologist to detect and diagnose insufficiency fractures as well as to differentiate them from malignant fractures. Radiographs are the basic modality used for screening of insufficiency fractures, yet depending on the location of the fractures sensitivity is limited. Magnetic resonance imaging (MRI) is a very sensitive tool to visualize bone marrow abnormalities associated with insufficiency fractures and has allowed differentiation of benign versus malignant fractures. Thin section Multidetector CT depicts subtle fracture lines allowing direct visualization of cortical and trabecular bone. Dedicated Mikro-CTs (Xtreme-CT) can detect subtle fractures reaching an in-plane resolution of 80 μm. Bone scintigraphy still plays a role in detecting fractures, with good sensitivity but unsatisfactory specificity. PET-CT with hybrid scanners has been the upcoming modality for the differentiation of benign from malignant fractures. Bone densitometry and clinical fracture history may determine the future risk of possible insufficiency fractures.

1   Introduction

1.1   Background

Insufficiency fractures are stress fractures that occur when stress is applied to abnormal, weakened bone with less than

C. R. Krestan (✉) · U. Nemec · S. Nemec
Department of Radiology,
Medical University of Vienna, Vienna General Hospital,
Waehringerstr. 18-20, 1090 Vienna, Austria
e-mail: christian.krestan@meduniwien.ac.at

G. Guglielmi (ed.), *Osteoporosis and Bone Densitometry Measurements*, Medical Radiology. Diagnostic Imaging,
DOI: 10.1007/174_2012_613, © Springer-Verlag Berlin Heidelberg 2013

the normal elastic resistance. The most prevalent disease leading to insufficiency fractures is postmenopausal osteoporosis, followed by osteomalacia. Unlike the other subtype of stress fractures fatigue fractures are due to normal or physiologic stress on weakened bone. They result from the application of abnormal stress or torque on a bone with normal elastic resistance and strength. Loss of bone trabeculae decreases the bone's elastic resistance. Awareness is increasing concerning the occurrence of these fractures among older persons. The prevalence of both osteoporosis and osteomalacia increases with age and, in subjects over the age of 90, osteoporosis is found in 71 % of patients and osteomalacia is found in 29 % of patients (Hordon and Peacock 1990). Insufficiency fractures occur most commonly at the pelvic girdle including the sacrum, followed by the proximal femur and the vertebral bodies in particular at the lumbar spine and the lower thoracic spine. Other sites frequently affected by insufficiency fractures are the tibia, fibula, and calcaneus and metatarsal bones (Soubrier et al. 2003). Insufficiency fractures of the femoral diaphyses are rare. Most frequently insufficiency fractures are due to undiagnosed or untreated osteoporosis.

1.2 Pathophysiology

A fracture represents the end result of the spectrum of a bone's response to an increasing level of stress. According to Wolff's law, stress that occurs beyond the bone's elastic range causes persistent plastic deformity as a result of microfractures. In this situation, osteoclastic resorption exceeds osteoblastic activity. A strong association exists between fractures of the sacrum and those of the pubic bone. They can often be found in a symmetrical fashion and are often due to osteomalacia. Pubic fractures may develop as a result of increased anterior arch strain secondary to initial failure of the posterior arch (sacrum). There are many causes of insufficiency fractures including postmenopausal osteoporosis, rheumatoid arthritis, Paget's disease, osteomalacia, hyperparathyroidism, renal osteodystrophy, osteogenesis imperfecta, osteopetrosis, and fibrous dysplasia. Other important causes are senile osteoporosis or pelvic irradiation and corticosteroid therapy leading to secondary osteoporosis. Also reported are total hip replacement, scurvy, osteopetrosis, primary biliary cirrhosis, organ transplantation, tabes dorsalis, and high dose fluoride therapy (Soubrier et al. 2003).

1.3 Frequency

Most patients with insufficiency fractures are older than 60 years. The mean age ranges from 62 to 74 years (Frey et al. 2007; Peh and Evans 1993; Grasland et al. 1996;

Soubrier et al. 2003). Women predominantly are affected especially in the postmenopausal state. On the average insufficiency fractures are estimated to occur in 1–5 % of the population, depending on the referral population (Kanis and Pitt 1992). In most patients, insufficiency fractures resolve or improve significantly with conservative management. However, in recent years interventional procedures using percutaneous cement application have been suggested, in particular of vertebral bodies and the sacrum (Brook et al. 2005; Cho et al. 2010).

1.4 Clinical Presentation

Typically, patients present with acute pain in the groin, back, or buttock, resp. foot or around the knee, depending on the site of the fracture. Twenty-five percent of patients have multiple sites of pain. In many patients, pain is severe enough to render the patient nonambulatory. Usually, patients present with either no history of trauma or a history of low impact trauma. On physical examination usually, signs of insufficiency fracture are nonspecific or nonexistent. Neurologic deficits are rarely found. Typically, a discordance exists between the severe symptoms and the mild or absent physical signs. Management is conservative and consists initially of bed rest, reduced weight bearing, and simple analgesics for pain relief. In severe cases a more aggressive approach can be performed. Imaging-guided sacroplasty for treatment of sacral insufficiency fractures has been described (Frey et al. 2007). Vertebroplasty or kyphoplasty to treat vertebral insufficiency fractures is a common procedure in radiology or orthopaedic departments.

1.5 Locations

1.5.1 Pelvis

Insufficiency fractures of the pelvis are being increasingly recognized as a major cause of low back pain in elderly women with osteoporosis (Fig. 1). Fractures in the sacrum are difficult to diagnose, as plain radiographic findings are sometimes unhelpful or misleading. Bone scintigraphy is very sensitive for the detection of fractures in the sacrum, with demonstration of the H-shaped (or butterfly) sacral pattern or the combination of concomitant sacral and parasymphyseal uptake being considered as a typical finding of insufficiency fractures (Fujii et al. 2005). MRI is a very sensitive method for detecting insufficiency fractures visualizing bone marrow edema pattern and frequently also fracture lines. It can be helpful in distinguishing insufficiency from pathologic fractures due to tumour infiltration (Figs. 2, 3). The majority of patients respond well to periods of enforced bed rest and administration of analgesics.

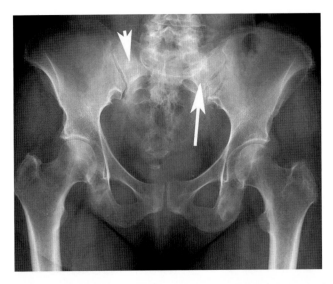

Fig. 1 Anteroposterior radiograph of the pelvis demonstrates areas of sclerosis in both sacral ala (*arrows*) consistent with insufficiency fractures

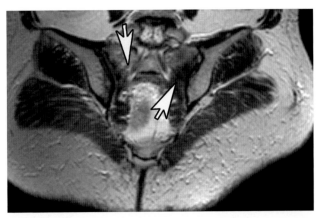

Fig. 3 Axial MRI (T1-w-sequence) demonstrating signal loss in both sacral ala compatible with bilateral insufficiency fractures in a 55-year-old woman after radiotherapy of the pelvis for cervical carcinoma

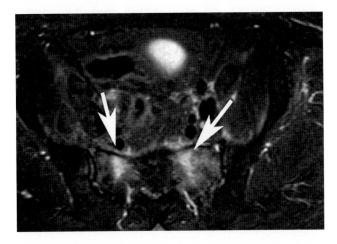

Fig. 2 Axial MRI (STIR-sequence) of the pelvis demonstrating bone marrow edema pattern in bilateral sacrum compatible with bilateral insufficiency fractures

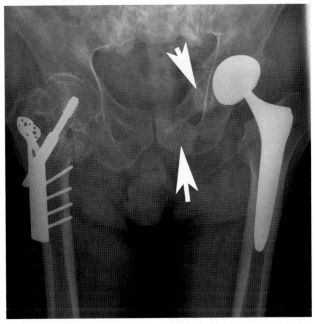

Fig. 4 AP radiograph of both hip joints shows insufficiency fractures (*arrows*) in the left parasymphyseal region and the left periacetabular region. Total hip replacement is an additional predisposing causative factor

Recognition of the spectrum of imaging findings for this entity should lead to its correct identification and the institution of appropriate treatment (Peh et al. 1996). Insufficiency fractures following total hip arthroplasty (THA) frequently occur in the superior and inferior pubic ramus, the puboischial rami, or the ischium around the obturator foramen, while they rarely occur in the medial wall of the acetabulum (Kanaji et al. 2007) (Fig. 4). Computed tomography (CT) is helpful for confirming the presence of fractures in cases with atypical scintigraphic patterns, particularly in those with a known primary malignant neoplasm. CT is especially useful in the further evaluation of parasymphyseal and pubic rami lesions

(Figs. 5, 6). Radiotherapy is a well-known risk factor for pelvic insufficiency fractures in postmenopausal women. Recognition of insufficiency fractures helps to avoid the pitfalls of misdiagnosing tumour recurrence or bony metastases (Peh et al. 1995) (Fig. 7).

It should also be noted that multiple pelvic insufficiency fractures are frequently found, particularly in the presence of pubic or acetabular fractures, and careful search for concomitant fractures is warranted. In a previous study in 70.3 % of cases with pelvic insufficiency fractures, multiple

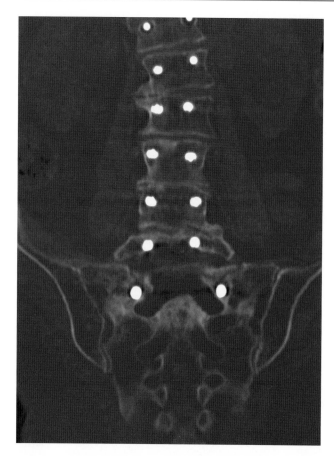

Fig. 5 Coronal CT-reformation of the sacrum demonstrates sacral insufficiency fractures at S1 with fracture lines and sclerosis. Posterior spinal fusion Th12-S1 with loosening of T12 pedicle screws

fracture sites were present. In the case of pubic fractures in 90 % concomitant fractures were present. Also, 76 % of acetabular fractures had concomitant fractures present (Cabarrus et al. 2008).

1.5.2 Lower Extremity

Insufficiency fractures of the fibula are typically found in patients with underlying rheumatic diseases, mainly rheumatoid arthritis (Alonso-Bartolome et al. 1999; Yamamoto et al. 2002) (Figs. 8, 9). Insufficiency fractures are also frequently found at the metatarsal bones in particular in the setting of inflammatory arthropathies (Fig. 10). Also these may be diagnosed in patients with severe osteoporosis, high-dose corticosteroids, or methotrexate therapy. Patients with marked joint deformity are also at high risk for developing insufficiency fractures (Maenpaa et al. 2002). Less frequently, in up to 25 %, insufficiency fractures at the femoral shaft can occur, predominately in elderly patients with osteoporosis (Martin-Hunyadi et al. 2000) (Fig. 11). Insufficiency fractures at the tibia (Fig. 12a–c) may be found as an early manifestation of bone failure in patients after renal transplantation as reported by a previous study

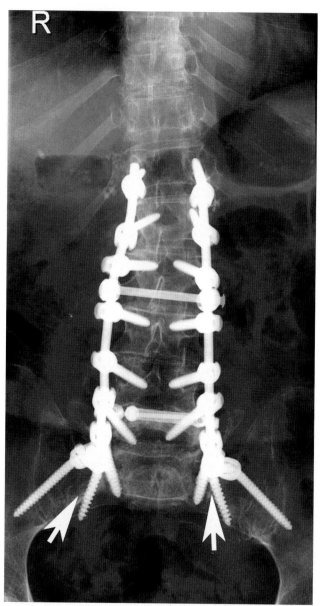

Fig. 6 AP radiograph of the sacrum after orthopaedic trans-sacroiliac screw fixation of bilateral sacral insufficiency fractures at the S1 level

(Franco et al. 2003). The main causes are preexisting renal osteodystrophy, glucocorticoid therapy, and hyperparathyroidism, whether residual or secondary to imperfect graft function (Franco et al. 2003). Longitudinal stress fractures of the tibia can also occur in patients with healed chronic osteomyelitis (Feydy et al. 2000). Even postpartum osteoporosis was found to be a cause of insufficiency fractures around the knee (Clemetson et al. 2004).

One of the important differential diagnoses of subchondral insufficiency fractures of the femoral head may include osteonecrosis. Typical MRI findings in insufficiency fractures include a pattern of bone marrow edema with a low-signal-intensity line (resp. fracture) on the T1-weighted

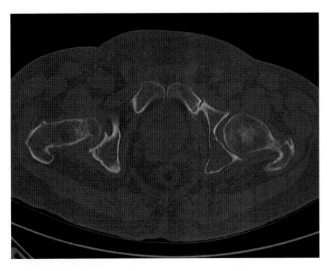

Fig. 7 Axial CT image at the level of the hip joints demonstrates insufficiency fracture of the left pubic bone (*arrow*), note also osteolysis of the left posterior acetabulum due to multiple myeloma in this 55-year-old male (*arrowhead*)

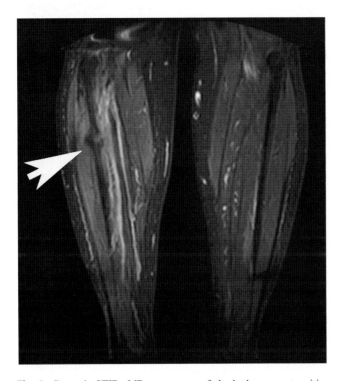

Fig. 8 Coronal STIR MR sequence of both lower extremities demonstrating marrow edema and subtle fracture line due to insufficiency fracture at the right fibula

Fig. 9 AP radiograph of the left knee demonstrating an old insufficiency fracture of the right fibula with callus formation after total knee replacement

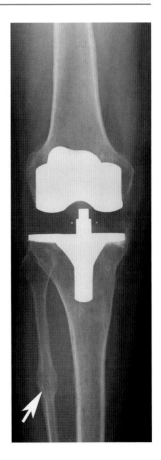

images parallel to the subchondral bone. In general, the circumscribed lesions on MRI, which are commonly observed in osteonecrosis, are not found (Yamamoto et al. 2007). Histopathologically fracture callus, reactive cartilage, and granulation tissue is seen without any evidence of antecedent osteonecrosis. The subchondral insufficiency fracture of the femoral head (SIF) is a recently recognized cause of acute onset arthritis mostly in elderly women, which previously had been commonly considered either as osteonecrosis or osteoarthritis.

1.5.3 Spine

Insufficiency fractures at the spine are a leading cause for acute low back pain without an acute traumatic event. Usually a concave or wedge-shaped deformity of the affected vertebra is found and a wide range of the vertebral height ratios and fracture distribution were reported (Kawaguchi et al. 2001). Once an initial vertebral fracture is sustained, the risk of subsequent vertebral fracture increases significantly. However, this effect cannot be explained by low bone mass alone, suggesting that factors independent of this parameter contribute to this occurrence (Briggs et al. 2007). The assessment of vertebral fractures using a semi-quantitative approach has been described, grading osteoporotic fractures into type 1 (20–25 % deformity), type 2 (25–40 %), and type 3 (>40 %) (Genant et al. 1993). Accurate radiographic diagnosis of osteoporotic vertebral fractures is important. Several studies indicated a false-negative rate of up to 34 % in reports of lateral radiographs of the thoracolumbar spine (Delmas et al. 2005). Radiologists

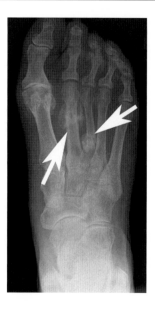

Fig. 10 Dorso-plantar radiograph of the right foot demonstrates insufficiency fracture of the second and third with massive callus formation in this 85-year-old female patient

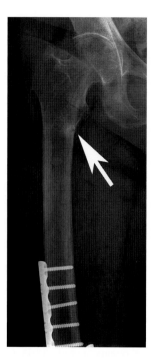

Fig. 11 AP radiograph of the right proximal femur with sclerosis and subtle fracture line at the medial aspect of the femur shaft below the lesser trochanter (*arrow*) indicating an old insufficiency fracture; note generalized osteopenia; and internal fixation hardware at the distal femur

1.5.4 Upper Extremity

A common site of fragility fractures is the distal forearm. In addition, fractures involving the wrist are known to be strongly associated with osteoporosis. It is well-known that patients with distal radius fracture who are otherwise healthy have a preferential bone loss at the distal forearm. Distal radius fractures are also associated with generally low bone mass and elevated fracture risk at other skeletal sites. In these subjects pharmacotherapy for osteoporosis is warranted (Mallmin and Ljunghall 1994). Interestingly in osteoporosis the proximal humerus may also be a fracture site at risk (Guggenbuhl et al. 2005).

1.6 Differential Diagnosis

An important differential diagnosis of a stress/insufficiency fracture is a fracture due to malignant disease. MRI features of a malignant fracture are diffusely or focally abnormal bone marrow signal which may be either well-defined or ill-defined and does not follow fracture lines. In addition abnormal intracortical, periosteal, or muscle signal intensity are found as well as endosteal scalloping and soft-tissue masses. The features seen on CT are bone marrow abnormality which may be well-defined, ill-defined, permeative or moth-eaten, endosteal scalloping, periosteal reaction, and a soft-tissue mass. Accuracy for differentiating malignant fractures from stress fractures was reported to be highest with MRI (93–98 %) followed by CT (82–88 %) and radiographs (88–94 %) (Fayad et al. 2005).

1.7 Imaging Methods and Limitations

Radiographs are the initial imaging test in patients with pain localized to the skeleton. If the radiographs are inconclusive and pain persists, either MRI or CT will be performed. Multidetector computed tomography (MDCT) is currently standard and allows multiplanar reconstruction, near isotropic 3D reconstructions of anatomical structures, reduction of artefacts as well as thin-section high-resolution imaging which is beneficial to visualizing also subtle fracture lines. It should be considered, however, that MRI is more sensitive and the imaging modality of choice if the patient history suggests malignant disease and metastasis may be responsible for fracture. Though MRI is very sensitive for detection of fractures, bone marrow changes, and related soft-tissue edema, it should be considered that in the absence of fractures lines or a typical history MRI may also be misleading and suggest other bone marrow pathology such as malignant infiltration. While MRI is the most sensitive technique in the visualization of insufficiency

should be aware of the importance of vertebral fracture diagnosis in assessing future osteoporotic fracture risk. Vertebral fractures incidental to radiologic examinations done for other reasons should be identified and reported, in particular vertebral fractures should be assessed in lateral chest radiographs. Proper training of radiologists is necessary to improve detection of vertebral fractures (Lentle et al. 2007). In oncologic patients differentiation from benign and malignant vertebral fractures is important and can be achieved by MRI or PET-CT (Figs. 13, 14).

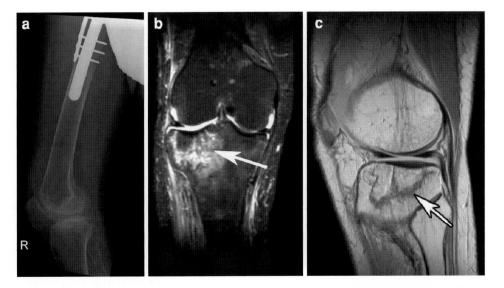

Fig. 12 Patient with history of tumor endoprosthesis at the proximal femur and insufficiency fracture at the proximal tibia. Lateral radiograph of the distal femur and knee shows severe osteopenia but no fracture **a**. The coronal STIR sequence shows significant bone marrow edema pattern and subtle fracture line at the lateral tibia **b**. The sagittal T1-w image better demonstrates the fracture line in the same patient **c**

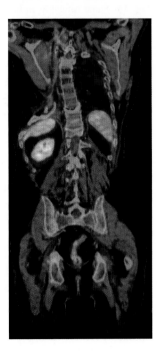

Fig. 13 61-year-old female patient with a history of bronchial carcinoma, FDG-PET-CT showing only moderate metabolic activity in the thoracic spine with several compression fractures. PET-CT excludes malignant fractures due to underlying disease

Fig. 14 Same patient as in Fig. 13 demonstrating multiple vertebral fractures with gibbus at the thoracic spine

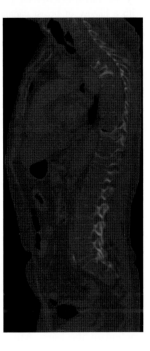

fractures, CT sometimes tends to depict the extent and stability of these fractures better. Bone scintigraphy is highly sensitive, but not specific. Atypical uptake patterns may be difficult to interpret and abnormal uptake may persist for several months.

1.7.1 Radiographs

Radiographic findings depend on the site of the fracture. Parasymphyseal and pubic ramus fractures may have an aggressive appearance that depends on the stage of fracture maturity. Findings include sclerosis, lytic fracture line, bone expansion, exuberant callus, and osteolysis. The most common finding is a sclerotic band or line. A lytic fracture line or cortical break rarely is observed. The degree of

confidence is low in sacral fractures because of osteoporosis, overlying bowel gas, and calcified vessels and is better at peripheral sites like in long bones and the metatarsal bones. Parasymphyseal and pubic ramus fractures often are misinterpreted as malignant lesions. Sacral, iliac, and supra-acetabular fractures often are difficult to detect.

1.7.2 Multidetector Computed Tomography

On CT images a linear fracture line with surrounding sclerosis may be observed, but depending on the age of the fracture sometimes only sclerosis may be demonstrated. Pubic fractures may be seen as a lytic fracture line often surrounded by callus. Typically, a soft-tissue mass is absent, bone destruction is lacking, and adjacent fascial planes are

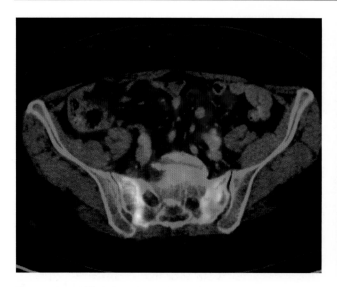

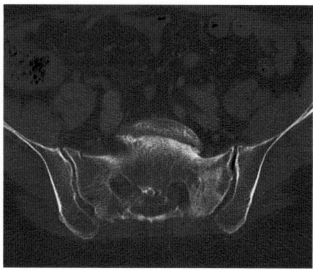

Fig. 15 Fused FDG-PET-CT images in a 69-year-old female patient with a history of breast carcinoma and bilateral elevated metabolic activity

Fig. 16 Same patient as in Fig. 13 shows bilateral sclerosis compatible with bilateral insufficiency fractures

preserved. MDCT also is useful for detecting large bony sacral defects such as Tarlov cysts and for the diagnosis of coexisting malignant lesions. MDCT is very specific for the definitive diagnosis of an insufficiency fractures of the pelvis but may have limitations with sensitivity. MDCT is useful as an alternative to bone scintigraphy when radiographs are inconclusive and MRI is not available (Soubrier et al. 2003). Multiplanar CT reformats are essential for the diagnosis of insufficiency fractures of the long bones and pelvic girdle (Junila et al. 1996). Dedicated MDCT-protocols using thin-section MPR's with adequate overlap and reconstruction kernels are essential for detecting even subtle fractures (Philipp et al. 2003).

In the diagnosis and staging of osteoporosis the 3D bone structure has been shown to be an important predictor of bone strength in addition to bone mass or the mineral content of the bone. Micro-CT scanning has shown promising results in the differentiation of osteoporotic and non-osteoporotic individuals with respect to histomorphometry and quality of trabecular fractures (Heiss et al. 2005).

1.7.3 Magnetic Resonance Imaging

MRI shows decreased signal on T1-weighted images and increased signal on T2-weighted images. In the sacrum, signal changes are seen as linear bands within the sacral ala and body and are parallel to the sacroiliac joints. On T2-weighted images, the fracture line may be seen if it is surrounded by adjacent marrow edema pattern. MRI is highly sensitive and highly specific. MRI cannot be used in patients with pacemakers, a significant limitation in the elderly population. Iliac and sacral bones are frequently involved in patients with osteomalacia. MRI can determine

the clinical activity of the disease, and can monitor the response to treatment of insufficiency fractures (Kanberoglu et al. 2005). Diffusion-weighted MRI pulse sequences are capable of differentiating malignant from benign lesions and may be the modality of choice in the near future (Byun et al. 2007).

1.7.4 Nuclear Medicine

In nuclear studies, the typical H-shaped or butterfly pattern of uptake in the sacrum is diagnostic of insufficiency fracture (Abe et al. 1992). The vertical limbs of the H lie within the sacral ala, parallel to the sacroiliac joints, while the transverse limb of the H extends across the sacral body. Other sacral variant uptake patterns occur frequently and include the unilateral ala, incomplete H, and horizontal linear dot patterns. Iliac fractures are seen as linear areas of uptake. PET-CT using F18-FDG combined with MDCT gives metabolic and morphologic information at the same time, allowing the differentiation of pathologic fractures and insufficiency fractures (Figs. 15, 16) (Tsuchida et al. 2006; Halac et al. 2007). Pubic and supra-acetabular fractures produce areas of linear or focal uptake. Concomitant findings of two or more areas of uptake in the sacrum and at another pelvic site are considered diagnostic of insufficiency fractures of the pelvis. Nuclear studies are highly sensitive and highly specific when a typical pattern of sacral uptake or concomitant sacral and pubic uptake is observed. If a typical pattern of abnormality is not present, the bone scan is much less specific. If abnormal or incomplete patterns of uptake are observed, findings may be mistaken for malignancy and other diseases. CT or MR imaging are useful in these cases.

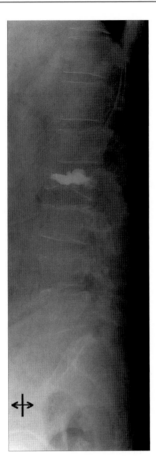

Fig. 17 Lateral radiograph of the lumbar spine demonstrating wedge fracture of L2 vertebral body with bone cement consistent with previous vertebroplasty

1.7.5 Interventional Radiology

Sacroplasty is a variation of the vertebroplasty technique for treatment of a sacral insufficiency fracture. Sacroplasty is a procedure in which polymethylacrylate, a quick-setting bone cement, is injected into the fractured bone. This technique appears to be useful in providing symptomatic relief to affected patients (Garant 2002). Other authors proposed a novel technique in which guidance with CT fluoroscopy allows placement of a transiliosacral bar in conjunction with sacroplasty combining the use of metallic hardware and bone cement for stabilization (Sciubba et al. 2007). There exist numerous publications about the treatment of vertebral fractures with vertebroplasty. Percutaneous vertebroplasty (PV) is a safe and effective treatment for relieving pain in patients complaining of severe back pain induced by osteoporotic compression fractures (Fig. 17). The success rate exceeds 90 % and the complication rate is lower than 1 % (Deramond and Mathis 2002). A substantial number of patients with osteoporosis develop new fractures after undergoing PV; two-thirds of these new fractures occur in vertebrae adjacent to those previously treated (Uppin et al. 2003).

1.8 Summary and Conclusion

Due to the increase in the average age of the population, the number of insufficiency fractures is steadily increasing. The majority of insufficiency fractures is due to weakened bone by osteoporosis. Usually, patients experience the acute onset of pain after an inadequate trauma. Insufficiency fractures can initially be missed on standard radiographs due to subtle findings. It is important to know the most commonly affected sites and the appearance with different radiological modalities. MDCT is superior to radiographs in the diagnosis of insufficiency fractures and should be used, in the case of negative radiographs exams, but high clinical suspicion of an insufficiency fracture. As insufficiency fractures usually occur in elderly patients, radiation dose is not a major concern. MRI should be used as a problem solver to distinguish between pathologic fractures and insufficiency or stress fractures and to monitor the bone marrow edema pattern. Radiographs can also be used for the follow-up of insufficiency fractures and the monitoring of callus formation and bone healing. Nuclear medicine studies gained a big role in the diagnosic work-up, due to the introduction of PET-CT with hybrid scanners in clinical routine. The radiologist's role nowadays also includes treatment of fractures with an increasing number of vertebroplasties performed each year. Other sites, such as the sacrum, have also been treated and the results seem promising.

References

Abe H et al (1992) Radiation-induced insufficiency fractures of the pelvis: evaluation with 99mTc-methylene diphosphonate scintigraphy. Am J Roentgenol 158(3):599–602

Alonso-Bartolome P et al (1999) Insufficiency fractures of the tibia and fibula. Semin Arthritis Rheum 28(6):413–420

Briggs AM, Greig AM, Wark JD (2007) The vertebral fracture cascade in osteoporosis: a review of aetiopathogenesis. Osteoporos Int 18(5):575–584

Brook AL, Mirsky DM, Bello JA (2005) Computerized tomography guided sacroplasty: a practical treatment for sacral insufficiency fracture: case report. Spine 30(15):E450–E454

Byun WM et al (2007) Diffusion-weighted magnetic resonance imaging of sacral insufficiency fractures: comparison with metastases of the sacrum. Spine 32(26):E820–E824

Cabarrus MC et al (2008) MRI and CT of pelvic insufficiency fractures: morphology, location and associated clinical findings. Am J Roentgenol 191(4):995–1001

Cho CH, Mathis JM, Ortiz O (2010) Sacral fractures and sacroplasty. Neuroimaging Clin N Am 20(2):179–186

Clemetson IA et al (2004) Postpartum osteoporosis associated with proximal tibial stress fracture. Skeletal Radiol 33(2):96–98

Delmas PD et al (2005) Underdiagnosis of vertebral fractures is a worldwide problem: the IMPACT study. J Bone Miner Res 20(4):557–563

Deramond H, Mathis JM (2002) Vertebroplasty in osteoporosis. Semin Musculoskelet Radiol 6(3):263–268

Fayad LM et al (2005) Distinction of long bone stress fractures from pathologic fractures on cross-sectional imaging: how successful are we? Am J Roentgenol 185(4):915–924

Feydy A et al (2000) A longitudinal insufficiency fracture of the tibia in association with a healed chronic osteomyelitis. Eur Radiol 10(12):1929–1931

Franco M et al (2003) Longitudinal bone insufficiency fracture of the tibia in a renal transplant recipient. Joint Bone Spine 70(4):296–299

Frey ME et al (2007) Percutaneous sacroplasty for osteoporotic sacral insufficiency fractures: a prospective, multicenter, observational pilot study. Spine J 8(2):367–373

Fujii M et al (2005) Honda sign and variants in patients suspected of having a sacral insufficiency fracture. Clin Nucl Med 30(3):165–169

Garant M (2002) Sacroplasty: a new treatment for sacral insufficiency fracture. J Vasc Interv Radiol 13(12):1265–1267

Genant HK et al (1993) Vertebral fracture assessment using a semiquantitative technique. J Bone Miner Res 8(9):1137–1148

Grasland A et al (1996) Sacral insufficiency fractures: an easily overlooked cause of back pain in elderly women. Arch Intern Med 156(6):668–674

Guggenbuhl P, Meadeb J, Chales G (2005) Osteoporotic fractures of the proximal humerus, pelvis, and ankle: epidemiology and diagnosis. Joint Bone Spine 72(5):372–375

Halac M et al (2007) Avoidance of misinterpretation of an FDG positive sacral insufficiency fracture using PET/CT scans in a patient with endometrial cancer: a case report. Clin Nucl Med 32(10):779–781

Heiss C et al (2005) Micro-CT analysis of cancellous bone fragments from the distal radius fracture zone in osteoporosis. Biomed Tech (Berl) 50(3):60–65

Hordon LD, Peacock M (1990) Osteomalacia and osteoporosis in femoral neck fracture. Bone Miner 11(2):247–259

Junila J, Lakovaara M, Lahde S (1996) Diagnosis of longitudinal stress fracture of the tibia with multiplanar CT reformats: a case report. Rofo 165(3):303–304

Kanaji A et al (2007) Insufficiency fracture in the medial wall of the acetabulum after total hip arthroplasty. J Arthroplasty 22(5):763–767

Kanberoglu K et al (2005) Magnetic resonance imaging in osteomalacic insufficiency fractures of the pelvis. Clin Radiol 60(1):105–111

Kanis JA, Pitt FA (1992) Epidemiology of osteoporosis. Bone 13(Suppl 1):S7–S15

Kawaguchi S et al (2001) Insufficiency fracture of the spine: a prospective analysis based on radiographic and scintigraphic diagnosis. J Bone Miner Metab 19(5):312–316

Lentle BC et al (2007) Recognizing and reporting vertebral fractures: reducing the risk of future osteoporotic fractures. Can Assoc Radiol J 58(1):27–36

Maenpaa HM et al (2002) Insufficiency fractures in patients with chronic inflammatory joint diseases. Clin Exp Rheumatol 20(1):77–79

Mallmin H, Ljunghall S (1994) Distal radius fracture is an early sign of general osteoporosis: bone mass measurements in a population-based study. Osteoporos Int 4(6):357–361

Martin-Hunyadi C et al (2000) Spontaneous insufficiency fractures of long bones: a prospective epidemiological survey in nursing home subjects. Arch Gerontol Geriatr 31(3):207–214

Peh WC, Evans NS (1993) Pelvic insufficiency fractures in the elderly. Ann Acad Med Singapore 22(5):818–822

Peh WC et al (1995) Sacral and pubic insufficiency fractures after irradiation of gynaecological malignancies. Clin Oncol (R Coll Radiol) 7(2):117–122

Peh WC et al (1996) Imaging of pelvic insufficiency fractures. Radiographics 16(2):335–348

Philipp MO et al (2003) Four-channel multidetector CT in facial fractures: do we need 2 × 0.5 mm collimation? Am J Roentgenol 180(6):1707–1713

Sciubba DM et al (2007) CT fluoroscopically guided percutaneous placement of transiliosacral rod for sacral insufficiency fracture: case report and technique. Am J Neuroradiol 28(8):1451–1454

Soubrier M et al (2003) Insufficiency fracture. A survey of 60 cases and review of the literature. Joint Bone Spine 70(3):209–218

Tsuchida T et al (2006) Sacral insufficiency fracture detected by FDG-PET/CT: report of 2 cases. Ann Nucl Med 20(6):445–448

Uppin AA et al (2003) Occurrence of new vertebral body fracture after percutaneous vertebroplasty in patients with osteoporosis. Radiology 226(1):119–124

Yamamoto T, Takabatake K, Iwamoto Y (2002) Subchondral insufficiency fracture of the femoral head resulting in rapid destruction of the hip joint: a sequential radiographic study. Am J Roentgenol 178(2):435–437

Yamamoto T et al (2007) Histopathologic prevalence of subchondral insufficiency fracture of the femoral head. Ann Rheum Dis 67(2):150–153

Identification of Vertebral Fractures

Mohamed Jarraya, Daichi Hayashi, James F. Griffith, Ali Guermazi, and Harry K. Genant

Contents

Abstract

Osteoporosis is characterized by reduced bone mass and microarchitectural deterioration of bone, leading to an increase in bone fragility and susceptibility to low-traumatic or atraumatic fractures, most commonly vertebral fractures. Osteoporotic vertebral fractures have a significant impact on morbidity, mortality, and healthcare costs. Vertebral fracture is an independent and significant predictor of increased risk for further fractures. The occurrence of vertebral fracture is often clinically asymptomatic, and many of these fractures, therefore, remain undiagnosed. Several techniques are available for their reliable identification on radiographs. The two most widely used methods are the semiquantitative (SQ) assessment, which is based on visual evaluation, and the quantitative approach, which is based on morphometric criteria. Genant's SQ approach is an accurate and reproducible method, tested and applied in many clinical studies. The newest generation of fan-beam dual energy X-ray absorptiometry (DXA) systems delivering lateral spine images of higher resolution offer a practical alternative to radiographs for vertebral fracture analysis. The advantages of DXA over radiography are its minimal radiation exposure and the practicalities of a one-step image acquisition allowing concurrent evaluation of vertebral fracture and bone mineral density, which are important criteria when assessing the risk of osteoporotic fracture. Standard computed tomography (CT) is not primarily used to detect vertebral fracture, though it often leads to the fortuitous detection of asymptomatic fracture. Magnetic resonance imaging (MRI) is an increasingly used modality for assessing the age and other important aspects of vertebral fracture.

M. Jarraya (✉) · D. Hayashi · J. F. Griffith · A. Guermazi · H. K. Genant
Department of Radiology, 820, Harrison Avenue, FGH building, 3rd floor, Boston, MA 02118, USA
e-mail: mjarraya@bu.edu

G. Guglielmi (ed.), *Osteoporosis and Bone Densitometry Measurements*, Medical Radiology. Diagnostic Imaging,
DOI: 10.1007/174_2012_701, © Springer-Verlag Berlin Heidelberg 2013

1 Significance of Vertebral Fracture

Osteoporosis is a progressive systemic skeletal disease characterized by a loss of bone quantity (low bone mass) and quality (microarchitectural deterioration), leading to increased bone fragility and susceptibility to low-energy traumatic or atraumatic fracture (Guermazi et al. 2002; Siris et al. 2012). Although osteoporotic vertebral fracture is often asymptomatic, it is a serious and irreversible outcome of osteoporosis (Cooper et al. 1992; Lindsay et al. 2001) associated with increased mortality (Ettinger et al. 1992) and morbidity (Ensrud et al. 2000). The decreased physical function and social isolation resulting from osteoporotic vertebral fractures has a significant impact on the patient's overall quality of life and self-esteem (Gold 2001). The economic toll is also considerable. With more than 432,000 hospital admissions, almost 2.5 million medical office visits, and about 180,000 nursing home admissions annually in the US, the cost to the healthcare system associated with osteoporosis-related fractures has been estimated at $17 billion for 2005 (Services. UDoHaH. Bone Health and Osteoporosis: A Report of the Surgeon General. In: Department of Health and Human Services OotSG, ed. Rockville, MD: US 2004). According to the United States Surgeon General, fractures and their associated costs could double or triple by the year 2040 (Services. UDoHaH 2004).

Vertebral fractures are the first osteoporotic fractures to occur and also the most common. The reported prevalence of vertebral fracture varies considerably according to the imaging criteria used to diagnose the fractures and the general health of the populations being studied. Thankfully, more stringent criteria on the reporting of vertebral fractures as well as greater recognition of their importance, are allowing a more reliable assessment of fracture rates in different populations. Fracture incidence increases with advancing age and is greater in women than men. Using comparable diagnostic criteria, vertebral fracture rates are rather similar worldwide (Table 1). Early and accurate recognition of vertebral fracture is essential to comprehensive clinical evaluation, determination of population prevalence, and fracture risk as well as evaluation of treatment efficacy. Although vertebral fractures are strongly linked to osteoporosis (DXA T-score at or below -2.5), almost half of them occur in patients with osteopenia (T-score at or below -1.0) or normal BMD (T-score above -1.0) (Siris et al. 2001; Sanders et al. 2006). Subjects with low-energy vertebral fracture indisputably have reduced bone strength, and are therefore osteoporotic irrespective of BMD measurement. For this reason, the National Osteoporosis Foundation has recommended that patients aged over 50 years with atraumatic new vertebral fractures receive appropriate bone protective/bone enhancing therapy, irrespective of DXA T-score (Foundation 2010).

It has been shown that the relative risk of new vertebral fracture increases with the number of baseline vertebral fractures (Black et al. 1999; Siris et al. 2007). Therefore, determining vertebral fracture status in addition to BMD, provides practical information when predicting fracture risk in post menopausal women (Siris et al. 2007). Over an 8-year period, subjects with pre-existing vertebral fractures had a 5-fold increased risk of further vertebral fractures and a 3-fold increased risk of proximal femoral fracture compared to those without a pre-existing vertebral fracture (Black et al. 1999). Incident vertebral fractures also increase risk of future vertebral fractures especially in the year following the fracture; 20 % of women with incidental vertebral fracture experience another fracture within a year (Lindsay et al. 2001). This demonstrates the need for identification and intervention of at-risk patients, especially as early treatment with appropriate anti-fracture medication significantly reduces the occurrence of new vertebral and nonvertebral fractures (Ensrud and Schousboe 2011).

Despite the importance of early vertebral fracture, under diagnosis is an appreciable problem worldwide. There are many reasons. First, vertebral fractures are often asymptomatic with only one-third of retrospectively diagnosed vertebral fractures relating to a clinically symptomatic period (Cooper et al. 1992). Second, the typical clinical symptoms of back pain and restricted movement are usually attributed to spondylosis rather than vertebral fracture so that most patients with vertebral fracture do not seek medical attention. Third, about one-third to one-half of vertebral fractures are under diagnosed in radiology reports (Delmas et al. 2005). Many vertebral fractures are clinically asymptomatic, and radiologists and clinicians who review imaging studies should look specifically for vertebral fractures (Lenchik et al. 2004; Adams et al. 2010). If a vertebral fracture is present, then it is imperative that it is reported clearly as a "vertebral fracture" and not with ambiguous descriptions such as "vertebral collapse", "compressed vertebral body", "loss of vertebral height", "wedging of vertebral body", "wedge deformity", "biconcavity" or "codfish deformity". The location and severity of any vertebral fracture should also be clearly stated.

2 Pathophysiology of Vertebral Fracture

Unlike the diaphyses of long bones, the vertebral body mainly relies on trabecular bone for its strength rather than cortical bone. However, trabecular bone surface area and thinness makes it particularly responsive to change in its microenvironment and, therefore, vertebral bodies are one of

Table 1 Comparison of age-specific vertebral fracture prevalence of women worldwide using comparable assessment methods

Age (years)	Chinese [a, f] (%)	Japanese [b, g] (%)	Latin American [c, g] (%)	European [d, g] (%)	American (white) [e, g] (%)
50 ~ 59		2.7	6.9	6.3	
60 ~ 69	10.8	13.8	10.2	11.7	14.5
70 ~ 79	17.4	17.5	18	20.9	22
80+	29.5		27.8		33.9

LAVOS Latin american vertebral osteoporosis study, EVOS European vertebral osteoporosis study

[a] Ms. OS (Hong Kong) study (Kwok et al. 2012)

[b] The japanese population-based osteoporosis study (Kadowaki et al. 2010)

[c] The latin american vertebral osteoporosis study (Clark et al. 2009)

[d] The European vertebral osteoporosis study (Johnell et al. 1997)

[e] The study of osteoporotic fractures (Clark et al. 2009; Black et al. 1999) (quoted from Table 5 in (Clark et al. 2009))

[f] Genant's SQ system

[g] Quantitative methods of McCloskey–Kanis criteria or McCloskey–Kanis criteria with mean—3SD criteria (population-based reference)

the first bones to be affected in osteoporosis (Griffith et al. in press). The vertebral body is particularly prone to early osteoporotic fracture. The weakest parts of the vertebral body are the central and antero-superior components of the end-plates where lower BMD is not compensated by higher trabecular strength (Banse et al. 2002). Other features such as microarchitecture, collagen composition, microdamage, mineralization, and osteocyte function may also play a role, although their relative contributions to vertebral strength remain ill-defined (Christiansen and Bouxsein 2010). Beside BMD, vertebral strength largely depends on vertebral size. An increase in vertebral body cross-sectional area will increase vertebral body strength (Griffith et al. in press). With age, vertebrae undergo periosteal apposition with resultant outward cortical displacement as a response to diminishing BMD. This enlarges the cross-sectional surface of the vertebral body and increases its resistance to compressive forces. These changes in vertebral body cross-sectional area can help somewhat to offset other changes occurring with age which have a cumulative deleterious effect, such as increased endocortical resorption, increased cortical porosity, and especially, decreased trabecular vertebral BMD (Riggs 2004). A greater lifelong decrease in trabecular and cortical vertebral bone mass coupled with a smaller bone size in women at the end of puberty compared to men helps to explain why osteoporotic fractures are more common in elderly women than in elderly men (Riggs 2004).

Changes in trabecular bone with age have been studied including assessment of the number and thickness of both vertical and horizontal trabeculae. While both horizontal and vertical trabeculae are removed with age, corresponding to a decrease in trabeculae number, only horizontal trabeculae display significant loss of thickness (Thomsen et al. 2002). The horizontal trabeculae are thought to be lost largely because of strain-adaptive resorption, while vertical trabeculae loss is due to perforation from microdamage resorption followed by rapid strain-adaptive resorption of the remaining unloaded trabeculae (Mc Donnell et al.

2009). The predominant loss of horizontal trabeculae and the preservation of the longitudinal trabeculae can result in the radiographic appearance of longitudinal striation (Fig. 1).

A vertebral fracture occurs when the force sustained by the vertebra exceeds its strength. Unlike long bones where fractures occur as a definite event, vertebral fractures often progress incrementally and this incremental nature is reflected in the overlapping of the various stages of fracture healing seen on histology (Diamond et al. 2007). Depending on the sustained force and inherent vertebral body strength, fracture severity can vary from a minor peripheral fracture to an almost complete vertebral body fracture. Most vertebral fractures occur in the mid-thoracic (T6-T8) and thoraco-lumbar (T11-L2) regions (Genant et al. 1996). Compressive loading is accentuated in the mid-thoracic spine during flexion when increased kyphosis is present, and also in the thoracolumbar region which is the transition zone between the relatively fixed thoracic, and the more mobile lumbar segments. Osteoporotic vertebral fractures are rare above the T4 level (Genant and Jergas 2003). Loading on the spine is determined by gravitational forces and muscle contracture which, in turn, are influenced by body weight, height, muscle action, coordination, and strength as well as spinal curvature and intervertebral disk characteristics (Christiansen and Bouxsein 2010). Fracture of a single vertebral body, particularly of the anterior wedge type, shifts compressive forces toward the anterior aspects of the vertebral bodies, potentially leading to a vertebral fracture "cascade", characterized by fractures in adjacent vertebrae occurring in rapid succession (Christiansen and Bouxsein 2010).

3 Clinical Diagnosis of Vertebral Fracture

Vertebral fractures are difficult to identify clinically. Recent large cohort studies of postmenopausal women with low BMD have shown that only about one-fourth of incident

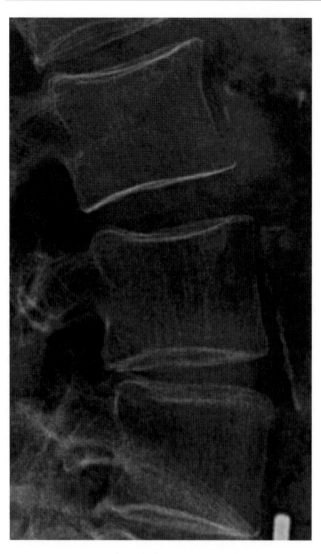

Fig. 1 Radiograph of osteoporotic lumbar vertebrae. The vertical striations of the spongiosa result from the loss of the horizontal trabeculae and preservation of remaining vertical trabeculae

radiographic vertebral deformities were clinically diagnosed as new vertebral fractures (Fink et al. 2005). Clinical recognition is better for more severe fractures (30 %) than mild fractures (15 %) (Fink et al. 2005). This low recognition rate can be attributed to the absence of specific symptoms and difficulty in determining the cause of symptoms such as pain or height loss. Less than 1 % of back pain episodes are related to vertebral fracture (Ettinger et al. 1995). Historical height loss is difficult to assess clinically. While some spinal height loss is expected with aging due to degenerative and attritional remodeling of the vertebral bodies, narrowing of intervertebral disks, and postural and scoliotic changes, loss of height can also be the result of vertebral fracture. Height loss is considered an unreliable indicator of fracture status until it exceeds 4 cm (Ettinger et al. 1992). Overall, clinical evaluation of vertebral fracture has poor sensitivity and specificity.

4 Radiographic Diagnosis of Vertebral Fracture

Although radiography of the thoracolumbar spine is the standard imaging approach for assessment of vertebral fracture, there is no agreed upon gold standard to define osteoporotic vertebral fracture. To resolve this issue, the first step is to define clearly what a "normal" vertebral body is, taking into account the wide range of intra- and inter-individual variation in vertebral body size and shape. Technical considerations, such as the oblique projection secondary to malpositioning of the patient, and the parallax effect caused by the divergent X-ray beam are additional factors that can create a misleading appearance (Hurxthal 1968). Once a vertebral body is recognized as "abnormal", the second step is to decide whether this abnormality actually indicates an osteoporotic fracture (Smith-Bindman et al. 1991; Cooper and Melton 1992; Herss Nielsen et al. 1991). Established methods rely mainly on the reduction of vertebral height to define a vertebral fracture. This is problematic especially for mild pre-existing (prevalent) fracture, since only a longitudinal comparison can identify true change in vertebral height (Ferrar et al. 2005).

Not every deformed vertebral body is a result of osteoporotic fracture. Radiologists should be aware of six common pitfalls that can be confused with mild vertebral fractures:

- *Physiologic wedging* is a normal feature as the spine changes from thoracic kyphosis to lumbar lordosis. All vertebrae, but particularly T5-T9, T12-L1, L4-L5 are physiologically wedged. The vertebral bodies of the lower thoracic and upper lumbar spine (T10-L2) are slightly anteriorly wedged, while the lower lumbar region is posteriorly wedged (L4 & L5) (Fig. 2) (Masharawi et al. 2008).
- *Short vertebral height (SVH)* is an important physiological feature that occurs with age and is commonly over-diagnosed as osteoporotic fracture. Differentiating SVH from a mild vertebral fracture is probably the most contentious and difficult area in vertebral fracture diagnosis. SVH is independent of osteoporosis and vertebral fracture, and is more important on the anterior aspect of the vertebrae than the middle and posterior parts, particularly with regard to thoracic kyphosis in the elderly (Diacinti et al. 1995). Women between 30 and 70 years of age show a decrease of the combined height of the anterior aspects of the vertebral bodies from T4 to L5 at a rate of about 1.5 mm/year, while the combined middle and posterior heights decline at about 1.2 mm/year (Diacinti et al. 1995). SVH refers to a reduction in vertebral height of up to 20 % of the expected height, but it is sometimes very hard to differentiate from a mild vertebral fracture

Fig. 2 Lateral *X*-rays of the lumbar spine in a 30-year-old woman and 25-year-old man, respectively. **a** Normal appearance of physiologic posterior wedging of L5. **b** Physiologic anterior wedging of L1 and L2

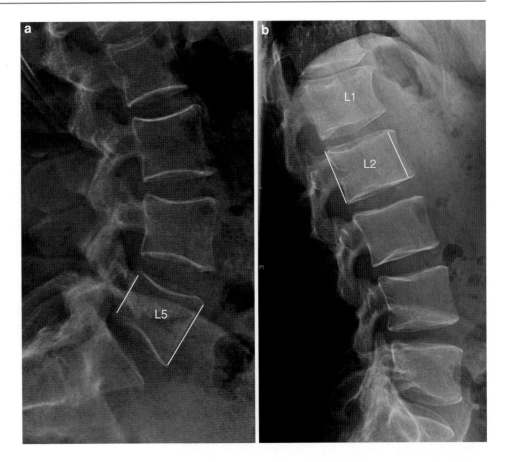

(20–25 % of height loss). However, the majority of evidence suggests that isolated SVH is not associated with low BMD or irregularity of the vertebral endplate (Ferrar et al. 2007). SVH, when isolated and when not associated with endplate irregularity or other features of fracture, is most likely the result of physiological wedging exacerbated by vertebral remodeling due to increasing age or spondylosis as discussed in the previous section (Fig. 3) (Griffith et al. in press).

- *Scheuermann disease* is a disorder that causes back pain in teenagers and young adults, and is likely related to compressive injuries to the cartilaginous endplates. It is identified by these criteria: (i) elongated vertebral bodies affecting at least three adjacent vertebrae; (ii) irregular wavy endplates with Schmorl nodes; (iii) accelerated degenerative changes (Ferrar et al. 2007). It can affect the thoracic or lumbar spine, mostly the former, leading to an exaggerated thoracic kyphosis and a decreased lumbar lordosis or both. An increased anteroposterior diameter of the vertebral body, small intervertebral disk, endplate irregularity, and premature disk degeneration are helpful features for diagnosing Scheuermann disease and distinguishing it from vertebral fracture.

- *Obliquity of vertebral bodies due to scoliosis* may lead to side-to-side discrepancy in vertebral body height. On the lateral projection, this obliquity gives a biconcave outline

to the vertebral endplates which may be misinterpreted as a vertebral fracture. On the anteroposterior view, the vertebral body is reduced on the concave side, and of normal height, or even increased, on the convex side. Degenerative-type scoliosis is quite common, particularly in the elderly lumbar spine. With experience, one can determine whether the degree of apparent loss of vertebral height is commensurate with the degree of scoliosis. Unilateral loss of vertebral height due to scoliosis should not be considered a vertebral fracture.

- *Schmorl node* is a displacement of intervertebral disk tissue into the vertebral body. Although Schmorl node is a manifestation of Scheuermann disease, it is far more commonly encountered in isolation (Pfirrmann and Resnick 2001), present in 40–75 % of imaging studies and sometimes associated with degenerative disease of the lumbar spine (Griffith et al. in press). Schmorl node only involves a segment of the endplate, and is seen as well-defined rounded contour, with an intact sclerotic margin (Fig. 4).

- *Cupid's bow deformity* is a common developmental endplate contour abnormality, most frequently affecting the inferior endplate of the fourth and fifth lumbar vertebral bodies. The more cephalad lumbar vertebrae, as well as thoracic vertebrae, may rarely be involved (Chan et al. 1997). It results from a lack of cartilage in the

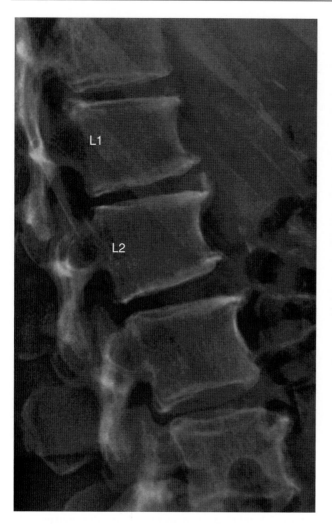

Fig. 3 SVH of L1 and L2 exaggerated by degenerative remodeling. Notice the presence of associated anterior osteophytes and L1-L2 disc space narrowing

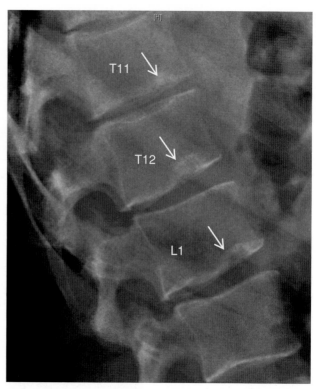

Fig. 4 Lateral *X*-ray of the lumbar spine showing Schmorl nodes of the inferior endplates of T11, T12, and L1. Notice their characteristic rounded contour with sclerotic margin (*arrows*)

5   Spinal Radiography

In clinical practice, radiographic diagnosis is the best way to identify osteoporotic vertebral fracture. The standardized radiographic protocol consists of anteroposterior (AP) and lateral views, including the C7-S1 vertebrae. A focus-film distance of 100 cm and an *X*-ray beam centered at T7 and L3, for the thoracic and lumbar spines respectively, are necessary for a good radiographic spinal examination. Because of the superimposition of the scapula and shoulder regions, the upper thoracic (T1-T3) vertebral bodies are often not clearly seen on lateral views. However, isolated osteoporotic fractures in this region are extremely uncommon. On the lateral projection, the spine must be parallel to the film so that the vertebral endplates at the level of the central *X*-ray beam are superimposed and seen as single dense, well-defined cortical lines. Since the *X*-ray beam is divergent, the endplates distant from the centering point appear concave ("bean can" effect) and must not be mistaken for vertebral fractures. Although a lateral view is usually sufficient, an AP projection may help detect scoliosis and determine the anatomical level of a vertebral fracture. For the thoracic spine, both an AP and a lateral projection are often undertaken, since the lateral view in isolation may not display the vertebral body outline as consistently as in the lumbar region. The typical effective doses

parasagittal endplate areas leading to impaired endochondral growth of the vertebral body with concave endplate depressions, resembling Cupid's bow on the anteroposterior radiograph. The nucleus pulposis tends to be enlarged and bilobed. On the lateral projection, the posterior two-thirds of the inferior endplate are indented, simulating a depressed endplate fracture (Griffith et al. in press) (Fig. 5).

In conclusion, "while all vertebral fractures result in vertebral deformity, not all vertebral deformities represent a vertebral fracture" (Genant and Jergas 2003). Radiologists should be aware of entities other than fracture that can change vertebral body shape. The term *deformity* is appropriate when reporting such nonfracture etiologies (Link et al. 2005). With careful scrutiny of imaging features, these vertebral deformities can usually be differentiated from vertebral fractures.

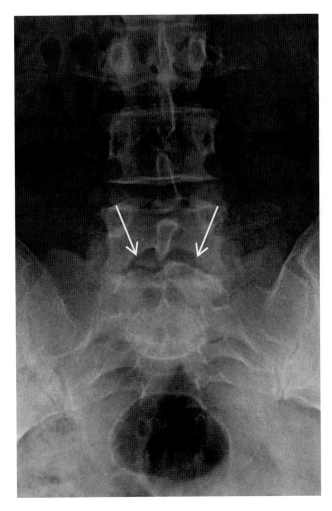

Fig. 5 AP *X*-ray of the lumbar spine in a 25-year-old woman displaying normal appearance of Cupid's bow of the inferior endplate of L5 (*arrows*)

Radiographic examinations of the thoracolumbar spine are usually evaluated by radiologists or clinicians with experience in viewing radiographs to identify vertebral fractures. This said, there is still no universally agreed definition of vertebral fracture. The importance of radiographic evaluation in the identification of vertebral fractures, and the susceptibility of radiographic output to bias, has prompted the quest for a standardized and objective visual assessment method of vertebral fracture identification. Different approaches have been proposed to facilitate both the detection and progression of osteoporotic fracture. These methods are presented in the next section.

6 Visual Assessment of Vertebral Fracture

Since the introduction of the first standardized approach by Smith et al. (1960), which graded only the most severely deformed vertebrae on lateral radiographs, further work has attempted to bring more precision and sensitivity to reporting vertebral fractures. Meunier proposed a grading method according to the shape and deformity of the vertebrae (Meunier 1968) (normal, biconcave, endplate fracture, wedged, or crushed vertebra). A "radiological vertebral index" was calculated as the sum of the vertebral grades, or as a quotient of this sum and the number of vertebrae. Kleerekoper and Nelson (1992) modified Meunier's radiological vertebral index and introduced the so-called "vertebral deformity score" in which a score was assigned to each vertebrae from T4 to L5 based on the reduction in the anterior, middle, and posterior heights (ha, hm, and hp respectively). A vertebral deformity was defined as a reduction of ha, hm, or hp by at least 4 mm or 15 %. These methods depend on vertebral shape and an incident vertebral fracture could only be detected if vertebral shape changed significantly. Genant et al. proposed a standardized visual approach to vertebral fracture identification and grading known as the semiquantitative (SQ) method (Fig. 6) (Genant et al. 1993, 1996; Genant and Jergas 2003). This method is based on the quantification of vertebral height reduction, as well as qualitative assessment which considers the integrity of the endplate, cortical borders, and other deformities such as biconcave, wedge, and compression. The SQ method is easy to apply and is more objective and reproducible than purely qualitative methods, resulting in better interobserver agreement. These clear advantages have made it a standard in several important epidemiological studies of osteoporosis (Ferrar et al. 2005; Siris et al. 2002; Harris et al. 1999) and in most clinical trials of osteoporosis therapies (Meunier et al. 2009; Matsumoto et al. 2009; Chesnut et al. 2004).

Genant's SQ approach consists of visually grading each vertebra from T4 to L4, without direct measurements, based on the apparent degree of vertebral height loss. Relative to

of ionizing radiation from a single lateral and AP projection of the thoracic spine are 0.3–0.4, while for the lumbar spine they are 0.3–0.7 mSv. By comparison, a 16-hour return transatlantic flight would amount to 0.07 mSv background radiation (Griffith et al. in press; Damilakis et al. 2010).

One global prospective study (the IMPACT study (Delmas et al. 2005)), compared the results of local radiographic reports from five continents with that of subsequent central readings in more than 2,000 postmenopausal women with osteoporosis. This study pointed out the significance of radiological under-diagnosis of vertebral fractures worldwide, with false-negative rates ranging from 27 to 45 %, despite a strict radiographic protocol that provided an unambiguous vertebral fracture definition and minimized the influence of inadequate film quality. It was concluded that the failure was a global problem attributable to either or both lack of radiographic detection and use of ambiguous terminology in reports.

Fig. 6 Genant's grading scheme for a semiquantitative evaluation of vertebral fracture. The drawings illustrate normal vertebrae (*top row*) and mild to severe fractures (respectively in the following *rows*). The size of the reduction in the anterior, middle, or posterior height is reflected in a corresponding fracture grade, from 1 (mild) to 3 (severe) (from Genant et al. 1993)

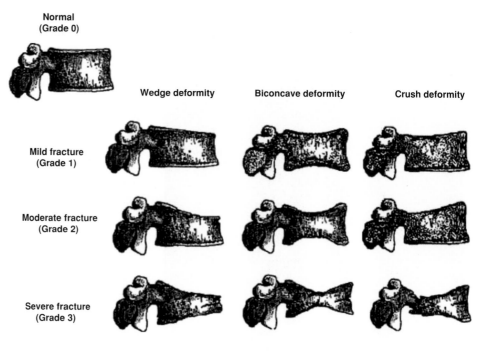

either normal appearing adjacent vertebrae or relative to what one would normally expect vertebral height to be at that level, the vertebrae are graded as normal (grade 0), mildly deformed (grade 1, reduction of ~ 20–25 % of height (Fig. 7), moderately deformed (grade 2, reduction of ~ 25–40 % of height), and severely deformed (grade 3, reduction $\sim >40$ % of height). Grade 0.5 is sometimes used and designates a borderline vertebral fracture that shows deformity but cannot clearly be assigned to grade 1. In addition, when using the SQ method, it is requisite that one also considers changes of the vertebral endplate and cortical margin, and lack of consistency with adjacent vertebrae, all of which help to distinguish fracture from SVH (Genant et al. 1993).

The SQ analysis of spinal radiographs for vertebral fracture is faster than other methods of vertebral fracture assessment, easy to implement, and suited to epidemiological research studies, clinical therapeutic efficacy trials, and everyday clinical practice. Vertebral fractures detected by SQ analysis are associated with low BMD and are predictive of future fracture, regardless of BMD (Siris et al. 2002, 2007; Delmas et al. 2005; Griffith et al. in press). For longitudinal studies, serial radiographs should be viewed in chronological order to fully appreciate changes in vertebral morphology. Although visual assessment methods of vertebral fractures are potentially more subjective than morphometric analysis, they do allow the experienced reader to address critical issues such as nonosteoporotic deformity and projectional artifacts. SQ analysis is also better suited to deal with errors introduced by radiographic technique such as magnification effects, which clearly would influence serial vertebral body measurements. The SQ method is a practical

and reproducible method of vertebral fracture assessment when performed by trained and experienced readers (Griffith in press; Ferrar et al. 2012; Buehring et al. 2010).

6.1 Vertebral Quantitative Morphometry

Vertebral quantitative morphometry (QM) is only used in a research setting (Guglielmi et al. 2008). The two main advantages of QM over other methods are that it can be performed by relatively inexperienced or nonmedical research staff, and it provides an objective measure of loss of vertebral height on serial images (Griffith in press). While the description and definition of the methodology is straightforward, the application in practice is often rather subjective. Vertebral QM consists of placement of six points delineating each vertebral body from T4 to L4. The four corner points and two additional points in the middle of the upper and lower endplates are used (Fig. 8). This technique was introduced in 1960 by Barnett and Nordin, who used a transparent ruler to measure vertebral heights on lateral radiographs of the thoracolumbar spine. Vertebral morphometry is performed on lateral radiographs (morphometric X-ray radiography or MRX) though it can also be applied to images obtained from dual X-ray absorptiometry (DXA) (morphometric X-ray absorptiometry or MXA). Currently, QM uses digital images displayed on a high-resolution workstation. Digitization allows magnification of images to a specific level, optimization of contrast and brightness levels, and digital archiving. Point placement may be done manually or automatically. Manual placement, proposed by Hurxthal (1968), excludes features such as

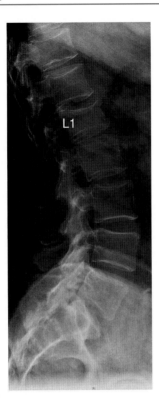

Fig. 7 Lateral *X*-ray of the lumbar spine showing a mild anterior fracture of L1 (grade 1 according to Genant's SQ assessment) in a 53-year-old man presenting with 1 week history of back pain

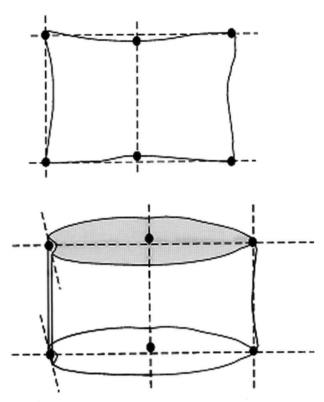

Fig. 8 Example of six-point placement for vertebral morphometry

Schmorl nodes and osteophytes from measurements. When the outer contours of the endplate are not superimposed (due to incorrect positioning or severe scoliosis), the middle point is placed centrally between the upper and the lower endplate contour (Guglielmi et al. 2008). With automatic placement, which brings more precision by reducing operator dependent errors (Nicholson et al. 1993; Kalidis et al. 1992), the endplates and the four corners of the vertebral bodies are highlighted by image post-processing. The software determines the midpoints between the posterior and anterior corner points of the upper and lower endplates, and then the reader selects the true midpoints by moving the caliper along the vertical midline joining the endplates (Guglielmi et al. 2008). Afterward, the computer calculates the posterior, anterior, and middle heights (ha, hm, and hp) of each vertebra from T4 to L5, as well as specific indices reflecting vertebral shape. These indices consist of A_H/P_H (anterior wedging), M_H/P_H (endplate concavity), and $P_H/P_{H'}$ of the adjacent normal vertebrae (posterior compression) (Griffith et al. in press; Grados et al. 2009). Prevalent vertebral fracture is defined as a reduction in one or more of the three vertebral height ratios (A_H/P_H, M_H/P_H, or $P_H/P_{H'}$) >20 % or 3 standard deviations from the mean of a reference population. Incident vertebral fracture is defined as a reduction in one of the three height ratios (A_H/P_H, M_H/P_H, or $P_H/P_{H'}$) >15–20 % or 3–4 mm compared to baseline (Griffith et al. in press; Melton et al. 1993; Eastell et al. 1991). While the reproducibility of QM is good in normal subjects, with an interobserver coefficient of variation of

<2 %, it is not as good in the very elderly and in those with osteoporotic fractures where the interobserver and intraobserver coefficients of variation are 5 and 6.3 % for M_H (Grados et al. 2001). Although QM parameters are objective, the approach has some significant limitations.

However, good the radiographic technique, even a mild degree of scoliosis will invariably lead to the endplate being visualized slightly en-face. In such situations, observer experience will influence reference point placement for baseline and sequential imaging examinations. Small differences in reference point placement on follow-up radiographs can result in an erroneous diagnosis of incident vertebral fracture by QM, though readily interpreted by the expert reader. QM also does not allow distinction between vertebral fracture and nonfracture vertebral deformity (such as SVH and physiological wedging) (Griffith et al. in press), resulting in false positive diagnoses (Grados et al. 2001; Grigoryan et al. 2003).

6.2 Algorithm-Based Qualitative Assessment

The algorithm-based qualitative (ABQ) method is a modified approach to qualitative assessment. It relies on the detection of vertebral endplate abnormalities related to fracture rather than height loss. The vertebrae are classified as either (i) normal, (ii) osteoporotic fracture, or (iii) nonosteoporotic deformity or SVH. The diagnosis of an osteoporotic vertebral fracture requires evidence of vertebral endplate fracture and/or loss of expected vertebral height but with no minimum threshold for apparent reduction in vertebral height (Jiang et al. 2004). If a fracture of the cortical margin is also visible radiographically, then there is a vertebral fracture present and it is likely to be of recent origin. Radiographically visible fracture lines in vertebral fracture are uncommon, however. When one or more vertebral heights (anterior, middle, or posterior) is shorter than expected, but without specific endplate abnormalities of fracture (altered texture adjacent to the endplate due to microfracture), it is designated as non-osteoporotic deformity (Griffith et al. in press). The ABQ method is specific but lacks sensitivity. The distinction between endplate fracture, the hallmark of the ABQ method, and other causes of endplate deformity such as Schmorl nodes and degenerative remodeling could be confounders here, especially if vertebral height loss is minimal.

6.3 Mild Vertebral Fracture

Practically, all of the current confusion in vertebral fracture identification is caused by the mild vertebral fracture. Diagnosis of moderate or severe fractures is so much more reliable that some investigators limit vertebral fracture diagnosis to these fractures alone. Such an approach clearly adds to the specificity but reduces the sensitivity of the study. Several studies have documented the clinical relevance of even mild fractures, albeit carrying less importance than moderate and severe SQ fractures (Delmas et al. 2003). When analyzing the findings of any study addressing vertebral fracture prevalence, one must pay careful attention to the criteria that were used to diagnose fracture. Over or under-diagnosing a small number of equivocal fractures will not make a great deal of difference if the population prevalence of vertebral fractures is high, such as in elderly at-risk women, but it will have a more noticeable effect if the vertebral fracture prevalence is low as in a younger population. Vertebral fracture prevalence is often the focus and point of pivotal interest in research studies and requires vigorous standardization to optimize accuracy of vertebral fracture diagnosis. Similarly, on an individual patient basis, diagnosing vertebral fracture at the earliest possible stage will have the most beneficial patient outcome. Conversely, over diagnosis of vertebral fracture may lead to the patient being incorrectly diagnosed as osteoporotic.

6.4 Standardization of Approach to Vertebral Fracture Assessment

In an effort to develop a standardized consensus protocol for the visual assessment of vertebral fracture, the United States National Osteoporosis Foundation Working Group on Vertebral Fractures suggested the following procedural requirements for qualitative (and SQ) assessment of vertebral fracture in osteoporosis research (Kiel 1995):

- Assessments should be performed by a radiologist or trained clinician with specific expertise in the radiology of osteoporosis.
- Qualitative and SQ assessments should be performed according to a written protocol of fracture definition, which is sufficiently detailed that it can be reproduced by other experts. Reference to an atlas of standard films or illustrations may be helpful. It is recommended that a standardized protocol be developed by a consensus of experts radiologists. For large clinical trials, either SQ should be employed in isolation or else QM should be used to support SQ of vertebrae with reduced height on QM assessment.
- The definition of fracture should include deformities of the endplates and anterior borders of vertebral bodies, as well as generalized collapse of the vertebral body.
- Grading of the degree of each fracture should employ discrete, mutually exclusive categories. Again, an atlas of standard film illustrations may help to assure consistency.

There is some subjectivity in each method, and segregating grading into exclusive categories may be problematic, especially for prevalent fractures. However, when assessing vertebral fractures as fracture/nonfracture, trained readers have achieved excellent results. Distinction of fracture from nonfracture is probably the most important step in the assessment, and the SQ standardized grading schemes are appropriate instruments to make this diagnosis reliable and valid. Ensuring reliability in interpretation of incident vertebral fractures on serial radiographs requires close attention to the imaging procedure. Serial radiographs of a patient should always be viewed together in chronological order to achieve a thorough and reliable analysis of all new fractures. Because a vertebral fracture is a permanent event that is not going to return to normal on follow-up radiographs, temporal blinding is not useful: most readers can identify the temporal sequence to a film series by new deformities as well as progressive degenerative changes (Grigoryan et al. 2003).

7 Dual X-ray Absorptiometry

Because of the difficulty in identifying vertebral fractures clinically, and the practicalities of routine radiographic assessment, vertebral fracture status is increasingly performed at the same time as the BMD evaluation by DXA. Imaging vertebral fractures using DXA is known as vertebral fracture assessment (VFA). VFA requires a fan-beam DXA scanner with appropriate software and can be performed either with the patient supine on a scanner with a rotating C arm gantry or with the patient in a lateral decubitus position on a scanner with a fixed gantry. Modern fan-beam DXA scanners can obtain single energy images of the spine from T4 to L4 in <10 s during suspended respiration. The T4-T6 vertebral bodies can be adequately visualized in 40–70 % of patients while vertebrae from T7 and below can be adequately identified in nearly all patients (Ferrar et al. 2000).

The advantages of VFA by DXA rather than radiographs are many and include a substantial reduction in patient dose (up to 100 times), lower cost, and the ability to perform the examination at the point of standard BMD assessment (Grigoryan et al. 2003). Fan-beam X-ray bone densitometry systems provide modest resolution lateral spine images, offering a practical alternative to radiographs for clinical VFA. The technology of fan-beam DXA systems with VFA capability is similar to computed tomography in providing a lateral spine image in as little as 10 s (Grigoryan et al. 2003). The DXA X-ray beam is orthogonal, rather than divergent, with less parallax and image distortion than radiography. VFA also shows all vertebrae on a single image allowing easier recognition of which vertebral body is fractured.

Once the DXA image is obtained, manual or automated vertebral morphometry known as MXA can be performed (Diacinti and Guglielmi 2010). Morphometric assessment of DXA spinal images assumes progression given the need for quantitative fracture evaluation in clinical trials. Demarcation of the vertebral body by reference points allows measurement of vertebral body height, and an automatic calculation of height ratios and average height. Automated assessment of fracture status based on comparison with normative data is also available (Diacinti and Guglielmi 2010). Superimposition of these baseline reference points on follow-up VFA spine images makes it simple to compare examinations (Diacinti and Guglielmi 2010). However, MXA alone is not recommended for fracture diagnosis. Visual inspection using the Genant SQ method is recommended by the International Society of Clinical Densitometry (ISCD) for diagnosing and grading the severity of vertebral fracture on VFA [http://www.iscd.org/Visitors/positions/OfficialPositionsText.cfm]. Even with current DXA systems, image quality is poorer than radiography, raising the question of how accurately VFA can identify vertebral fracture compared to radiography. Fuerst compared VFA by DXA and radiography, and showed that VFA has only moderate sensitivity for diagnosis of mild vertebral fracture, but a much higher sensitivity/specificity (>90 %) for detecting moderate or severe vertebral fractures (Fuerst et al. 2009). VFA will, certainly, have an increasingly important role in the diagnosis of vertebral fractures and in osteoporosis evaluation. In one DXA-based study, VFA detected unknown vertebral fractures in 1 of 5 patients (Jager et al. 2010).

While DXA-measured BMD is predictive of absolute risk and relative vertebral fracture risk, the degree of risk is difficult to apply on an individual patient basis in clinical practice. FRAX is a computer-based algorithm (http://www.shef.ac.uk/FRAX) developed by the World Health Organization Collaborating Centre for Metabolic Bone Diseases. The algorithm is mainly designed for primary care and calculates the fracture probability from easily obtained clinical risk factors (Kanis et al. 2008). The output of FRAX is the 10-year probability of a major osteoporotic fracture (hip, clinical spine, humerus, or wrist) and the 10-year probability of a hip fracture (Kanis et al. 2011). FRAX aids fracture prediction and such an assessment is needed to make rational treatment decisions, although it does not define any particular interventional threshold, which can vary from country to country.

8 Computed Tomography

Computed tomography (CT) technology includes from multidetector spiral whole-body CT (MDCT) to high-resolution peripheral quantitative CT to microCT. Thanks to its wide availability and ease of midline sagittal reformation, MDCT allows the thoracic/lumbar spine to be evaluated on all CT studies of the thorax/abdomen regardless of clinical indications. This allows the fortuitous detection of vertebral fracture (Fig. 9). In a recent study of patients older than 55 years who had thoracic CT, one-fifth had a moderate or severe thoracic vertebral fracture but less than one-fifth of these fractures had been reported. This same study showed a higher sensitivity of sagittal reformation for the detection of vertebral fracture compared with axial images (Williams et al. 2009). The CT scout views should also be scrutinized routinely for vertebral fractures, since these usually will include more of the spine than is covered by axial sections (Samelson et al. 2011). The major limitation to more widespread primary use and evaluation of CT in vertebral fracture diagnosis is the cost and radiation dose. The effective dose for DXA examination is 0.01–0.05, for 2D QCT of the lumbar spine it is 0.06–0.3 mSv, and for high-resolution volumetric CT to examine vertebral microarchitecture is 3 mSv (equivalent to 1.5 years of background radiation) (Krug et al. 2010).

9 Magnetic Resonance Imaging

Magnetic resonance imaging (MRI) has several advantages for assessing bone compared to CT, such as the lack of ionizing radiation, direct orthogonal plane imaging, and the ability to investigate aspects of bone physiology beyond structure, such as marrow fat content, marrow diffusion, and marrow perfusion. Its known disadvantages include the cost and complexity of the MRI equipment and analyses. While a vertebral fracture is generally diagnosed on radiography

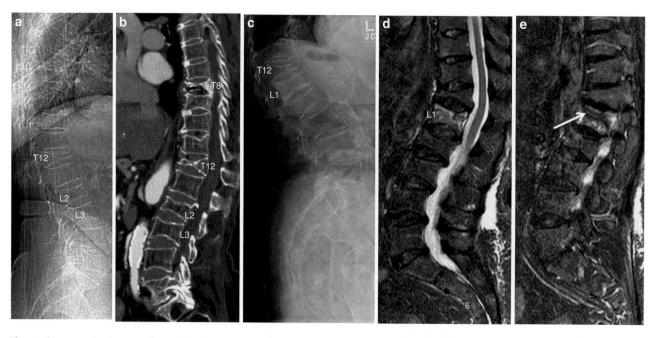

Fig. 9 Osteoporotic fractures in an 85-year-old woman presenting with a new onset of back pain. **a** and **b** Scout view and sagittal reformation of angio CT in 2006 fortuitously show vertebral fracture in T8 (Grade 3), T12 (Grade 3), L2 (Grade 2), and L3 (Grade 1) according to Genant's SQ assessment. Note the nonunion of T8 fracture with intravertebral vacuum and the normal appearance and height of L1. **c** Lateral X-ray of the lumbar spine, 5 years later,

performed for a new onset of back pain showing a new vertebral fracture of L1 (Grade 2). **d** and **e** Sagittal T2-weighted images with fat suppression displaying diffuse high signal intensity of the vertebral body of L1. No hyperintensity in the fractured vertebrae T12 and L2, indicates older fractures. **e** Linear hypointense fracture line parallel to the superior endplate of L1 (*arrow*)

when there is more than 20 % loss of vertebral height, MRI allows detection of true vertebral fracture without significant height loss, by demonstrating marrow edema in even mild fractures. This is particularly helpful in symptomatic patients without evidence of vertebral fracture on radiography. As MRI scanners have become more widely available, the use of MRI in the assessment of acute vertebral fractures has increased (Griffith et al. in press). Moreover, MRI is an important tool in determining the age of vertebral fracture by detecting marrow edema on fat-suppressed MRI. The presence and degree of edema on T2-weighted fat-suppressed MRI is a reliable guide to the age of a vertebral fracture (Fig. 9). Conversely, vertebral fractures which lack marrow edema are not recent fractures, and unlikely to be symptomatic. These old fractures are much less likely to respond to percutaneous vertebroplasty or balloon kyphoplasty (Griffith et al. in press).

Metastatic vertebral fracture is often the first manifestation of malignancy. Conversely, up to one-third of vertebral fractures in patients with known malignancy are osteoporotic rather than metastatic (Fornasier and Czitrom 1978). Accurate distinction between acute/subacute vertebral fracture and metastatic fracture is often not easy radiographically. The high contrast resolution of MRI makes it very useful in clinical practice for differentiating between osteoporotic and malignant vertebral fracture. By applying a variety of

imaging criteria, the distinction can be made with a high degree of accuracy, avoiding any need for percutaneous biopsy (Griffith and Guglielmi 2010).

Nonunion affects about 10 % of acute osteoporotic vertebral fractures. Nonunion is particularly prevalent in the T12 and L1 vertebrae and is evident radiographically as a vacuum cleft extending horizontally across the vertebral body (Fig. 9). These nonunited vertebral fractures are associated with more severe back pain than united fractures (Tsujio et al. 1976). Risk of nonunion is increased significantly if there is retropulsion of the posterior vertebral cortex, with areas of localized high intensity on T2-weighted images or diffuse low intensity within the vertebral body on T2-weighted images (Tsujio et al. 1976). MRI may have the potential to distinguish acute vertebral fractures particularly susceptible to progression or nonunion, which are more likely to benefit from aggressive treatment such as vertebroplasty (Griffith et al. in press).

10   Conclusion

Vertebral fracture is the most common consequence of osteoporosis, occurring in a substantial number of the elderly population. Most vertebral fracture, however, remains clinically unrecognized. The presence, number, and severity of vertebral fracture are strong risk factors for the development of subsequent osteoporotic fracture. Large-scale clinical trials have demonstrated that osteoporosis therapy can reverse bone loss and reduce the fracture rate, and that these benefits are most pronounced in patients with low BMD and pre-existing vertebral fracture. Clinical guidelines published by the National Osteoporosis Foundation, International Osteoporosis Foundation, and others recognize the importance of vertebral fracture along with BMD as key risk factors for evaluating osteoporosis. Although BMD is widely used in patient evaluation, radiological assessment of vertebral fracture is much less common, or if it is used, it is not well standardized and interpreted. Good radiographic technique and a high level of observer experience in image interpretation are important for the reliable diagnosis of vertebral fracture. VFA by DXA is increasingly being used for vertebral fracture identification. Vertebral fracture diagnosis may be made fortuitously from any imaging method in which the spine is included. In the future, virtual estimation of vertebral body strength with high-resolution imaging techniques may enable patients at risk of vertebral fracture to be identified more effectively. MRI can detect relatively minor acute or subacute vertebral fracture or re-fracture, assess fracture age, and distinguish between osteoporotic and neoplastic fracture with greater sensitivity than other imaging techniques.

References

Adams JE, Lenchik L, Roux C, Genant HK (2010) Radiological assessment of vertebral fracture. International osteoporosis foundation vertebral fracture initiative resource document part II 2010, pp 1–49. http://www.iofbonehealth.org/health-professionals/educational-tools-and-slide-kits/vertebral-fracture-teaching-program.html

Banse X, Devogelaer JP, Grynpas M (2002) Patient-specific microarchitecture of vertebral cancellous bone: a peripheral quantitative computed tomographic and histological study. Bone 30(6):829–835

Black DM, Arden NK, Palermo L, Pearson J, Cummings SR (1999a) Prevalent vertebral deformities predict hip fractures and new vertebral deformities but not wrist fractures. Study of osteoporotic fractures research group. J Bone Miner Res 14(5):821–828

Black DM, Palermo L, Nevitt MC, Genant HK, Christensen L, Cummings SR (1999b) Defining incident vertebral deformity: a prospective comparison of several approaches. the study of osteoporotic fractures research group. J Bone Miner Res 14(1):90–101

Buehring B, Krueger D, Checovich M, Gemar D, Vallarta-Ast N, Genant HK et al (2010) Vertebral fracture assessment: impact of instrument and reader. Osteoporos Int 21(3):487–494

Chan KK, Sartoris DJ, Haghighi P, Sledge P, Barrett-Connor E, Trudell DT et al (1997) Cupid's bow contour of the vertebral body: evaluation of pathogenesis with bone densitometry and imaging-histopathologic correlation. Radiology 202(1):253–256

Chesnut IC, Skag A, Christiansen C, Recker R, Stakkestad JA, Hoiseth A et al (2004) Effects of oral ibandronate administered daily or intermittently on fracture risk in postmenopausal osteoporosis. J Bone Miner Res 19(8):1241–1249

Christiansen BA, Bouxsein ML (2010) Biomechanics of vertebral fractures and the vertebral fracture cascade. Curr Osteoporos Rep 8(4):198–204

Clark P, Cons-Molina F, Deleze M, Ragi S, Haddock L, Zanchetta JR et al (2009) The prevalence of radiographic vertebral fractures in Latin American countries: the Latin American vertebral osteoporosis study (LAVOS). Osteoporos Int 20(2):275–282

Cooper C, Melton LJ 3rd (1992) Vertebral fractures. BMJ 304(6842):1634–1635

Cooper C, Atkinson EJ, O'Fallon WM, Melton LJ 3rd (1992) Incidence of clinically diagnosed vertebral fractures: a population-based study in Rochester, Minnesota, 1985–1989. J Bone Miner Res 7(2):221–227

Damilakis J, Adams JE, Guglielmi G, Link TM (2010) Radiation exposure in X-ray-based imaging techniques used in osteoporosis. Eur Radiol 20(11):2707–2714

Delmas PD, Genant HK, Crans GG, Stock JL, Wong M, Siris E et al (2003) Severity of prevalent vertebral and nonvertebral fractures and the risk of subsequent vertebral and nonvertebral fractures: results from the MORE trial. Bone 33(4):522–532

Delmas PD, Van de Langerijt L, Watts NB, Eastell R, Genant H, Grauer A, Cahall DL (2005) Underdiagnosis of vertebral fractures is a worldwide problem: The IMPACT study. J Bone Miner Res 20(4):557–563

Diacinti D, Guglielmi G (2010) Vertebral morphometry. Radiol Clin North Am 48(3):561–575

Diacinti D, Acca M, D'Erasmo E, Tomei E, Mazzuoli GF (1995) Aging changes in vertebral morphometry. Calcif Tissue Int 57(6):426–429

Diamond TH, Clark WA, Kumar SV (2007) Histomorphometric analysis of fracture healing cascade in acute osteoporotic vertebral body fractures. Bone 40(3):775–780

Eastell R, Cedel SL, Wahner HW, Riggs BL, Melton LJ 3rd (1991) Classification of vertebral fractures. J Bone Miner Res 6(3):207–215

Ensrud KE, Schousboe JT (2011) Clinical practice. Vertebral fractures. N Engl J Med 364(17):1634–1642

Ensrud KE, Thompson DE, Cauley JA, Nevitt MC, Kado DM, Hochberg MC et al (2000) Prevalent vertebral deformities predict mortality and hospitalization in older women with low bone mass. Fracture intervention trial research group. J Am Geriatr Soc 48(3):241–249

Ettinger B, Cooper C (1995) Clinical assessment of osteoporotic vertebral fractures. In: Genant HK, Jergas M, van Kuijk C (ed.) Vertebral fracture in osteoporosis. Radiology Research and Education Foundation Publishers, San Francisco, pp 15–20

Ettinger B, Black DM, Nevitt MC, Rundle AC, Cauley JA, Cummings SR et al (1992) Contribution of vertebral deformities to chronic back pain and disability. The study of osteoporotic fractures research group. J Bone Miner Res 7(4):449–456

Ferrar L, Jiang G, Barrington NA, Eastell R (2000) Identification of vertebral deformities in women: comparison of radiological assessment and quantitative morphometry using morphometric radiography and morphometric X-ray absorptiometry. J Bone Miner Res 15(3):575–585

Ferrar L, Jiang G, Adams J, Eastell R (2005) Identification of vertebral fractures: an update. Osteoporos Int 16(7):717–728

Ferrar L, Jiang G, Armbrecht G, Reid DM, Roux C, Gluer CC et al (2007) Is short vertebral height always an osteoporotic fracture? The osteoporosis and ultrasound study (OPUS). Bone 41(1):5–12

Ferrar L, Roux C, Reid DM, Felsenberg D, Gluer CC, Eastell R (2012) Prevalence of non-fracture short vertebral height is similar in premenopausal and postmenopausal women: the osteoporosis and ultrasound study. Osteoporos Int 23(3):1035–1040

Fink HA, Milavetz DL, Palermo L, Nevitt MC, Cauley JA, Genant HK et al (2005) What proportion of incident radiographic vertebral deformities is clinically diagnosed and vice versa? J Bone Miner Res 20(7):1216–1222

Fornasier VL, Czitrom AA (1978) Collapsed vertebrae: a review of 659 autopsies. Clin Orthop Relat Res 131:261–265

Foundation NO (2010) Clinician's guide to prevention and treatment of osteoporosis. National Osteoporosis Foundation, Washington

Fuerst T, Wu C, Genant HK, von Ingersleben G, Chen Y, Johnston C et al (2009) Evaluation of vertebral fracture assessment by dual X-ray absorptiometry in a multicenter setting. Osteoporos Int 20(7):1199–1205

Genant HK, Jergas M (2003) Assessment of prevalent and incident vertebral fractures in osteoporosis research. Osteoporos Int 14(Suppl 3):S43–S55

Genant HK, Wu CY, van Kuijk C, Nevitt MC (1993) Vertebral fracture assessment using a semiquantitative technique. J Bone Miner Res 8(9):1137–1148

Genant HK, Jergas M, Palermo L, Nevitt M, Valentin RS, Black D et al (1996) Comparison of semiquantitative visual and quantitative morphometric assessment of prevalent and incident vertebral fractures in osteoporosis. The study of osteoporotic fractures research group. J Bone Miner Res 11(7):984–996

Gold DT (2001) The nonskeletal consequences of osteoporotic fractures. Psychologic and social outcomes. Rheum Dis Clin North Am 27(1):255–262

Grados F, Roux C, de Vernejoul MC, Utard G, Sebert JL, Fardellone P (2001) Comparison of four morphometric definitions and a semiquantitative consensus reading for assessing prevalent vertebral fractures. Osteoporos Int 12(9):716–722

Grados F, Fechtenbaum J, Flipon E, Kolta S, Roux C, Fardellone P (2009) Radiographic methods for evaluating osteoporotic vertebral fractures. Jt Bone Spine 76(3):241–247

Griffith JF, Guglielmi G (2010) Vertebral fracture. Radiol Clin North Am 48(3):519–529

Griffith JF, Adams JE, Genant HK Diagnosis and classification of vertebral fracture. Primer metabolic bone disease and disorders of mineral metabolism, 8th edn. in press

Grigoryan M, Guermazi A, Roemer FW, Delmas PD, Genant HK (2003) Recognizing and reporting osteoporotic vertebral fractures. Eur Spine J 12(Suppl 2):S104–S112

Guermazi A, Mohr A, Grigorian M, Taouli B, Genant HK (2002) Identification of vertebral fractures in osteoporosis. Semin Musculoskelet Radiol 6(3):241–252

Guglielmi G, Diacinti D, van Kuijk C, Aparisi F, Krestan C, Adams JE et al (2008) Vertebral morphometry: current methods and recent advances. Eur Radiol 18(7):1484–1496

Harris ST, Watts NB, Genant HK, McKeever CD, Hangartner T, Keller M et al (1999) Effects of risedronate treatment on vertebral and nonvertebral fractures in women with postmenopausal osteoporosis: a randomized controlled trial. Vertebral efficacy with risedronate therapy (VERT) study group. JAMA 282(14):1344–1352

Herss Nielsen VA, Podenphant J, Martens S, Gotfredsen A, Riis BJ (1991) Precision in assessment of osteoporosis from spine radiographs. Eur J Radiol 13(1):11–14

Hurxthal LM (1968) Measurement of anterior vertebral compressions and biconcave vertebrae. Am J Roentgenol Radium Ther Nucl Med. 103(3):635–644

Jager PL, Slart RH, Webber CL, Adachi JD, Papaioannou AL, Gulenchyn KY (2010) Combined vertebral fracture assessment and bone mineral density measurement: a patient-friendly new tool with an important impact on the Canadian risk fracture classification. Can Assoc Radiol J 61(4):194–200

Jiang G, Eastell R, Barrington NA, Ferrar L (2004) Comparison of methods for the visual identification of prevalent vertebral fracture in osteoporosis. Osteoporos Int 15(11):887–896

Johnell O, O'Neill T, Felsenberg D, Kanis J, Cooper C, Silman AJ (1997) Anthropometric measurements and vertebral deformities. European vertebral osteoporosis study (EVOS) group. Am J Epidemiol 146(4):287–293

Kadowaki E, Tamaki J, Iki M, Sato Y, Chiba Y, Kajita E et al (2010) Prevalent vertebral deformity independently increases incident vertebral fracture risk in middle-aged and elderly Japanese women: the Japanese population-based osteoporosis (JPOS) cohort study. Osteoporos Int 21(9):1513–1522

Kalidis L, Felsenberg D, Kalender WA, et al. (1992) Morphometric analysis of digitized radiographs: description of automatic evaluation. In: EFJ R (ed.) Current research in osteoporosis and bone mineral measurement II. British Institute of Radiology, London, pp 4–16

Kanis JA, Johnell O, Oden A, Johansson H, McCloskey E (2008) FRAX and the assessment of fracture probability in men and women from the UK. Osteoporos Int 19(4):385–397

Kanis JA, Hans D, Cooper C, Baim S, Bilezikian JP, Binkley N et al (2011) Interpretation and use of FRAX in clinical practice. Osteoporos Int 22(9):2395–2411

Kiel D (1995) Assessing vertebral fractures. national osteoporosis foundation working group on vertebral fractures. J Bone Miner Res 10(4):518–523

Kleerekoper M, Nelson DA (1992) Vertebral fracture or vertebral deformity. Calcif Tissue Int 50(1):5–6

Krug R, Burghardt AJ, Majumdar S, Link TM (2010) High-resolution imaging techniques for the assessment of osteoporosis. Radiol Clin North Am 48(3):601–621

Kwok AWL, Gong J-S, Wang Y-X J, Leung JCS, Kwok T, Griffith JF, Leung PC (2012) Prevalence and risk factors of radiographic vertebral fractures in elderly Chinese men and women: results of Mr. OS (Hong Kong) and Ms. OS (Hong Kong) studies. Osteoporos Int In press doi: 10.1007/s00198-012-2040-8

Lenchik L, Rogers LF, Delmas PD, Genant HK (2004) Diagnosis of osteoporotic vertebral fractures: importance of recognition and description by radiologists. AJR Am J Roentgenol 183(4):949–958

Lindsay R, Silverman SL, Cooper C, Hanley DA, Barton I, Broy SB et al (2001) Risk of new vertebral fracture in the year following a fracture. JAMA 285(3):320–323

Link TM, Guglielmi G, van Kuijk C, Adams JE (2005) Radiologic assessment of osteoporotic vertebral fractures: diagnostic and prognostic implications. Eur Radiol 15(8):1521–1532

Masharawi Y, Salame K, Mirovsky Y, Peleg S, Dar G, Steinberg N et al (2008) Vertebral body shape variation in the thoracic and lumbar spine: characterization of its asymmetry and wedging. Clin Anat 21(1):46–54

Matsumoto T, Hagino H, Shiraki M, Fukunaga M, Nakano T, Takaoka K et al (2009) Effect of daily oral minodronate on vertebral fractures in Japanese postmenopausal women with established osteoporosis: a randomized placebo-controlled double-blind study. Osteoporos Int 20(8):1429–1437

Mc Donnell P, Harrison N, Liebschner MA, Mc Hugh PE (2009) Simulation of vertebral trabecular bone loss using voxel finite element analysis. J Biomech 42(16):2789–2796

Melton LJ 3rd, Lane AW, Cooper C, Eastell R, O'Fallon WM, Riggs BL (1993) Prevalence and incidence of vertebral deformities. Osteoporos Int 3(3):113–119

Meunier P (1968) La dynamique du remaniement osseux humain, etudiee par lecture quantitative de la biopsie osseuse. Lyon

Meunier PJ, Roux C, Ortolani S, Diaz-Curiel M, Compston J, Marquis P et al (2009) Effects of long-term strontium ranelate treatment on vertebral fracture risk in postmenopausal women with osteoporosis. Osteoporos Int 20(10):1663–1673

Nicholson PH, Haddaway MJ, Davie MW, Evans SF (1993) A computerized technique for vertebral morphometry. Physiol Meas 14(2):195–204

Pfirrmann CW, Resnick D (2001) Schmorl nodes of the thoracic and lumbar spine: radiographic-pathologic study of prevalence, characterization, and correlation with degenerative changes of 1,650 spinal levels in 100 cadavers. Radiology 219(2):368–374

Riggs BL, Melton III LJ, 3rd, Robb RA, Camp JJ, Atkinson EJ, Peterson JM et al. (2004) Population-based study of age and sex differences in bone volumetric density, size, geometry, and structure at different skeletal sites. J Bone Miner Res 19(12):1945–1954

Samelson EJ, Christiansen BA, Demissie S, Broe KE, Zhou Y, Meng CA et al (2011) Reliability of vertebral fracture assessment using multidetector CT lateral scout views: the framingham osteoporosis study. Osteoporos Int 22(4):1123–1131

Sanders KM, Nicholson GC, Watts JJ, Pasco JA, Henry MJ, Kotowicz MA et al (2006) Half the burden of fragility fractures in the community occur in women without osteoporosis. When is fracture prevention cost-effective? Bone 38(5):694–700

US Department of Health and Human Services (2004). Bone health and osteoporosis: a report of the surgeon general. In: Rockville MD (ed.)

Siris ES, Miller PD, Barrett-Connor E, Faulkner KG, Wehren LE, Abbott TA et al (2001) Identification and fracture outcomes of undiagnosed low bone mineral density in postmenopausal women: results from the national osteoporosis risk assessment. JAMA 286(22):2815–2822

Siris E, Adachi JD, Lu Y, Fuerst T, Crans GG, Wong M et al (2002) Effects of raloxifene on fracture severity in postmenopausal women with osteoporosis: results from the MORE study. multiple outcomes of raloxifene evaluation. Osteoporos Int 13(11):907–913

Siris ES, Genant HK, Laster AJ, Chen P, Misurski DA, Krege JH (2007) Enhanced prediction of fracture risk combining vertebral fracture status and BMD. Osteoporos Int 18(6):761–770

Siris ES, Boonen S, Mitchell PJ, Bilezikian J, Silverman S (2012) What's in a name? What constitutes the clinical diagnosis of osteoporosis? Osteoporos Int In press doi:10.1007/s00198-012-1991-0

Smith RW, Eyler WR, Mellinger RC (1960) On the incidence of osteoporosis. Ann Intern Med 52:773–781

Smith-Bindman R, Cummings SR, Steiger P, Genant HK (1991) A comparison of morphometric definitions of vertebral fracture. J Bone Miner Res 6(1):25–34

Thomsen JS, Ebbesen EN, Mosekilde LI (2002) Age-related differences between thinning of horizontal and vertical trabeculae in human lumbar bone as assessed by a new computerized method. Bone 31(1):136–142

Tsujio T, Nakamura H, Terai H, Hoshino M, Namikawa T, Matsumura A, et al. (2011) Characteristic radiographic or magnetic resonance images of fresh osteoporotic vertebral fractures predicting potential risk for nonunion: a prospective multicenter study. Spine (Phila Pa 1976) 36(15):1229–1235

Williams AL, Al-Busaidi A, Sparrow PJ, Adams JE, Whitehouse RW (2009) Under-reporting of osteoporotic vertebral fractures on computed tomography. Eur J Radiol 69(1):179–183

Benign and Malignant Vertebral Fractures

Anastasia N. Fotiadou

Contents

Abstract

Vertebral compression fractures are a common clinical problem, particularly in elderly patients. Osteoporosis is the most common cause in this age group. However, malignancy can also be a cause of vertebral collapse in the same age group. The diagnostic challenge is even greater when vertebral fractures are detected in patients with a history of cancer. In all these patients, determining the cause of vertebral collapse is crucial for the management, treatment planning and prognosis. The purpose of this chapter is to analyze the imaging features used to differentiate malignant from benign causes.

1 Introduction

The most frequent benign causes of vertebral collapse include osteoporosis, trauma and infection. In patients with minimal or no trauma and without clinical and radiological features of infection, osteoporosis is thought to be the most common cause. On the other hand, the spine is a common site of malignant disease, which may result in a pathologic fracture (Yuh et al. 1989). Distinguishing malignant from benign vertebral compression fractures based on clinical findings, radiography, bone scans and computed tomography (CT) may not be adequate, especially in patients with no trauma or known malignancy. Magnetic resonance imaging (MRI) has proven to be superior to other diagnostic tools by using morphologic and signal intensity criteria (Uetani et al. 2004; Tan et al. 2002). The aim of this chapter is to analyze the imaging features used to differentiate benign from malignant vertebral fractures.

2 Conventional Radiography

For the accurate assessment of vertebral collapse it is crucial to obtain spinal radiographs of good quality. In order to acquire optimum lateral images, it is very important to

A. N. Fotiadou (✉)
Hinchingbrooke Hospital NHS Trust, Hinchingbrooke Park,
PE29 6NT, Huntingdon, Cambridgeshire, UK
e-mail: natfot@yahoo.gr

G. Guglielmi (ed.), *Osteoporosis and Bone Densitometry Measurements*, Medical Radiology. Diagnostic Imaging,
DOI: 10.1007/174_2012_611, © Springer-Verlag Berlin Heidelberg 2013

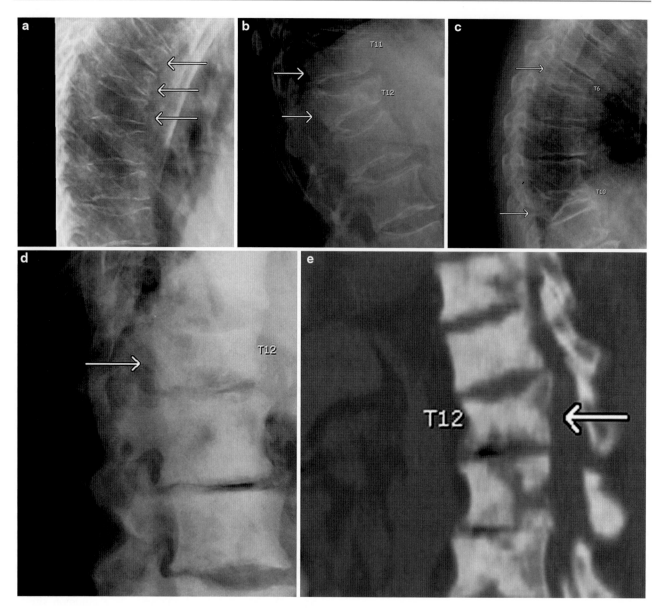

Fig. 1 Conventional lateral thoracic spine radiographs demonstrating vertebral fractures. **a** Osteoporotic fractures at the mid thoracic spine with slight anterior wedging of the vertebral bodies (*arrows*). **b** Mild anterior wedging of the T11 and T12 vertebral bodies with convex posterior vertebral border suggestive of malignant disease (*arrows*). **c** Significant loss of height of the T10 vertebral body and wedge deformity of approximately 50 % of the T6 vertebral body, with associated pedicle involvement (*arrows*). These features are in keeping with malignant compression fractures. **d** Patient with a history of prostate cancer. The lateral radiograph shows biconcave shape of the T12 vertebral body (*arrow*). Moreover, there is diffuse sclerosis noted at this level and the adjacent vertebral bodies, findings consistent with metastatic disease. **e** Same patient as in **d**. Sagittal CT reformat demonstrating the extent of sclerotic change

ensure that the spine is as parallel as possible to the radiographic table. In good quality radiographic images, the endplates of each vertebra should not be superimposed, since this obliquity might exaggerate a vertebral deformity.

In patients with pathologic spinal curvature, such as scoliosis, severe kyphosis or lordosis, there are certain technical limitations. In mild scoliosis, obtaining radiographs with the convexity of the scoliosis directed towards the X-ray table might prove to be useful (Rea et al. 1998). Nowadays, in most centres conventional radiographs are performed and viewed digitally, which allows adjustment of the windowing as well as filtering.

2.1 Findings Suggestive of Benign Vertebral Fracture

A concave posterior vertebral border is most likely associated with benign osteoporotic fractures, especially if there is some retropulsion of the bony parts into the spinal canal (Fig. 1a).

2.2 Findings Suggestive of Malignant Vertebral Fracture

Location of the fracture above the T7 level, presence of an epidural or paravertebral mass, osseous destruction and involvement of the posterior part of the vertebral body are most frequently features of malignant aetiology. In particular, pedicle involvement has been described as specific for malignant lesions (Baur-Melnyk and Reiser 2004). In addition, a convex posterior vertebral border suggests malignant disease (Fig. 1b–e).

2.3 Vertebral Collapse Associated with Specific Diseases

Vertebral fractures due to osteomalacia in adults (Fig. 2) are demonstrated as a biconcave deformity of the endplates ("cod fish" vertebrae) and are similar to those encountered in osteoporosis (Resnick 1982). Other characteristic radiographic findings in association with benign vertebral collapse include the "H" deformity in sickle cell anaemia and Gaucher's disease. This type of deformity is visualized as a step-like depression of the superior and inferior vertebral margins and can also be found in thalassemia and congenital hereditary spherocytosis. In Scheuermann's disease Schmorl's nodes are seen. These are localised depressions of the endplate as a result of invagination of disc material into the subchondral vertebral body. Lastly, infection is a cause of endplate erosion and loss of disc height. In these cases MRI is used for the diagnosis, since it has been shown to have good to excellent sensitivity. Nonetheless, it should be pointed out that pathologic fractures can complicate infectious spondylitis (Ledermann et al. 2003).

3 Computed Tomography

The use of multislice spiral CT has significantly improved the image quality and spatial resolution. CT is less sensitive than MRI in depicting abnormalities of the bone marrow. Nonetheless, CT may provide more detailed information than MRI on the margins of a lesion and matrix alterations, which is vital for the differentiation between benign and malignant vertebral fractures (Yuzawa et al. 2005). In addition, CT is more sensitive in demonstrating the vacuum phenomenon, which is a sign of benign disease. Lastly, CT is superior in visualising the bony structures and in demonstrating the fracture lines (Laredo et al. 1995; Stäbler et al. 1999).

3.1 CT Findings Suggestive of Benign Vertebral Fracture

The intravertebral vacuum phenomenon, which is commonly visualised following vertebral fractures, is associated

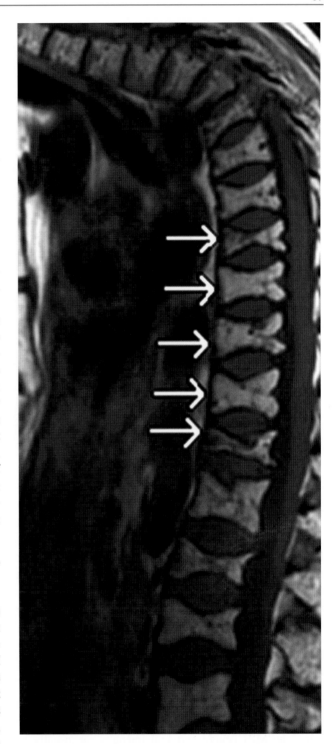

Fig. 2 Sagittal T1-weighted image shows multiple thoracic vertebral fractures due to osteomalacia (*arrows*) in a 68-year-old female patient. Biconcave deformity of the endplates ("cod fish" vertebrae) and kyphotic deformity are visualised

with osteoporotic collapse and increase in frequency with age (Stäbler et al. 1999). Furthermore, benign vertebral compression fractures usually show retropulsion of a posterior bone fragment into the spinal canal or intravertebral fluid (Fig. 3a–c).

Fig. 3 Sagittal CT reformats.
a Osteoporotic fractures of the T8 and T11 vertebral bodies (*arrows*) with anterior wedging, which is more pronounced at the T11 level. **b** Anterior wedging of the T5 vertebral body (*long arrow*) with retropulsion of its posterior inferior part, in keeping with an osteoporotic fracture. Also, Schmorl's node is noticed at the inferior endplate of the T6 vertebra (*short arrow*). **c** Benign fracture of the T12 vertebral body (*arrow*) with slight retropulsion of its posterior superior part. **d** Loss of height of the L1 vertebral body with associated convex posterior cortex (*long arrow*), suggestive of malignant cause. Also, there is a lytic lesion noted at the posterior part of the T12 vertebral body (*short arrow*)

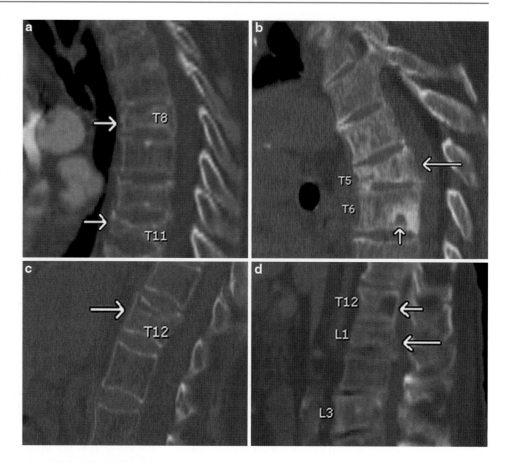

3.2 CT Findings Suggestive of Malignant Vertebral Fracture

In malignant vertebral fractures, the vertebral bodies have a convex posterior cortex and associated paravertebral or epidural masses might be found (Fig. 3d). Another highly specific finding is the posterior element infiltration, in particular that of the pedicle.

4 Magnetic Resonance Imaging

Although several recent studies have applied new MRI techniques in assessing vertebral collapse, on conventional spin echo MRI benign vertebral fractures can usually be distinguished from malignant ones (Baker et al. 1990). The reported sensitivity, specificity and accuracy of MRI for the diagnosis of metastatic compression fractures is 100, 93, and 95 %, respectively (Shih et al. 1999). In elderly patients, because of the almost complete replacement of the bone marrow by fatty tissue, fat suppression is thought to be necessary for the evaluation of the diseased vertebrae.

4.1 MRI Findings Suggestive of Benign Vertebral Fracture

4.1.1 Patterns of Signal Intensity and Enhancement

The signal intensity patterns of benign osteoporotic compression fractures are usually variable. In the majority of cases, the signal-intensity changes are localised (Fig. 4a) and normal bone marrow is visualised in at least one area within the vertebral body (Sugimura et al. 1987). Indeed, most vertebral metastases do not result in compression fractures until the entire body is infiltrated by the tumour (Fig. 4b), causing destruction of the trabeculae, the cortex or both (Yuh et al. 1989). However, it has been reported that in 15 % of acute osteoporotic compression fractures (Fig. 4c) there is complete replacement with abnormal signal intensity (Shih et al. 1999). This might be due to spread to the entire vertebra of a reactive process induced by the fracture. Therefore, in acute osteoporotic fractures, when the height of the vertebral body is preserved and diffused signal-intensity changes are seen on T1-weighted, STIR, and contrast-enhanced T1-weighted images, the diagnosis may be very difficult, since these imaging features mimic those encountered in malignant

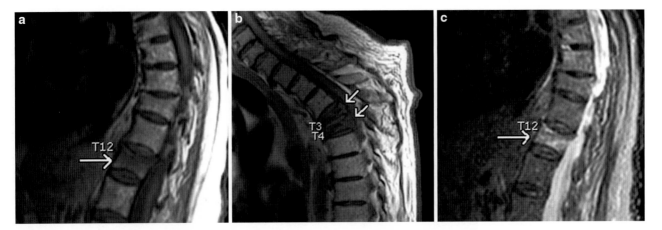

Fig. 4 **a** Sagittal T1-weighted image showing biconcave morphology and diffuse low signal-intensity within the T12 vertebral body. However, at least one area of normal bone marrow is detected (*arrow*). Also, retropulsion of the posterior superior part of the vertebra is seen. These features are in keeping with benign aetiology. **b** Sagittal T1-weighted image demonstrating anterior wedging of the T3 and T4 vertebral bodies, with complete replacement of the normal bone marrow by low signal intensity. Also, there is slight convexity of the posterior part of the vertebrae (*arrows*) noticed. These findings are in keeping with malignant disease. **c** Same patient as in a. STIR sagittal image. Almost complete and diffuse replacement of the bone marrow with high signal intensity (*arrow*) is detected, representing bone marrow oedema

Fig. 5 Fluid sign in osteoporotic fractures. **a** Linear area of high signal intensity is seen at the anterior endplate (long arrow) on this sagittal T2-weighted image. There is some retropulsion of the posterior superior part of the vertebral body within the spinal canal also noticed at this level (*short arrow*). **b** Sagittal STIR sequence demonstrating the "fluid sign"

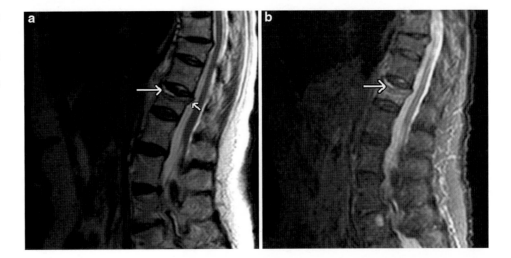

compression fractures. In chronic osteoporotic fractures there is no abnormal signal intensity identified in the bone marrow of the compressed vertebra (Tan et al. 2002).

4.1.2 Fluid Sign

A cleft of fluid (demonstrated as a linear area of high signal-intensity) or gas within the vertebral body on T2-weighted and STIR images (Fig. 5a, b), have been described in association with osteoporotic fractures (Baur et al. 2002). These are considered to represent avascular necrosis or pseudoarthrosis. In particular, the "fluid sign" is seen adjacent to the fractured endplates and the signal is isointense to that of cerebrospinal fluid (Oka et al. 2005).

4.1.3 Low Signal Intensity Band

In acute benign compression fractures, a band like low signal intensity area on T1-weighted and T2-weighted images is commonly seen (Fig. 6a, b). This area is sited adjacent to the collapsed

endplate and is encountered in 93 % of acute osteoporotic fractures as opposed to 44 % of metastatic ones (Jung et al. 2003).

4.1.4 Retropulsion of a Posterior Bone Fragment

Retropulsion of a posterior bone fragment is believed to be sensitive and specific for osteoporotic fractures. It is detected in 60 % of acute osteoporotic fractures as opposed to 11 % of metastatic collapses (Fig. 7). In cases of metastatic disease, retropulsion might be due to preexisting compression fractures that were secondarily involved by metastatic disease. It is also possible that metastatic disease can sometimes be associated with retropulsion of bone fragments (Kaplan et al. 1987).

4.1.5 Pedicle Involvement

Pedicle involvement has been reported as specific for malignancy (Fig. 8a–d). However, it can be found in many patients with osteoporotic fractures, particularly in the early

Fig. 6 Low signal intensity band in benign vertebral compression fractures. **a** Sagittal T1-weighted MR image showing a band-like low signal intensity area adjacent to the collapsed endplate of the T12 vertebral body (*arrow*). **b** Sagittal T2-weighted image. There is a subtle low signal intensity band demonstrated at the level of the collapsed superior endplate (*arrow*)

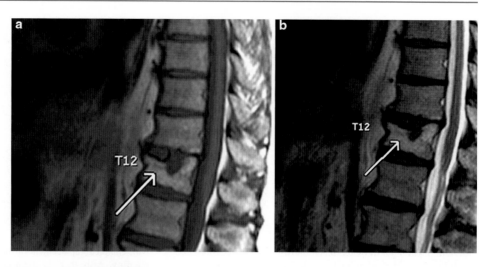

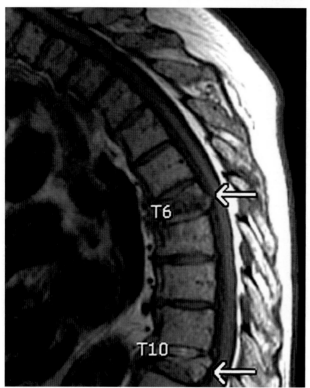

Fig. 7 Osteoporotic vertebral collapse. Retropulsion of a posterior bone fragment is noted at the level of the T6 and T10 vertebral bodies on this sagittal T1-weighted image (*arrows*)

phase. It has been reported that pedicle abnormal signal intensity and contrast enhancement are seen in 64 % of benign compression fractures and in 84.2 % of malignant ones, with no significant difference between groups (Ishiyama et al. 2010). In general, the criteria of pedicle infiltration by tumour include the presence of inhomogeneous diffuse signal-intensity changes or a mass effect.

Nonetheless, it should be stressed that signal-intensity changes in osteoporotic fractures are often focal and inhomogeneous as well. When pedicle involvement is the only

sign, a diagnosis of malignant pathologic fracture should not be assumed. Sclerosis of the pedicle is seen during the healing process of microfractures and is considered to represent reactive change. This reflects the signal intensity patterns noted on MRI, which represent infiltration by inflammatory cells, granulation tissue or fibrosis.

4.1.6 Multiple Compression Fractures

Multiple compression fractures (Fig. 9) have not been shown to be a useful finding for the differentiation of osteoporotic aetiology from malignancy (Rupp et al. 1995). Nevertheless, in the study by Jung et al. (2003) multiple compression fractures were detected in 58 % of acute osteoporotic fractures as opposed to 33 % of metastatic fractures. In this study, however, multiple myeloma which frequently manifests as multiple compression fractures, was excluded.

4.2 MRI Findings Suggestive of Malignant Vertebral Fracture

4.2.1 Patterns of Signal Intensity and Enhancement

It has been reported that in all cases of metastatic compression fractures, hypointense to isointense signal intensity is noticed within the collapsed vertebral body on T1-weighted images (Cuénod et al. 1996). Also, round areas of low signal intensity may be found in adjacent non collapsed vertebrae (Fig. 10a). Furthermore, areas of high or inhomogeneous signal intensity within the diseased vertebrae on T2-weighted and contrast-enhanced conventional spin-echo MR images (Fig. 10b) are significantly more common in metastatic compression fractures (Baker et al. 1990; Shih et al. 1999).

In the study by Jung et al. (2003) the signal intensity on fast spin-echo T2-weighted images played little role in differentiating between acute osteoporotic and metastatic compression fractures. They also concluded that the signal

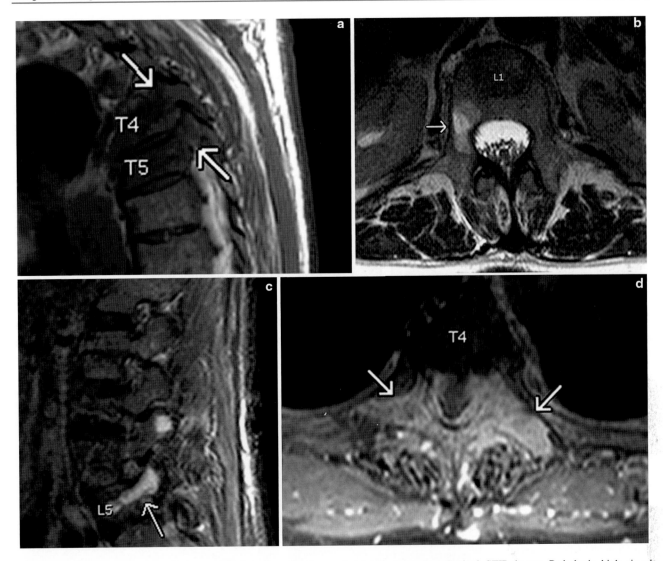

Fig. 8 Pedicle involvement in malignant vertebral compression fractures. **a** Sagittal T1-weighted image showing diffuse abnormal low signal intensity within the pedicles and the vertebral bodies at the T4 and T5 levels (*arrows*). **b** Axial T2-weighted image demonstrating abnormal high signal intensity within the pedicle of the L1 vertebra on the right hand side (*arrow*). **c** Sagittal STIR image. Pathologic high signal intensity is noted within the pedicle of the L5 vertebra. **d** Contrast-enhanced axial T1-weighted image with fat suppression. There is enhancement of the pedicles and the transverse processes (*arrows*) of the T4 vertebra seen. Enhancement of the spinous process is noticed as well

intensity on fat suppressed contrast-enhanced T1-weighted images is not useful either, since all acute osteoporotic fractures showed intense enhancement, which was heterogeneous in the vast majority of them.

In multiple myeloma, pathologic fractures and diffuse bone marrow infiltration are visualised on conventional MRI. In these cases, the bone marrow returns diffuse low signal intensity on T1-weighted images and high signal intensity on T2-weighted images (Fig. 11a, b).

4.2.2 Convex Posterior Border of the Vertebral Body

A convex posterior border of the vertebral body (Fig. 12a–c) is more frequently detected in metastatic compression

fractures than in acute osteoporotic ones (Tan et al. 1991; Cuénod et al. 1996). It has been reported that this feature is demonstrated in 74 % of metastatic involvement versus 20 % of acute osteoporotic fractures (Jung et al. 2003).

4.2.3 Pedicle and Posterior Element Involvement

In most malignant compression fractures, before collapse takes place, the tumour has already spread from the bone marrow of the vertebral body to the pedicles and neural arch. In osteoporotic compression fractures, reactive bone marrow changes usually spare the pedicles (Kaplan et al. 1987; Tan et al. 1991). Thus, the frequency of pedicle abnormal signal intensity is higher in metastatic fractures than in acute

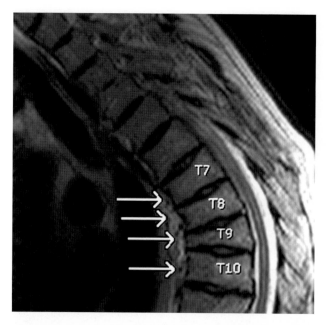

Fig. 9 Sagittal T2-weighted image that shows multiple osteoporotic compression fractures (*arrows*)

osteoporotic ones (Fig. 8a–d). Posterior element involvement is also more frequently observed in metastatic fractures.

It should be taken into consideration that abnormal signal intensity at the pedicle and posterior element can be detected in about one-half of acute osteoporotic compression fractures, and the conspicuity increases when contrast-enhanced T1-weighted imaging with fat suppression is used (Jung et al. 2003). These patterns do not apply to chronic compression fractures.

4.2.4 Epidural Mass

An epidural soft tissue mass is suggestive of malignant vertebral collapse (Fig. 13) and is observed in 74 % of metastatic fractures versus 25 % of acute osteoporotic fractures, particularly when the epidural mass is encasing (Jung et al. 2003).

4.2.5 Focal Paraspinal Mass

It has been reported that the demonstration of a paraspinal mass (Fig. 14) is not helpful in depicting the cause of vertebral collapse (Rupp et al. 1995). However, it has been shown that this finding is significantly more frequent in

Fig. 10 a Patient with metastatic disease. Sagittal T2-weighted image, showing collapse of the superior endplate of the L3 vertebral body and inhomogeneous bone marrow signal intensity (*long arrow*). Moreover, round areas of low signal intensity are found in the L1 and L5 vertebrae (*short arrows*). **b** Axial T2-weighted image through the T7 vertebral body demonstrating multiple foci of high signal intensity at the body and the pedicle on the left hand side (*arrow*), in keeping with metastases

Fig. 11 Patient with multiple myeloma. **a** Pathologic fracture of the T1 vertebral body (*arrow*) is seen on this sagittal T1-weighted image. Diffuse bone marrow infiltration, demonstrated as low signal intensity at all visualized levels, is noticed also. **b** Sagittal T2-weighted image showing significant collapse of the T1 vertebral body (*arrow*)

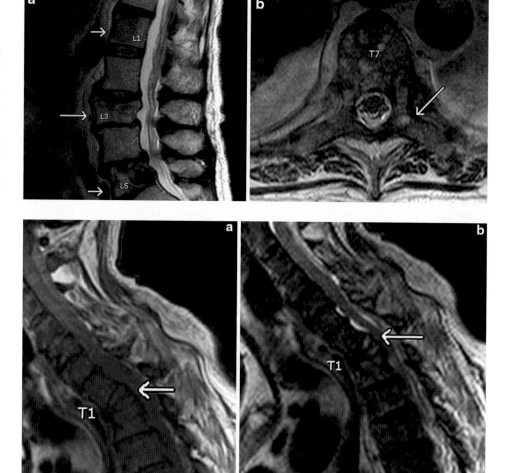

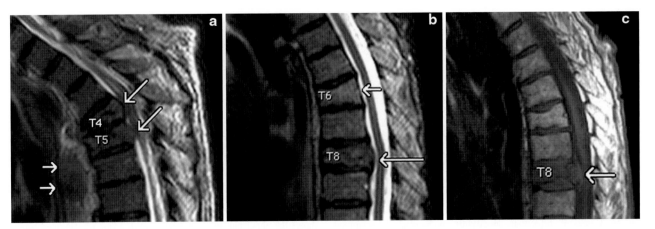

Fig. 12 Convex posterior border of the vertebral body in malignant collapse. **a** Sagittal T2-weighted image showing metastatic compression fractures of the T4 and T5 vertebral bodies (*long arrows*). The convex posterior part of the diseased vertebrae appears to impinge upon the spinal cord. Mediastinal lymphadenopathy (*short arrows*) is also detected. **b** Sagittal T2-weighted image demonstrating loss of height of the T8 vertebral body with associated convexity of its posterior border (*long arrow*). There is anterior wedging of the T6 vertebral body (*short arrow*) without convexity, visualised as well. **c** Significant convexity of the collapsed T8 vertebral body (*arrow*) is detected on this sagittal T1-weighted image

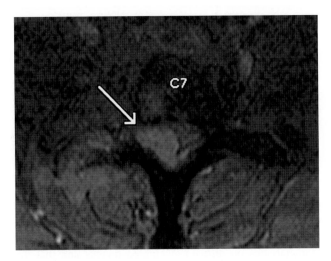

Fig. 13 Epidural mass is depicted on the right hand side at the level of the C7 (*arrow*) on this axial T2-weighted image. The right pedicle is surrounded by a soft tissue mass also

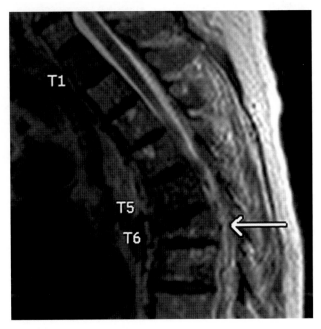

Fig. 15 Sagittal T2-weighted image showing multiple spinal metastases. There are bone marrow signal intensity abnormalities seen in vertebrae other than the collapsed T6 (*arrow*)

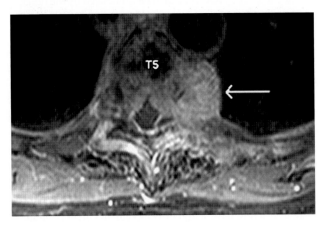

Fig. 14 Axial gadolinium enhanced T1-weighted fat suppressed image, which demonstrates an avidly enhancing left paraspinal mass (*arrow*), with associated destruction of the vertebral cortex. Involvement of the rib is noted also

metastatic compression fractures than in acute benign fractures. The same principle does not apply to a diffuse paraspinal mass.

4.2.6 Other Spinal Metastasis

Bone marrow signal intensity abnormalities in vertebrae other than the collapsed one, are more frequently seen in metastatic compression fractures than in acute benign compression fractures. These abnormalities more commonly indicate other spinal metastases (Fig. 15).

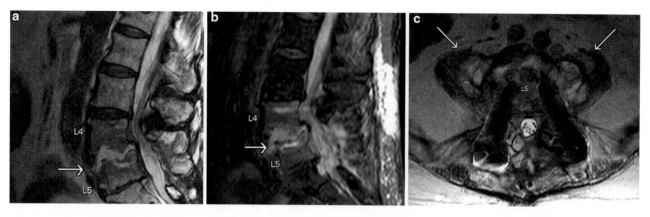

Fig. 16 Cases of infectious spondylitis. **a** Sagittal T2-weighted image. Pathologic bone marrow signal intensity is seen at L4 and L5. Also, there is destruction of the endplates and the disc space is of water-equivalent signal intensity (*arrow*). **b** Sagittal STIR image that shows the abnormal disc space (*arrow*). **c** Axial T2-weighted image. Abscess formation within the psoas muscle on both sides (*arrows*) at the level of L5 is visualized

Fig. 17 a Sagittal T2-weighted image showing malignant collapse of the T8 vertebral body. The posterior border of the vertebral body appears to be convex (*arrow*). **b** Diffusion image showing hyperintensity at the level of the diseased vertebra (*arrow*)

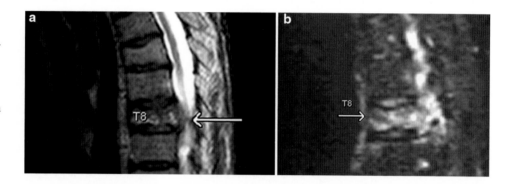

4.3   Differential Diagnosis from Spondylitis

In some cases pathologic spinal fractures need to be differentiated from infectious spondylitis. In the later, bone marrow oedema of two adjacent vertebrae and early destruction of the endplates are visualised. Additionally, the disc space is of water-equivalent signal intensity on T2-weighted and STIR images and enhances post intravenous gadolinium administration (Fig. 16a, b). Abscess formation (Fig. 16c) and enhancement of the surrounding granulation tissue are commonly encountered also (Stäbler and Reiser 2001).

4.4   Diffusion Imaging and ADC mapping

On diffusion-weighted MR images obtained with a b value of 165 s/mm^2, it has been reported that benign compression fractures are hypo- to isointense in comparison to adjacent normal vertebral bodies (Fig. 17a, b), whereas malignant compression fractures are hyperintense (Baur et al. 1998). However, in the study by Castillo et al. (2000) diffusion-weighted imaging was found to offer no advantage over conventional unenhanced MR imaging for the detection of vertebral metastases. They concluded that the T2 shine-through effect can significantly influence signal intensity characteristics on diffusion-weighted images and that this effect should be eliminated by using quantitative ADC mapping.

The measured ADCs can also be influenced by the range of b-values used, with b-values greater than 600 s/mm^2 probably resulting in an underestimation (Baur-Melnyk 2009).

4.5   Other Imaging Techniques

There has been research on MRI techniques with potential value in the distinction between benign and malignant acute vertebral compression fractures. These techniques include gadolinium-enhanced dynamic MRI studies and in-phased/opposed-phased imaging (Chen et al. 2002; Erly et al. 2006). It has been shown that metastatic vertebral lesions with or without fracture have a higher peak enhancement percentage and steeper enhancement slope than those of chronic compression fractures, but no difference when compared to those of acute compression fractures (Chen et al. 2002). Moreover, in-phase/opposed-phase imaging of the spine has been proposed to be a sensitive and specific way to differentiate benign from malignant spine signal intensity abnormalities (Zampa et al. 2002; Erly et al. 2006).

Finally, it has been reported that fluorodeoxyglucose (FDG) PET-CT is a useful tool for the distinction between benign and malignant vertebral collapse. Increased FDG uptake (standardized uptake value >3) has been related to a malignant cause (Mulligan et al. 2011).

5 Biopsy

Biopsy is considered to be the gold standard for the final diagnosis of vertebral compression fractures. There have been reports on patients with provisional diagnosis of osteoporotic fractures, which in biopsy during vertebroplasty and kyphoplasty were proven to be malignant ones (Shindle et al. 2006; Schoenfeld et al. 2008). On the other hand, it has also been reported that in 11 % of biopsy cases suggestive of chronic osteomyelitis, a diagnosis of osteoporotic spinal fractures was made (Allen et al. 2009).

6 Conclusion

In conclusion, morphologic criteria constitute the most important diagnostic tool for the differentiation between benign and malignant vertebral collapse. The findings of low-signal-intensity band, spared normal bone marrow signal intensity, retropulsion and other spinal metastasis have been shown to add predictive information (Jung et al. 2003). New techniques such as diffusion-weighted MR imaging, FDG PET-CT and MRI perfusion might prove helpful in equivocal cases.

References

Allen RT, Kum JB, Weidner N, Hulst JB, Garfin SR (2009) Biopsy of osteoporotic vertebral compression fractures during kyphoplasty: unsuspected histologic findings of chronic osteitis without clinical evidence of osteomyelitis. Spine (Phila Pa 1976) 34(14):1486–1491

Baker LL, Goodman SB, Perkash I, Lane B, Enzmann DR (1990) Benign versus pathologic compression fractures of vertebral bodies: assessment with conventional spin-echo, chemical shift, and STIR MR imaging. Radiology 174(2):495–502

Baur-Melnyk A (2009) Malignant versus benign vertebral collapse: are new imaging techniques useful? Cancer Imagig 9 (Spec No A): S49–S51

Baur-Melnyk A, Reiser M (2004) Staging of multiple myeloma with MRI: comparison to MSCT and conventional radiography. Radiologe 44(9):874–881

Baur A, Stäbler A, Brüning R et al (1998) Diffusion-weighted MR imaging of bone marrow: differentiation of benign versus pathologic compression fractures. Radiology 201(2):349–356

Baur A, Stäbler A, Arbogast S, Duerr HR, Bartl R, Reiser M (2002) Acute osteoporotic and neoplastic vertebral compression fractures: fluid sign at MR imaging. Radiology 225(3):730–735

Castillo M, Arbelaez A, Smith JK, Fisher LL (2000) Diffusion-weighted MR imaging offers no advantage over routine noncontrast MR imaging in the detection of vertebral metastases. Am J Neuroradiol 21(5):948–953

Chen WT, Shih TT, Chen RC et al (2002) Blood perfusion of vertebral lesions evaluated with gadolinium-enhanced dynamic MRI: in comparison with compression fracture and metastasis. J Magn Reson Imaging 15(3):308–314

Cuénod CA, Laredo JD, Chevret S et al (1996) Acute vertebral collapse due to osteoporosis or malignancy: appearance on unenhanced and gadolinium-enhanced MR images. Radiology 199(2):541–549

Erly WK, Oh ES, Outwater EK (2006) The utility of in-phase/opposed-phase imaging in differentiating malignancy from acute benign compression fractures of the spine. Am J Neuroradiol 27(6):1183–1188

Ishiyama M, Fuwa S, Numaguchi Y, Kobayashi N, Saida Y (2010) Am J Neuroradiol 31(4):668–673

Jung HS, Jee WH, McCauley TR, Ha KY, Choi KH (2003) Discrimination of metastatic from acute osteoporotic compression spinal fractures with MR imaging. Radiographics 23(1): 179–187

Kaplan PA, Orton DF, Asleson RJ (1987) Osteoporosis with vertebral compression fractures, retropulsed fragments, and neurologic compromise. Radiology 165(2):533–535

Laredo JD, Lakhdari K, Bella L, Hamze B, Janklewicz P, Tubiana JM (1995) Acute vertebral collapse: CT findings in benign and malignant nontraumatic cases. Radiology 194(1):41–48

Ledermann HP, Schweitzer ME, Morrison WB, Carrino JA (2003) MR imaging findings in spinal infections: rules or myths? Radiology 228(2):506–514

Mulligan M, Chirindel A, Karchevsky M (2011) Characterizing and predicting pathologic spine fractures in myeloma patients with FDG PET/CT and MR imaging. Cancer Invest 29(5):370–376

Oka M, Matsusako M, Kobayashi N, Uemura A, Numaguchi Y (2005) Intravertebral cleft sign on fat-suppressed contrast-enhanced MR: correlation with cement distribution pattern on percutaneous vertebroplasty. Acad Radiol 12(8):992–999

Rea JA, Steiger P, Blake GM, Fogelman I (1998) Optimizing data acquisition and analysis of morphometric X-ray absorptiometry. Osteoporos Int 8(2):177–183

Resnick DL (1982) Fish vertebrae. Arthritis Rheum 25(9):1073–1077

Rupp RE, Ebraheim NA, Coombs RJ (1995) Magnetic resonance imaging differentiation of compression spine fractures or vertebral lesions caused by osteoporosis or tumor. Spine 20(23):2499–2504

Schoenfeld AJ, Dinicola NJ, Ehrler DM et al (2008) Retrospective review of biopsy results following percutaneous fixation of vertebral compression fractures. Injury 39(3):327–333

Shih TT, Huang KM, Li YW (1999) Solitary vertebral collapse: distinction between benign and malignant causes using MR patterns. J Magn Reson Imaging 9(5):635–642

Shindle MK, Tyler W, Edobor-Osula F et al (2006) Unsuspected lymphoma diagnosed with use of biopsy during kyphoplasty. J Bone Joint Surg Am 88(12):2721–2724

Stäbler A, Reiser MF (2001) Imaging of spinal infection. Radiol Clin North Am 39(1):115–135

Stäbler A, Schneider P, Link TM et al (1999) Intravertebral vacuum phenomenon following fractures: CT study on frequency and etiology. J Comput Assist Tomogr 23(6):976–980

Sugimura K, Yamasaki K, Kitagaki H, Tanaka Y, Kono M (1987) Bone marrow diseases of the spine: differentiation with T1 and T2 relaxation times in MR imaging. Radiology 165(2):541–544

Tan SB, Kozak JA, Mawad ME (1991) The limitations of magnetic resonance imaging in the diagnosis of pathologic vertebral fractures. Spine 16(8):919–923

Tan DY, Tsou IY, Chee TS (2002) Differentiation of malignant vertebral collapse from osteoporotic and other benign causes using magnetic resonance imaging. Ann Acad Med Singapore 31(1):8–14

Uetani M, Hashmi R, Hayashi K (2004) Malignant and benign compression fractures: differentiation and diagnostic pitfalls on MRI. Clin Radiol 59(2):124–131

Yuh WT, Zachar CK, Barloon TJ, Sato Y, Sickels WJ, Hawes DR (1989) Vertebral compression fractures: distinction between benign and malignant causes with MR imaging. Radiology 172(1):215–218

Yuzawa Y, Ebara S, Kamimura M et al (2005) Magnetic resonance and computed tomography-based scoring system for the differential diagnosis of vertebral fractures caused by osteoporosis and malignant tumors. J Orthop Sci 10(4):345–352

Zampa V, Cosottini M, Michelassi C, Ortori S, Bruschini L, Bartolozzi C (2002) Value of opposed-phase gradient-echo technique in distinguishing between benign and malignant vertebral lesions. Eur Radiol 12(7):1811–1818

Bone Marrow Changes in Osteoporosis

James F. Griffith

Contents

J. F. Griffith (✉)
Department of Imaging and Interventional Radiology,
The Chinese University of Hong Kong,
Shatin, Hong Kong, People's Republic of China
e-mail: griffith@cuhk.edu.hk

Abstract

Bone research in osteoporosis has quite rightly focused on the mineralised component of bone as this is the component that is ultimately responsible for bone strength. However, the non-mineralised component of bone, i.e. the bone marrow, is many times more metabolically active and responsive than the mineralised component of bone. Despite this, the bone marrow has been relatively overlooked with regard to the pathogenesis of osteoporosis and related conditions. This has changed with magnetic resonance imaging and positron emission tomography allowing non-invasive quantification of bone marrow physiology and pathology on a large scale. Aspects of the bone marrow that can be evaluated on imaging are marrow fat content, perfusion, molecular diffusion and metabolic activity. There are many ways in which bone marrow metabolism may potentially influence bone metabolism. For example, the bone marrow forms the microenvironment of biologically relevant endosteal and trabecular bone and this bone may be responding to changes in the bone marrow. Similarly, the bone marrow contains pluripotent mesenchymal stem cells with the ability to differentiate preferentially along either haematopoetic, adipocytic or osteoblastic cell lines. Preliminary research has shown how bone loss in senile osteoporosis mass is accompanied by scalar changes in marrow fat content, marrow perfusion and marrow diffusion. Similar to the bone loss of osteoporosis, the bone marrow changes in osteoporosis represent an exaggeration of physiological age-related change. Bone marrow changes occur in synchrony rather than pre- or post-date changes in the mineralised component of bone. Whether the bone marrow is an active contributor or a passive bystander to physiological and osteoporotic bone loss remains to be seen.

G. Guglielmi (ed.), *Osteoporosis and Bone Densitometry Measurements*, Medical Radiology. Diagnostic Imaging,
DOI: 10.1007/174_2012_614, © Springer-Verlag Berlin Heidelberg 2013

1 Background

Bone densitometry, high resolution imaging techniques to access bone architecture and advanced image analytic platforms have greatly improved our understanding of osteoporosis particularly with respect to bone structure and strength prediction over the past three decades (Link 2012). This osteoporotic research has quite rightly focused on the hard tissue component of bone as this is the component that ultimately gives bone its strength. The marrow cavity, nevertheless, also forms a major constituent of bone and has, until recently, received relatively less attention regarding osteoporotic research. Yet, bone marrow is a more metabolically active tissue than mineralised bone tissue and several plausible mechanisms existing through which the bone marrow may influence bone metabolism. Our knowledge of bone marrow metabolism has been greatly assisted by MR and PET-CT technology which allows, for the first time, a quantitative non-invasive study of the bone marrow. This study has focused on lifelong physiological changes in the bone marrow as well as how the bone marrow is affected in common musculoskeletal disorders such as osteoporosis, marrow infiltration, osteoarthritis and disc degeneration. The bone marrow is one of the most voluminous and metabolically active organs in the human body, that undergoes progressive change throughout life and is involved in perfusion or nutrition of adjacent structures. It is hoped that the bone marrow may provide some answers that exist regarding the pathogenesis of these common musculoskeletal diseases.

For example, with respect to osteoporosis, one could argue that current densitometry techniques and even high resolution imaging techniques are diagnosing osteoporosis too late (Griffith et al. 2010). By the time osteoporosis is recognised by densitometric techniques, bone strength is already significantly impaired. Pharmaceutical agents can stall or retard the osteoporotic process but will not return bone strength to normal. Thinned cortices and trabeculae may thicken with osteoporotic treatment, but those trabeculae that have absorbed will not return such that impaired bone strength persists even with a good treatment response. Also, for subjects with normal bone density or low bone mass (osteopenia), prediction of which subjects will progress to more severe degrees of bone loss and impairment of bone strength, is not sufficiently accurate to select those patients which will particularly benefit from osteoporotic treatment. In addition, osteoporosis is associated with several other conditions such as steroid use, atherosclerosis, vascular calcification, diabetes, dyslipidaemia and Alzheimer's disease though the pathogenetic mechanisms linking these diseases to osteoporosis are not fully understood (Manolagas and Almeida 2007). One can appreciate that finding a contributory link between these diseases and osteoporosis would be a significant step towards the development of a common single therapy.

2 Bone Marrow

The bone marrow is supported by trabeculae and a fibrous tissue retinaculum and surrounded by a bone cortex of variable thickness ranging from approximately 1 to 5.5 mm. The actual composition of the bone marrow varies with anatomical location, physiological well-being and age (Hwang and Panicek 2007) though in general is made up of trabecular bone (approx 20 %), fatty marrow (approx 50 %), non-fatty functioning marrow (approx 25 %) and vascular channels (approx 5 %). Non-fatty functioning marrow comprises cells derived from the haematopoetic cell line (erythrocytes, granulocytes, lymphocytes, monocytes, platelets and osteoclasts) as well as stem cells.

At birth, the bone marrow is nearly entirely haematopoetic except for the epiphyses and apophyses which are mainly fat. With maturation, the haematopoetic appendicular marrow converts to a predominantly fatty marrow in a symmetrical centripetal fashion from the periphery to the central skeleton (Hwang and Panicek 2007). Superimposed on this centripedal conversion, haematopoetic marrow converts to fatty marrow in the tubular bones proceeding from the diaphysis to metaphysis (Hwang and Panicek 2007; Hartsock et al. 1965) (Fig. 1). At 10 years of age, marrow conversion of red to fatty marrow has begun in the diaphyses (Hwang and Panicek 2007). By 30 years of age, some red marrow remains only in the proximal metaphyses, and the axial skeletal (pelvis, spine, scapulae, clavicles, sternum and skull). In the event of an increased functional demand for haematopoesis such as smoking or malignancy, this sequence of events can reconvert with fatty marrow reconverting to red marrow in a reverse, symmetrical centrifugal manner (Poulton et al. 1993).

Red and yellow marrow areas are not composed purely of either non-fatty cells or fat cells, respectively. 'Red marrow' typically contains about 60 % haematopoetic cells and about 40 % fat cells (Fig. 2a, b) while 'fatty marrow' contains about 5 % haematopoetic cells and about 95 % adipocytes (Hwang and Panicek 2007; Steiner et al. 1993). In other words, 'fatty marrow' tends to be more 'pure' than haematopoetic marrow. Fat cells (adipocytes) as expected contain more lipid than haematopoetic cells while haematopoetic cells contain slightly more water and protein than adipocytes. The approximate chemical composition of fatty marrow is about 80 % lipid, 15 % water and 5 % protein while that of red marrow is about 50 % lipid, 35 % water and 15 % protein (Hwang and Panicek 2007; Steiner et al. 1993) (Fig. 3). This is relevant since quantification techniques such as MR spectroscopy (MRS) use the fat: water ratio to determine the % marrow fat fraction [also referred to as marrow fat content (%)].

Fig. 1 From birth, red marrow converts to fatty marrow from the periphery to the central skeleton. Superimposed on this centripedal pattern, red marrow converts to fatty marrow in the tubular bones proceeding from diaphysis to metaphysis until by the age of 20 years only the proximal metaphyseal area contains appreciable red marrow

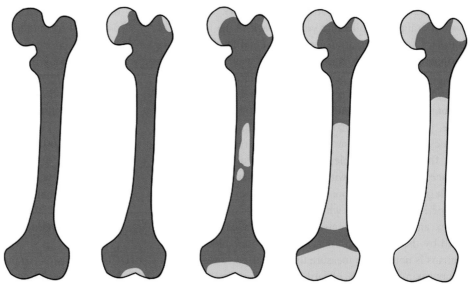

Fig. 2 **a** Histology of predominantly red marrow. There is still quite an abundance of fat cells present. **b** Histology of predominantly fatty marrow. There are only a few red cells present. In other words fatty marrow is more fatty than red marrow is red

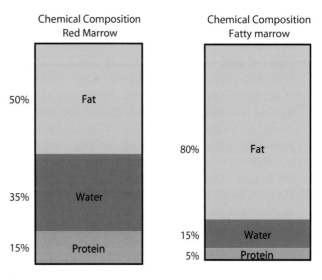

The pH of the marrow cavity is not known though the pH of extravascular tissues is generally lower than that of arterial blood (pH 7.4) and venous blood (pH 7.36) (Arnett 2010). The oxygen tension of normal bone marrow is about 52 mmHg (6.6 %) which is lower than that of arterial blood (95 mmHg, $\sim$12 %) and higher than that of veno-capillary blood (40 mmHg, $\sim$5 %) (Arnett 2010). In normal tissues other than the bone marrow, median interstitial oxygen tension levels measure $\sim$3–9 % (Arnett 2010).

The marrow cavity is supplied by large nutrient arteries that pass through the cortex into the medullary canal (Travlos 2006). Ascending and descending nutrient branches give rise to small thin-walled arterioles that extend towards the periphery where they give rise to capillaries piercing the bone cortex and also merge with thin venous sinuses lined by flat endothelial cells. These endothelial cells lack a tight junction though may overlap or interdigitate facilitating two-way passage of haematopoetic cells

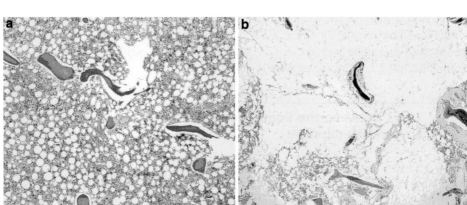

Fig. 3 Chemical composition of red marrow and fatty marrow. Haematopoetic marrow contains more water than fatty marrow

(Travlos 2006; Lichtman 1981; Brookes 1974). The venous system drains via collecting venules back to the nutrient or emissary veins. This arrangement of vessel from central to peripheral, leads to a higher number of vascular channels and slower flow at the periphery of the marrow cavity. The thin (50–150 μm) trabeculae do not possess a Haversian system or capillary system though do, similar to cortical bone, posses a fine canalicular network linking embedded osteocytes to the bone surface. The cortex receives its blood flow from capillaries piercing its endosteal and periosteal surfaces and running within the Haversian system. As a rough guide, the outer one-third of the cortex is supplied by the periosteal arteries while the inner two-thirds of the cortex and the constituents of the marrow cavity are supplied by the nutrient arteries. Absolute bone blood flow in humans is not easy to measure though has been estimated to be approximately 11 % of cardiac output or 7 ml/min/100 g in humans (Brookes 1974; Van Dyke et al. 1971). More recently, in a study of ten young patients, lower vertebral body blood flow measured by PET and a ^{15}O-labelled CO^2 steady-state technique was deemed to be approximately 15 ml/min/100 g bone marrow (Kahn et al. 1994).

3 Links Between the Bone Marrow to Bone Metabolism

There are many tens of ways in which bone marrow properties may affect bone metabolism. From the imaging perspective, these following seem to be the most relevant.

(1) There exists in the bone marrow, pluripotent mesenchymal stem cells that have the potential to differentiate along osteoblastic, adipocytic and haematological cell lines (Gimble and Nuttall 2004). Reduction in estrogen and oxidative stress may cause a drift in mesenchymal stem cell differentiation towards adipocytosis and away from osteoblastogenesis or haematopoesis (D'Ippolito et al. 2006; Fatokun et al. 2006; Shouhed et al. 2005; Kha et al. 2004; Duque 2008; Rosen and Klibanski 2009). Also adipocytes once formed are potentially self promotive whilst simultaneously actively suppressing osteoblastogenesis (Gimble and Nuttall 2004; Duque 2008; Lecka-Czernik et al. 2002).

(2) Bone receives much of its signalling from the bone marrow and the most metabolically active bone areas are those in immediate contact with the bone marrow. The most metabolically active component of bone is the endosteal surface of the cortex with trabeculae bone being the next most metabolically active area (Parfitt 2002). The active unit of bone metabolism, i.e. the basic multicellular unit also lies in close contact with the marrow. Bone metabolism is possibly influenced by changes in the marrow microenvironment. For example,

decreased Ph and deceased oxygenation will increase osteoclast formation and activity (Arnett 2010).

(3) Mechano conduction and mechano sensation are terms which embody the principle of bone metabolism being influenced by interstitial fluid flow along osteocytes. Reduced bone blood flow will lead to reduced interstitial fluid flow and reduced shear stresses between osteocytes (Letechipia et al. 2010; Cowin 2002; McCarthy 2005, 2011). These shear stresses stimulate local release of bone remodelling mediators such as NO and PGI2 with the functionally important bone remodelling units and may be related to the rapid loss on bone (and muscle) mass seen microgravity. Osteocytes also produce VEGF which may stimulate bone perfusion.

(4) Good perfusion is a pre-requisite for fracture healing and most bone perfusion comes from the marrow. In contrast, compromised perfusion may aggravate microfracture accumulation which is an integral part of insufficiency fracture development.

(5) Long chain polyunsaturated fatty acids, or a change in the $n − 6/n − 3$ ratio, can affect bone metabolism. For example, long chain $n − 6$ fatty acids such as arachidonic acid and its metabolite prostaglandin PGE2 are pro-inflammatory with PGE_2 being a potent stimulator of RANKL expression. This can reduce the OPG/RANKL ratio and may increase osteoclastogenesis (Coetzee et al. 2007). Alternatively, long chain $n − 3$ fatty acids such as eicosapentaenoic acid, docosahexaenoic acid and γ-linolenic have anti-inflammatory activity and may inhibit this PGE2-stimulated increase in RANKL expression (Poulsen et al. 2008). In other words, a change in the fatty acid milieu of bone may affect bone metabolism.

(6) Bone and vasculature metabolism are so closely connected that, at a molecular level, there exists well over a hundred potential mechanisms whereby arteries can interact with bone and vice versa (Demer and Tintut 2009; Hamerman 2005). Broadly speaking, an arterial disorder may be affecting bone; a bone disorder may be affecting arteries or both tissues may be influenced by common extraneous factor or factors. For example, endothelial dysfunction itself has a potent downstream effect on bone metabolism by decreasing local production of nitric oxide and prostaglandin E_2 (PGE_2) (both of which stimulate osteoblasts and inhibit osteoclasts), decreasing production of PGI_2 (which inhibits osteoclasts) and decreasing production of the bone matrix protein osteopontin (Bloomfield et al. 2002). In other words, endothelial dysfunction may, through local mediators, reduce osteoblastic and increase osteoclastic activity (Bloomfield et al. 2002; Wimalawansa 2010).

Fig. 4 ^{1}H MR spectroscopy examination. **a** Sagittal T2-weighted MR image showing positioning of volume of interest (VOI) for proton spectroscopy of L3 vertebral body. **b** Coronal oblique T1-weighted image of proximal femur showing VOI's used to measure fat content (%) in the femoral head, neck, and shaft

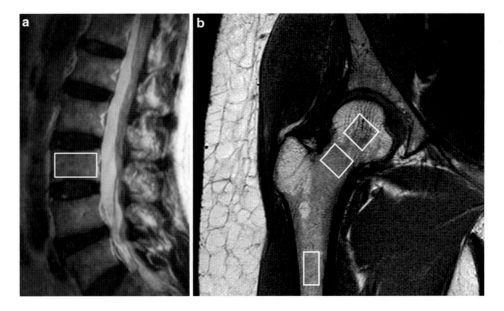

The remaining part of this chapter will address functional imaging techniques used to assess changes in the bone marrow, will look at what is known about lifelong changes in marrow fat, perfusion and diffusion and will look at how these processes are greatly affected in osteoporosis.

4   Bone Marrow Fat

4.1   Measurement of Marrow Fat

Proton MRS is the most widely used method to quantitatively assess marrow fat. MRS uses the fat: water ratio to determine the fat content (Figs. 4, 5). An obvious limitation is that a constant water content (%) is assumed. In other words, fat: water ratios may change due to a change in water content rather than fat content. MRS requires a minimal volume of approximately 1 cm^2 to acquire a sufficient signal to noise ratio. Other non-spectroscopic yet precise methods of quantifying fat fraction are available such as the two-point Dixon method which involves sequential suppression or fat and water, the three-point Iterative Decomposition of water and fat with Echo Asymmetry and Least-squares estimation (IDEAL) (Gerdes et al. 2007), or the analogous Gradient-Echo Sampling of the Free Induction Decay and Echo method (Wehrli et al. 2000). The accuracy of MRI spectroscopic and non-spectroscopic methods in detecting the relative amounts of water and fat has been tested against 11 different emulsions of increasing fat content. This study confirmed a high correlation ($r^2 > 0.92$) between MR methods of fat quantification and the % fat volume fraction within test bottles (Bernard

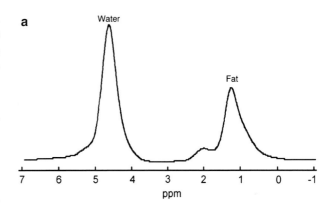

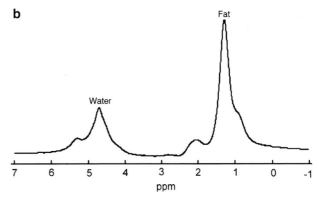

Fig. 5 Typical ^{1}H MR spectra in **a** normal subject with little marrow fat and **b** osteoporotic subject with a large amount of marrow fat

et al. 2008). Also, reproducibility of proton MRS in a clinical setting is high, ranging from 0.78 to 0.85, with the highest reproducibility being in those areas with the highest inherent fat content, i.e. the femoral head and lowest in the femoral neck (Griffith et al. 2009).

Table 1 Fat content of lumbar vertebral bone marrow (%) grouped according to age (years) and sex

Age	10–20	21–30	31–40*	41–50*	51–60*	61–70*	71–80*	81–90*
Males (%)	24.6	33.5	41.4	47.6	47.7	52.0	53.8	64.0
Females (%)	23.5	27.5	29.7	37.0	41.8	64.2	64.7	73.2

*Significant difference between groups $P < 0.05$ (Kugel et al. 2001; Griffith et al. 2012)

4.2 Physiological Changes in Bone Marrow Fat Content

An inverse relationship between increasing marrow fat and trabecular bone loss in senile osteoporosis has been recognised histologically for 40 years (Dunnill et al. 1967). However, it is only recently, though MRS and other MR-based techniques that marrow fat content can be quantified non-invasively on a large scale (De Bisschop et al. 1993; Schellinger et al. 2000; Kugel et al. 2001; Jung et al. 2000; Wehrli et al. 2000; Shih et al. 2004; Chen and Shih 2006; Liney et al. 2007) and at different anatomical sites (Duda et al. 1995) There is a gradual physiological increase in percentage marrow fat content with advancing years (Kugel et al. 2001; Griffith et al. 2012). An easy approximation to remember is that vertebral body marrow fat content is 25 % at 25 years and 65 % at 65 years of age (Kugel et al. 2001; Griffith et al. 2012).

There is also a distinct sex difference does exist in marrow fat content (Kugel et al. 2001; Griffith et al. 2012). Young males have about 10 % more fat in their marrow than females of equivalent age up to about 50 years of age (Kugel et al. 2001). Males show a gradual steady increase in marrow fat content of 7 % per decade throughout life from young to old (Kugel et al. 2001; Griffith et al. 2012) (Table 1, Fig. 6). Females, in contrast, show a less steep increase in marrow fat of about 2–7 % up to 55 years and then a dramatic increase between the ages of 55 and 65 years (Kugel et al. 2001; Griffith et al. 2012) (Table 1, Fig. 6). By 60 years of age, healthy females tend to possess about 10 % more marrow fat in their vertebrae than males (Griffith et al. 2012) (Table 1, Fig. 6).

The sharp rise in marrow fat content with the menopause may be due to a reduced haematopoietic requirement with cessation of menstruation. This may not, however,be the only cause given that menstrual blood loss is generally quite low (median of about 43 ml per menstrual cycle) (Gao et al. 1987). The sharp increase in marrow fat content in early post-menopausal females may be a more direct effect of estrogen deficiency influencing fat deposition (or stem-cell differentiation) both inside and outside the skeleton. In this respect, the increase in marrow fat content does tally with changes in female extra-skeletal fat distribution recognised to occur at this time.

Androgen and estrogen levels both decline in later years, though estrogen levels fall more sharply in menopausal

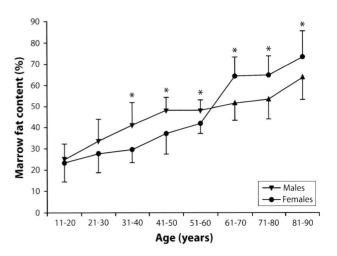

Fig. 6 Marrow fat content (%) of lumbar vertebral body stratified for age and sex (Kugel et al. 2001; Griffith et al. 2012)

females leading to a higher circulating androgen: estrogen ratio. This, and other factors, promotes greater intra-abdominal or visceral fat, i.e. an 'android' pattern of fat deposition in post-menopausal females (Toth et al. 2000; Blouin et al. 2008). This is different to the gynoid-pattern of fat distribution seen in pre-menopausal women when fat accumulates in the gluteal and thigh areas (Toth et al. 2000; Blouin et al. 2008). Whilst there is no specific literature available on the relationship between estrogen and marrow fat content, it is known that visceral fat content (i.e. an android pattern of fat distribution) does correlate positively with marrow fat content (Bredella et al. 2011). It is feasible, therefore, that the increased marrow fat content seen in females in the post-menopausal era may be the bone-equivalent of android fat deposition. Android fat deposition is also associated with increased risk of cardiovascular disease and metabolic syndrome (Bredella et al. 2011).

Similar findings are found using multivoxel chemical shift registration MR imaging to measure variation in the water fraction of the lumbar vertebral bone marrow with age and sex (Ishijima et al. 1996). The water fraction for males was 75 % for young males, decreased to about 50 % for middle-aged males and remained almost constant for later years (Table 2, Fig. 7) (Ishijima et al. 1996). Conversely, in females, the water fraction for young females remained fairly constant at around 70 % but decreases quite rapidly around the time of menopause such that it is lower than in males during later

Table 2 Water fraction of lumbar vertebral bone marrow (%) grouped according to age (years) and sex

Age	5–14	15–24	25–34*	35–44*	45–54*	55–64	65–74	75–84*
Males	75.2	69.0	53.7	51.1	52.9	48.8	48.1	48.2
Females	78.9	75.0	69.3	70.9	61.1	49.7	46.0	39.7

*Significant difference between groups $P < 0.05$ (Ishijima et al. 1996)

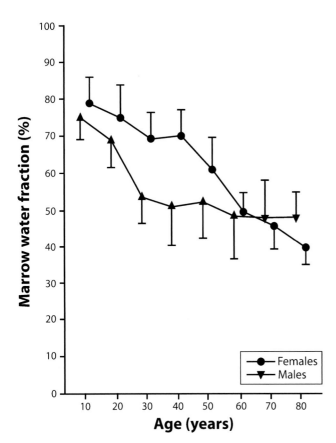

Fig. 7 Marrow water content (%) stratified for age and sex (Ishijima 1996)

years (Table 2, Fig. 7) (Ishijima et al. 1996). This tallies with the previously noted lifelong changes in % fat content since fatty marrow contains much less water (~ 5 %) than red marrow (~ 35 %) (Hwang and Panicek 2007).

Overall, there is at least a 40–50 % increase in fat cell content with increasing age. This increase in fat cell volume will occur at the expense of functioning marrow volume. Trabecular volume decreases by about one-third to one-half with increasing age, though the relative percentage of the marrow space occupied by trabecular bone is small. Since, the marrow cavity is a defined space and vascular sinusoids do not seem to expand with age, one can infer that an increase in marrow fat content is really a marker for a decrease in the amount of functioning marrow, i.e. a decrease in red marrow volume.

4.3 Changes in Marrow Fat Content in Osteoporosis

Over and above the physiological increase in marrow fat content with age, osteoporosis is associated with an even greater increase in marrow fat content. In the third lumbar vertebral body, for example, post-menopausal subjects with normal bone mineral density (BMD) have less marrow fat content than subjects with osteopenia. Similarly, subjects with osteopenia have less marrow fat content than this with osteoporosis (De Bisschop et al. 1993; Schellinger et al. 2000; Kugel et al. 2001; Jung et al. 2000; Wehrli et al. 2000; Shih et al. 2004; Chen and Shih 2006; Liney et al. 2007; Griffith et al. 2005, 2006; Shen et al. 2007; Tang et al. 2010; Liu et al. 2010) (Table 3). The proximal femur, which has a higher fat content than the vertebral body, also shows similar changes in increasing marrow fat content as the bone becomes more osteoporotic (Griffith et al. 2008) (Table 3). Even the femoral head, which has a very high intrinsic fat content, also shows an increase in marrow fat content with decreasing BMD though this increase is not as pronounced as in other areas.

4.4 Possible Erroneous Effect of Increasing Marrow Fat

It is possible that the aforementioned findings of increasing marrow fat content with decreasing BMD as measured by dual X-ray absorptiometry (DXA) may be spurious due to the effect of increasing marrow fat on BMD estimation by DXA. Increase in marrow fat content may cause an erroneous reduction in BMD measurements made by DXA (Sorenson 1990; Bolotin 1998; Bolotin et al. 2001; Bolotin 2007). This is because DXA evaluates BMD by measuring the transmission of X-rays at two different photon energies (Blake et al. 2009). The mathematical theory of DXA (basis set decomposition) holds that across a broad range of photon energies, the X-ray transmission factor through any physical object can be decomposed into the equivalent areal densities (g/cm^2) of any two designated materials (Blake et al. 2009). For DXA scans, the two materials chosen are bone mineral (hydroxyapatite) and lean tissue. As a result, DXA measurements will only accurately reflect true BMD

Table 3 Bone marrow fat content (%) in elderly male and female subjects (mean age 73 years) for the lumbar spine and proximal femur

Marrow fat content	Normal	Osteopenia	Osteoporosis	P value
L3 vertebral body (male)	50.1 ± 8.7	55.7 ± 10.2	58.2 ± 7.8	0.002
L3 vertebral body (female)	59.2 ± 10.0	63.3 ± 9.5	67.7 ± 8.5	0.002
Femoral head (female)	86.3 ± 5.7	89.1 ± 3.8	89.9 ± 3.3	0.001
Femoral neck (female)	80.8 ± 9.3	86.2 ± 6.5	88.4 ± 4.8	<0.001
Sub-trochanteric (female)	80.0 ± 6.0	84.5 ± 6.3	87.2 ± 4.4	0.001

One can appreciate the greater bone marrow fat content (%) of the proximal femur. P value refers to difference between any of the three groups

if the object being examined is composed entirely of hydroxyapatite and lean tissue. In practice, the human body is made up of not two but three main types of tissue, namely bone, lean tissue and fat. Neglecting the difference between lean and fat may lead to a spurious reduction in DXA–BMD measurement. When marrow fat content is known, DXA estimation of BMD needs to be corrected by 0.0014 g/cm^2 in women and 0.0016 g/cm^2 in men for every 1 % increase in marrow fat about zero (Blake et al. 2009). Applying this correction, the aforementioned results of increasing marrow fat with decreasing BMD still hold true.

4.5 Does Marrow Fat Composition Change with Reducing BMD?

Since changes in marrow fat composition can affect bone metabolism in vivo, and diets rich in polyunsaturated fats can affect BMD, it is conceivable that changes in marrow fat composition can affect bone metabolism (Yeung et al. 2005). To address, this question samples of marrow fat and subcutaneous fat from 126 subjects (98 females, 34 males, mean age 69.7 ± 10.5 years) undergoing orthopaedic surgery were analysed for fatty acid composition using gas chromatography and results correlated with BMD–DXA (Griffith et al. 2009; Yeung et al. 2008) (Fig. 8a, b). A total of 22 fatty acids were identified in marrow and subcutaneous fat. Significant differences existed between marrow and subcutaneous fat fatty acid composition as well as between marrow fat samples obtained from the relatively haematopoietic proximal femur and relatively fatty proximal tibia. Other than cis-7-hexadecenoic acid [C16:1 ($n = 9$)] and docosanoic acid [C22:0], no difference in marrow fatty acid composition was evident between subject groups of varying BMD (normal, low bone mass and osteoporosis). In particular, the overall polyunsaturated fatty acid content, the $n − 6/n − 3$ ratio and the percentage composition of those fatty acids most frequently implicated in bone remodelling, namely docosahexaenoic acid, arachidonic acid, γ-linolenic acid and eicosapentaenoic acid, were unchanged in subjects with normal BMD, low bone mass or osteoporosis (Griffith et al. 2009). Overall, it seems less likely that a change in marrow fat composition is directly affecting bone

metabolism. The two associations found between fatty acid composition and BMD may be inconsequential given that they account for <1 % (for C16:1($n − 9$)) and <0.1 % (for C22:0) of the total marrow fatty acid composition and they do not have any known effect on bone metabolism (Griffith et al. 2009).

5 Bone Marrow Perfusion

5.1 Measurement of Bone Marrow Perfusion

Dynamic contrast-enhanced magnetic resonance imaging (DCE-MRI), also known as MR perfusion imaging, measures bone marrow perfusion as opposed to bone marrow blood flow (Griffith and Genant 2011). DCE-MRI is a robust technique that yields empirical indices of perfusion such as maximal signal intensity enhancement (E^{max}) and enhancement slope (E^{slope}) (Figs. 9, 10). E^{slope} and E^{max} are derived from the first-pass phase of signal intensity enhancement and have been shown to be strongly predictive of tissue vascularity, microvessel density and tissue necrosis. In simple terms, E^{slope} can be thought of as gadolinium delivery to the bone marrow and is a feature of blood supply, vascular sinusoidal size and permeability. E^{max} is dependent on these factors though also on the perfusion requirements (i.e. metabolic activity) of the bone marrow. Reproducibility of bone marrow DCE-MRI is moderate to high ranging from 0.59 to 0.98 with best reproducibility in those areas with the highest inherent bone marrow perfusion (Griffith et al. 2009).

Perfusion data acquired from dynamic contrast-enhanced MR imaging is also amenable to two-compartment pharmacokinetic modelling using models such as the Tufts or Brix model (Fig. 11). The Tufts model uses a combination of arterial input function (AIF), and rate constants K^{trans}, K^{ex} and K^{el}. AIF is assessed by analyzing the first pass intensity profile of the feeding artery. K^{trans} refers to the transport constant and is influenced primarily by blood flow. K^{ex} refers to capillary exchange and is influenced by capillary space, permeability, interstitial pressure and extracellular space. K^{el} refers to elimination or wash-out and is influenced by venous return. The Brix model does not rely

Fig. 8 **a** Aspiration of marrow fat from proximal tibia during knee replacement. **b** Gas chromatography spectrum of marrow fat. Each fatty acid methyl ester is quantified based on peak high relative to internal standard

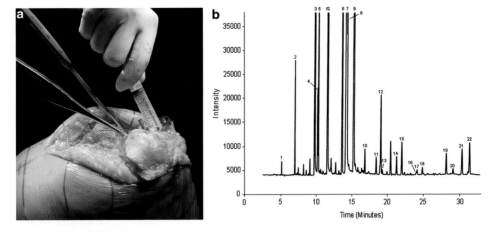

Fig. 9 Dynamic contrast-enhanced MR imaging **a** Sagittal T2-weighted MR image showing positioning of region of interest (ROI) for perfusion imaging of L3 vertebral body. **b** Coronal oblique T1-weighted image of proximal femur showing ROI's used to measure marrow perfusion in the femoral head, neck and shaft

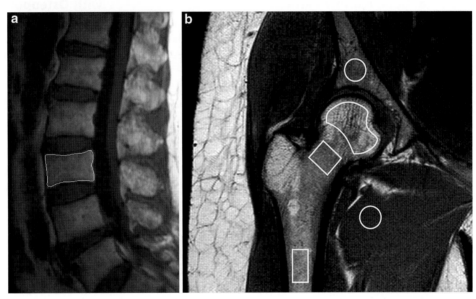

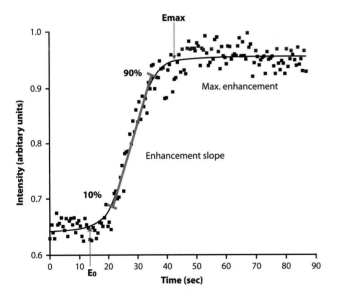

Fig. 10 Time-intensity curve with E^{max} and E^{slope}. E^{max} represents maximum enhancement while E^{slope} represents the slope of the rapidly up-rising part of the curve

on AIF or K^{trans} but still considers K^{ex} and K^{el}. It assumes a linear relationship between MR signal enhancement and tissue contrast concentration or, in other words, it assumes that tissue contrast concentration directly correlates with perfusion. No specific pharmacokinetic model to reflect the unique characteristics of marrow perfusion has been developed. Measurement of bone marrow perfusion can also be undertaken by PET-CT imaging undertaken using ^{18}F-fluoride which has a half-life of 112 min. Since this tracer is metabolised in bone, ^{18}F-fluoride imaging is a combined measure of both bone perfusion and bone metabolism as compared to MR perfusion imaging which only measures bone perfusion. Pure bone perfusion can be evaluated by PET using the freely diffusible tracer $^{15}OH_2O$. However, these studies are difficult to perform as $^{15}OH_2O$ has a half-life of only 122 s and thus requires an on-site cyclotron. Nevertheless, a highly significant correlation between blood perfusion measured using ^{18}F-fluoride and true bone perfusion using $^{15}OH_2O$ has been reported (Piert et al. 2002).

Fig. 11 Schematic diagram of **a** Tofts model and **b** Brix model

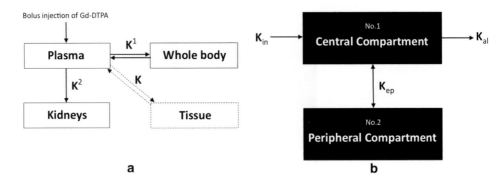

5.2 Physiological Age-Related Changes in Bone Marrow Perfusion

Bone marrow perfusion deceases with increasing age (Chen et al. 2001; Montazel et al. 2003; Baur et al. 1997). Subjects aged more than 50 years have a 62 % lower E^{max} (21.88 ± 14.77) that those aged less than 50 years (58.21 ± 44.65, $P < 0.005$) (Chen et al. 2001). When this is further analysed according to sex, a greater discrepancy is observed. In women, E^{slope} decreased by 80 % (from 87.17 ± 54.13 to 17.98 ± 13.80) in those older than age 50 years ($P < 0.005$). A similar trend is seen in men with E^{slope} decreases by 33 % from 38.16 ± 21.69 to 25.38 ± 15.43 in subjects more than 50 years though this change did not reach statistical significance ($P > 0.05$) (Chen et al. 2001). Overall, vertebral bone marrow perfusion is higher in young females than young males (Chen et al. 2001). However, the rate of decrease of perfusion is less in males, which leads to vertebral bone marrow perfusion being higher in elderly males than elderly females (Chen et al. 2001). Similar findings were shown by Montazel JL et al. E^{max} values being significantly higher in patients younger than 40 years than in those aged more than 40 years ($P < 0.001$). Perfusion parameters decreased with increasing age in a logarithmic relationship ($r = 0.71$) and correlated with increase in marrow fat content (Montazel et al. 2003). Savvopoulou et al. (2008) showed how the upper (L1, L2) lumbar vertebral bodies were better perfused than the lower (L3, L4, L5) vertebral bodies. In elderly subjects with normal BMD, E^{max} was lower in females (32.3 ± 8.5 %) than males (34.5 ± 13 %) while E^{slope} was higher in females (1.70 ± 5.2 %/s) than males (1.48 ± 0.7 %/s) (Griffith et al. 2005, 2006). To summarise, vertebral marrow perfusion is higher in young females than young males. However, perfusion decreases to a greater degree in females than males. Elderly females have reduced E^{max} but not E^{slope} compared to elderly males.

5.3 Changes in Bone Marrow Perfusion with Osteoporosis

Osteoporosis is associated with a decrease in bone perfusion over and above that accountable for by age alone. Normal BMD subjects have better bone marrow perfusion than osteopenic subjects, while osteopenic subjects have better bone marrow perfusion than osteoporotic subjects (Shih et al. 2004; Griffith et al. 2005, 2006, 2008) (Fig. 12) (Table 4). Similar changes occur in the proximal femur as in the vertebral body (Griffith et al. 2008; Wang et al. 2009). In the proximal femur, reduction in perfusion parameters is most pronounced in the biologically relevant femoral neck than the femoral head or sub-trochanteric regions (Wang et al. 2009).

5.4 Causes of Marrow Perfusion Changes with Ageing and Osteoporosis

The reduction in marrow perfusion seen with advancing age and osteoporosis is most likely a feature of the marrow per se rather than due to a more generalised vascular or circulatory disturbance since any perfusion changes only occur in the marrow and are not seen in extra-osseous skeletal muscle with the same blood supply (Griffith et al. 2005, 2006, 2008) (Fig. 13).

Overall, the most scenario is that a decrease in the more metabolically active functioning marrow content that is driving the marrow perfusion change seen in ageing and osteoporotic bone (Griffith et al. 2010). Using a combination of MRI and FDG-PET imaging data, the metabolic activity of red marrow as assessed by maximum SUV (standardised uptake value), was estimated to be seven times higher than that of fatty marrow (Basu et al. 2007). Observed changes in marrow fat and trabecular bone fraction with increasing age and osteoporosis essentially mirror a decrease in functioning marrow

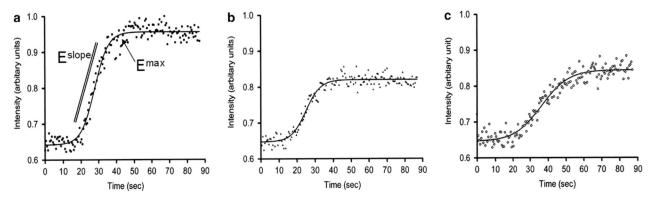

Fig. 12 Typical time-intensity curves for subjects with **a** normal BMD, **b** osteopenia and **c** osteoporosis

Table 4 Bone marrow perfusion parameters, maximum enhancement E^{max} and enhancement slope E^{slope} in elderly (mean age 73 years) male and female subjects with normal BMD, osteopenia and osteoporosis

	Normal	Osteopenia	Osteoporosis	P value
Enhancement maximum				
L3 vertebral body (male)	34.9 ± 13.0	28.4 ± 10.8	23.5 ± 9.9	<0.001
L3 vertebral body (female)	32.3 ± 8.5	26.9 ± 9.5	22.4 ± 8.2	<0.001
Acetabulum (female)	24.6 ± 9.7	16.8 ± 8.4	11.6 ± 5.7	<0.001
Femoral head (female)	4.7 ± 2.5	4.0 ± 1.8	3.2 ± 1.2	0.017
Femoral neck (female)	16.1 ± 9.8	10.5 ± 5.7	8.1 ± 5.2	0.010
Sub-trochanteric (female)	17.5 ± 13.7	14.2 ± 8.6	10.2 ± 7.8	0.010
Enhancement slope				
L3 vertebral body (male)	1.48 ± 0.7	1.15 ± 0.6	0.78 ± 0.3	0.0001
L3 vertebral body (female)	1.70 ± 0.5	1.45 ± 0.5	1.10 ± 0.5	<0.001
Acetabulum (female)	1.26 ± 0.5	0.91 ± 0.5	0.64 ± 0.4	<0.001
Femoral head (female)	0.20 ± 0.1	0.13 ± 0.1	0.11 ± 0.0	0.001
Femoral neck (female)	0.64 ± 0.4	0.42 ± 0.3	0.32 ± 0.3	<0.001
Sub-trochanteric (female)	0.59 ± 0.4	0.60 ± 0.5	0.42 ± 0.4	0.010

One can appreciate how bone marrow perfusion indices diminish as BMD decreases and how perfusion indices are generally lower in the proximal femur than the lumbar spine. *P* value refers to difference between any of the three groups

content. The percentage of the marrow cavity occupied by marrow fat increases from about 25 % in young females to about 70 % in elderly females while over the same period, the percentage occupied by trabecular bone decreases from about 20 to 15 % due to physiological age-related bone loss (Griffith et al. 2012; Müller et al. 1998) (Fig. 6). Within the size restraints of the marrow cavity, one can appreciate that, in line with these changes, the amount of functioning marrow should decrease from 55 to 20 % with ageing (Fig. 6). This reduction in functioning marrow content is manifested clinically as the 'anaemia of old age' and an impaired ability of older people to deal with biological stress. Similarly, because functioning marrow also comprises cells of the immune system, this decrease in functioning marrow may also contribute to the 'immunosenescence' of old age (Gameiro et al. 2010).

Atherosclerosis and endothelial function may also be related to the compromised bone perfusion seen with ageing and osteoporosis. Increasing age and osteoporosis are strongly associated with arthrosclerosis and, in particular, vascular calcification (Griffith et al. 2012; Nordström et al. 2010; Marcovitz et al. 2005; Collins et al. 2009). Low BMD independently predicts coronary artery disease in women undergoing coronary angiography better than traditional risk factors such as age, hypertension, diabetes, smoking, family history or dyslipidemia (Marcovitz et al. 2005). Histological studies have shown how progressive occlusion of intraosseous arteries, arterioles or arterial capillaries occurs with increasing age (Bridgeman and Brookes 1996) and in patients with proximal femoral osteoporosis (Laroche et al. 1995). Angiographic study has shown how arterioles within the centre of the vertebral body decrease in number, elongate and coil with advancing age (Ratcliffe 1986). A weak negative correlation ($r = -0.33$, $P = 0.0018$) was found between vertebral body E^{max} and carotid artery intima-media

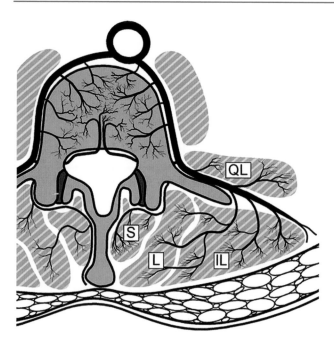

Fig. 13 Schematic representation of vertebral body arterial supply. Each lumbar artery divides to send a nutrient artery to the posterior aspect of the vertebral body and additional arteries to supply the paravertebral muscles. *L* lumbar artery, *QL* quadratus lumborum, *S* spinalis, *L* longissimus, *IL* iliocostalis

thickness age after adjusting for the effect of sex, age, blood pressure, BMI, total cholesterol, high density lipoprotein and triglycerol level in a linear regression model ($P = 0.008$) (Chen et al. 2004). Vertebral body E^{max} was significantly lower in those subjects with carotid intimal thickening group compared to those with normal intimal thickness (73 ± 23 vs. 90 ± 27, $P = 0.0023$) (Chen et al. 2004).

Endothelial dysfunction is one of the earliest manifestations of atherosclerosis and may be aggravated by sex hormone depletion. Endothelial dysfunction leads to impaired vascular reactivity and seems to effect all arteries, including very likely the nutrient arteries of bones. Impaired endothelial function has been observed in young diabetics and overweight children (Khan et al. 2003). After adjusting for age and years since the menopause, women with low bone mass or osteoporosis had significantly impaired endothelial function that those of normal BMD (Sumino et al. 2007; Sanada et al. 2004; Samuels et al. 2001). Endothelium-dependent vasodilatation is about 20–25 % lower in the femoral nutrient arteries of aged experimental male rats (Prisby et al. 2007). Since blood flow is directly dependent on the vessel radius to the fourth power (Pouiseuille's Law), a 25 % reduction of vessel diameter due to either arthrosclerosis and/or endothelial dysfunction could potentially reduce volumetric blood flow to the medullary canal by 33 % (Pfitzner 1976).

6 Bone Marrow Diffusion

The free movement of water molecules within the extracellular fluid of the bone marrow is affected by the cells that they encounter. The more closely packed the cells, the more restricted the water motion. Although cell packing is likely to be one of the main modulators, extracellular water motion is also dependent on other factors such as blood flow, capillary permeability, interstitial pressure, temperature and the viscosity of interstitial fluid. Diffusion-weighted MR imaging measures water diffusivity by applying 'diffusion sensitising gradients' to T2-weighted spin echo sequences using echoplanar readouts (Khoo et al. 2011). The strength and duration of diffusion sensitising gradients is indicated by their '*b*-value' with a range of '*b*-values'. The '*b*-values' applied to clinical diffusion-weighted imaging are such that extracellular and not the intracellular water diffusivity is being measured.

'Apparent diffusion coefficient' (ADC) provides a measure of water diffusivity. The ADC of water is 3×10^{-3} mm^2/s (Mills 1973). The ADC of fat is close to zero with values of $0.011–0.012 \times 10^{-3}$ for subcutaneous fat (Lehnert et al. 2004). ADC values of 0.2×10^{-3} and 0.1×10^{-3} have been reported for red and yellow marrow, respectively (Ward et al. 2000).

7 Age-Related Physiological Changes in Bone Marrow Diffusion

Age-related changes in bone marrow diffusion has only been addressed in a few diffusion-weighted studies (Hillengass et al. 2011; Yeung et al. 2004). Bone marrow ADC values in young (mean age 28 years) females were shown to be significantly higher ($0.49 \pm 0.08 \times 10^{-3}$ mm^2/s) than elderly (mean age 70 years) females ($43 \pm 0.08 \times 10^{-3}$ mm^2/s, $P = 0.029$) (Yeung et al. 2004). This is reflective of increased fat packing of bone marrow fat reducing water diffusivity (Nonomura et al. 2001). Against this, in another study of 36 healthy subjects (16 men, 14 women), mean age 56 years, no relationship was found between vertebral marrow ADC and age applying b values of 400 and 750 s/mm^2 (Hillengass et al. 2011).

7.1 Diffusion Changes in Osteoporosis

Only a few studies have applied quantitative DWI to the study of bone marrow in patients with and without osteoporosis (Table 4) (Griffith et al. 2006; Liu et al. 2010; Yeung et al. 2004; Hatipoglu et al. 2007). In general, there is a reducing trend in molecular diffusion (as judged by

Table 5 Mean and standard deviation of lumbar bone marrow ADC values from different studies

References	Age	Normal	Osteopenia	Osteoporosis	Pulse
Yeung et al. (2004)	70 (no data)	0.43 ± 0.08	0.41 ± 0.10		SS-EPI
Griffith et al. (2006)	72.1 (67–84)	0.46 ± 0.08	0.41 ± 0.12	0.43 ± 0.12	SS-EPI
Hatipoglu et al. (2007)	52 (20–86)	0.46 ± 0.02	0.41 ± 0.05	0.38 ± 0.25	SS-EPI
Liu et al. (2010)	67.3 (55–83)	0.47 ± 0.03	0.42 ± 0.02	0.39 ± 0.03	SS-EPI

Bone marrow ADC consistently decreases as BMD decreases

Table 6 Mean and standard deviation of ADC values from different studies assessing whether quantitative diffusion MRI can distinguish benign from malignant vertebral fracture

References	Normal	Benign	Malignant	Pulse	Fat-sup
Zhou et al. (2002)	–	0.32 ± 0.03	0.19 ± 0.03	FSE DWI	No
Chan et al. (2002)	0.23 ± 0.05	1.94 ± 0.35	0.19 ± 0.03	SSH-EPI	Yes
Herneth et al. (2002)	1.66 ± 0.37	1.61 ± 0.37	0.71 ± 0.27	MS-EPI	Yes
Maeda et al. (2003)	–	1.21 ± 0.17	0.92 ± 0.20	LS	No
Balliu et al. (2009)	–	1.9 ± 0.39	0.92 ± 0.13	MS-EPI	Yes
Tang et al. (2007)	–	2.23 ± 0.21	1.04 ± 0.03	SSH-EPI	Yes
Biffar et al. (2010)	0.58 ± 0.17	1.74 ± 0.25	1.35 ± 0.41	SS-TSE	Yes
	0.31 ± 0.15	1.17 ± 0.37	1.06 ± 0.19	MS-EPI	Yes

Considerable variability exists in actual values obtained though bone marrow ADC is consistently lower in malignant fractures

ADC) with diminishing BMD most likely to fat packing of marrow reducing molecular diffusion. One can appreciate that the values obtained from different centres are quite comparable (Table 5).

More studies have applied quantitative DWI to distinguish between fractured osteoporotic and metastatic vertebral bodies (Zhou et al. 2002; Chan et al. 2002; Herneth et al. 2002; Maeda et al. 2003; Balliu et al. 2009; Tang et al. 2007; Biffar et al. 2010) occasionally using adjacent normal appearing vertebra as an internal control (Chan et al. 2002; Herneth et al. 2002; Maeda et al. 2003; Balliu et al. 2009; Tang et al. 2007; Biffar et al. 2010). One can appreciate that the values obtained for normal vertebrae in these studies are different from though reported in non-fractured spines (Table 6).

In general, osteoporotic vertebral fractures tend to have higher ADC values than metastatic vertebral fractures (Table 6). No particular ADC threshold to make this distinction has been adopted (Thawait et al. 2011). There is quite an overlap between reported ADC measurements for benign and metastatic fractures (Table 6). This may relate to selection criteria (such as fracture duration, fracture location, fracture severity, presence of intervertebral clefts, metastatic cell type, sclerotic or non-sclerotic type) or technical factors such as pulse sequencing and b values employed. With respect to differentiation from infectious lesions, reported mean ADC values from infectious vertebral lesions ($0.963 \pm 0.491 \times 10^{-3}$ mm^2/s) were not statistically different from those obtained from malignant lesions ($0.917 \pm 0.13 \times 10^{-3}$ mm^2/s) (Balliu et al. 2009).

Tang et al. have reported that the best differentiation of vertebral fracture type can be achieved at b values of around 300 s/mm^2 (Tang et al. 2007) while Biffar et al. (2010) report that single shot TSE sequences proved more discriminatory than multi-shot echo planar imaging sequences.

Chemical shift imaging (or opposed phase imaging) has also been used to distinguish between benign and malignant vertebral fractures (Erly et al. 2006; Zampa et al. 2002). If a SIR threshold of 0.80 with >0.8 defined as malignant and <0.8 defined as a benign, in-phase/opposed-phase imaging had a sensitivity of 0.95 and specificity, of 0.89 in discriminating benign from malignant fractures (Erly et al. 2006). Another study has recommended an SIR threshold of 1.2, re-emphasising the variability in choosing the optimal threshold to distinguish benign from metastatic vertebral fracture.

7.2 Predictive Potential of Marrow Parameters

Currently, our ability to select subjects most prone to bone loss is limited, with clinical risk factors such as age, weight, weight loss over 2 years and baseline BMD being the best-recognised markers of future bone loss (Hannan et al. 2000; Lau et al. 2006; Dennison et al. 1999). To address the value of MR marrow parameters in predicting bone loss, a group of subjects with baseline MRS and perfusion imaging of the hip were followed up with hip densitometry at 2 and 4

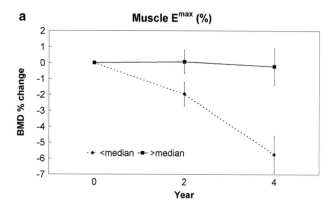

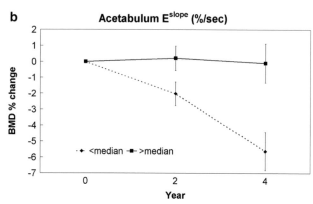

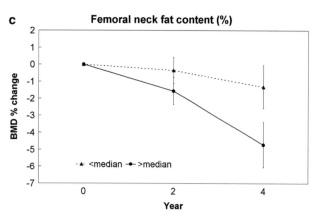

Fig. 14 Bone loss over 4 years. Best MR predictors of bone loss in the femoral neck over 4 years when adjusted for covariates, were **a** muscle E^{max}, **b** acetabulum E^{slope} and **c** femoral neck fat content

practice. Nevertheless, the results were sufficiently encouraging to suggest that further refinement of marrow parameters may improve their ability to predict bone loss (Griffith and Genant 2011).

7.3 Changes in the Extra-osseous Soft Tissues

Although beyond the scope of this chapter, osteoporosis and the menopause is also known to be associated with exaggerated disc degeneration (Wang and Griffith 2010), skeletal muscle loss (Crepaldi et al. 2007) and changes in fat distribution (Bredella et al. 2011; Bredella 2010).

8 Summary

MRI and PET-CT have allowed, the for first time, a quantitative non-invasive assessment of the bone marrow providing us with more information on how the bone marrow changes in health and disease. We can now begin to more fully appreciate physiological age-related changes in the bone marrow that differ between sexes. One can also appreciate that osteoporosis is a disease associated with an exaggeration of physiological age-related changes not just with respect to bone loss but also marrow fat accumulation with a decrease in functioning marrow content and reduced bone perfusion. To fully comprehend the osteoporotic process, we should move away from simply thinking about osteoporosis as a disease of reduced bone density to a more encompassing paradigm which considers bone changes in conjunction with marrow changes, and changes in the extraossoeus soft tissues, particularly muscle. The MR imaging techniques we use to evaluate the bone marrow are still very much a work in progress. Radiologists are in an ideal position to move this bone marrow research forward and help explore in a wider sense connection between systemic diseases, the bone marrow and bone metabolism.

years. Percentage reduction in femoral neck BMD at 4 years post-baseline was significantly greater in subjects with below median selected marrow or muscle perfusion parameters at baseline compared to those with above median perfusion parameters at baseline (Griffith and Genant 2011) (Fig. 14a–c). Similarly, subjects with more marrow fat at baseline had significantly greater BMD loss over the ensuing 2–4 years (Griffith and Genant 2011) (Fig. 14a–c). However, MR parameters where not sufficiently more predictive of bone loss than traditional risk factors to warrant using MRI to this effect in clinical

References

Arnett TR (2010) Acidosis, hypoxia and bone. Arch Biochem Biophys 1(503):103–119

Balliu E, Vilanova JC, Peláez I, Puig J, Remollo S, Barceló C, Barceló J, Pedraza S (2009) Diagnostic value of apparent diffusion coefficients to differentiate benign from malignant vertebral bone marrow lesions. Eur J Radiol 69:560–566

Basu S, Houseni M, Bural G, Chamroonat W, Udupa J, Mishra S, Alavi A (2007) Magnetic resonance imaging based bone marrow segmentation for quantitative calculation of pure red marrow metabolism using

2-deoxy-2-[F-18] fluoro-D-glucose-positron emission tomography: a novel application with significant implications for combined structure-function approach. Mol Imaging Biol 9:361–365

Baur A, Stabler A, Bartl R, Lamerz R, Scheidler J, Reiser M (1997) MRI gadolinium enhancement of bone marrow: age-related changes in normals and in diffuse neoplastic infiltration. Skeletal Radiol 26:414–418

Bernard C, Liney G, Manton D, Turnbull L, Langton C (2008) Comparison of fat quantification methods: a phantom study at 3.0 T. J Magn Reson Imaging 27:192–197

Biffar A, Baur-Melnyk A, Schmidt GP, Reiser MF, Dietrich O (2010) Multiparameter MRI assessment of normal-appearing and diseased vertebral bone marrow. Eur Radiol 20:2679–2689

Blake GM, Griffith JF, Yeung DK, Leung PC, Fogelman I (2009) Effect of increasing vertebral marrow fat content on BMD measurement, T-score status and fracture risk prediction by DXA. Bone 44:495–501

Bloomfield SA, Hogan HA, Delp MD (2002) Decreases in bone blood flow and bone material properties in aging Fischer-344 rats. Clin Orthop 396:248–257

Blouin K, Boivin A, Tchernof A (2008) Androgens and body fat distribution. J Steroid Biochem Mol Biol 108:272–280

Bolotin HH (1998) Analytic and quantitative exposition of patient-specific systematic inaccuracies inherent in planar DXA-derived in vivo BMD measurements. Med Phys 25:139–151

Bolotin HH (2007) DXA in vivo BMD methodology: an erroneous and misleading research and clinical gauge of bone mineral status, bone fragility and bone remodelling. Bone 41:138–154

Bolotin HH, Sievansen H, Grashuis JL, Kuiper JW, Jarvinen TL (2001) Inaccuracies inherent in patient-specific dual-energy x-ray absorptiometry bone mineral density measurements: comprehensive phantom-based evaluation. J Bone Miner Res 16:417–426

Bredella MA (2010) Perspective: the bone-fat connection. Skeletal Radiol 39:729–731

Bredella MA, Torriani M, Ghomi RH, Thomas BJ, Brick DJ, Gerweck AV, Rosen CJ, Klibanski A, Miller KK (2011) Vertebral bone marrow fat is positively associated with visceral fat and inversely associated with IGF-1 in obese women. Obesity (Silver Spring) 19:49–53

Bridgeman G, Brookes M (1996) Blood supply to the human femoral diaphysis in youth and senescence. J Anat 188:611–621

Brookes M (1974) Approaches to non-invasive blood flow measurement in bone. Biomed Eng 9:342–347

Chan JH, Peh WC, Tsui EY, Chau LF, Cheung KK, Chan KB, Yuen MK, Wong ET, Wong KP (2002) Acute vertebral body compression fractures: discrimination between benign and malignant causes using apparent diffusion coefficients. Br J Radiol 75:207–214

Chen WT, Shih TT (2006) Correlation between the bone marrow blood perfusion and lipid water content on the lumbar spine in female subjects. J Magn Reson Imaging 24:176–181

Chen WT, Shih TT, Chen RC, Lo SY, Chou CT, Lee JM, Tu HY (2001) Vertebral bone marrow perfusion evaluated with dynamic contrast-enhanced MR imaging: significance of aging and sex. Radiology 220:213–238

Chen WT, Ting-Fang Shih T, Hu CJ, Chen RC, Tu HY (2004) Relationship between vertebral bone marrow blood perfusion and common carotid intima-media thickness in aging adults. J Magn Reson Imaging 20:811–816

Coetzee M, Haag M, Kruger MC (2007) Effects of arachidonic acid, docosahexaenoic acid, prostaglandin E(2) and parathyroid hormone on osteoprotegerin and RANKL secretion by MC3T3-E1 osteoblast-like cells. J Nutr Biochem 18:54–63

Collins TC, Ewing SK, Diem SJ, Taylor BC, Orwoll ES, Cummings SR, Strotmeyer ES, Osteoporotic Fractures in Men (MrOS) Study Group (2009) Peripheral arterial disease is associated with higher rates of hip bone loss and increased fracture risk in older men. Circulation 119:2305–2312

Cowin SC (2002) Mechanosensation and fluid transport in living bone. J Musculoskelet Neuronal Interact 2:256–260

Crepaldi G, Romanato G, Tonin P, Maggi S (2007) Osteoporosis and body composition. J Endocrinol Invest 30:42–47

D'Ippolito G, Diabira S, Howard GA, Roos BA, Schiller PC (2006) Low oxygen tension inhibits osteogenic differentiation and enhances stemness of human MIAMI cells. Bone 39:513–522

De Bisschop E, Luypaert R, Louis O, Osteaux M (1993) Fat fraction of lumbar bone marrow using in vivo proton nuclear magnetic resonance spectroscopy. Bone 14:133–136

Demer LL, Tintut Y (2009) Mechanisms linking osteoporosis with cardiovascular calcification. Curr Osteoporos Rep 7:42–46

Dennison E, Eastell R, Fall CH, Kellingray S, Wood PJ, Cooper C (1999) Determinants of bone loss in elderly men and women: a prospective population-based study. Osteoporos Int 10:384–391

Duda SH, Laniado M, Schick F, Strayle M, Claussen CD (1995) Normal bone marrow in the sacrum of young adults: differences between the sexes seen on chemical-shift MR imaging. AJR Am J Roentgenol 164:935–940

Dunnill MS, Anderson JA, Whitehead R (1967) Quantitative histological studies on age changes in bone. J Pathol Bacteriol 94:275–291

Duque G (2008) Bone and fat connection in aging bone. Curr Opin Rheumatol 20:429–434

Erly WK, Oh ES, Outwater EK (2006) The utility of in-phase/opposed-phase imaging in differentiating malignancy from acute benign compression fractures of the spine. AJNR Am J Neuroradiol 27:1183–1188

Fatokun AA, Stone TW, Smith RA (2006) Hydrogen peroxide-induced oxidative stress in MC3T3-E1 cells: the effects of glutamate and protection by purines. Bone 39:542–551

Gameiro CM, Romão F, Castelo-Branco C (2010) Menopause and aging: changes in the immune system—a review. Maturitas 67:316–320

Gao J, Zeng S, Sun BL, Fan HM, Han LH (1987) Menstrual blood loss and hematologic indices in healthy Chinese women. J Reprod Med 32:822–826

Gerdes CM, Kijowski R, Reeder SB (2007) IDEAL imaging of the musculoskeletal system: robust water fat separation for uniform fat suppression, marrow evaluation, and cartilage imaging. AJR Am J Roentgenol 189:W284–W291

Gimble JM, Nuttall ME (2004) Bone and fat: old questions, new insights. Endocrine 23:183–188

Griffith JF, Genant HK (2011) New imaging modalities in bone. Curr Rheumatol Rep 13:241–250

Griffith JF, Yeung DK, Antonio GE, Lee FK, Hong AW, Wong SY, Lau EM, Leung PC (2005) Vertebral bone mineral density, marrow perfusion, and fat content in healthy men and men with osteoporosis: dynamic contrast-enhanced MR imaging and MR spectroscopy. Radiology 236:945–951

Griffith JF, Yeung DK, Antonio GE, Wong SY, Kwok TC, Woo J, Leung PC (2006) Vertebral marrow fat content and diffusion and perfusion indexes in women with varying bone density: MR evaluation. Radiology 241:831–838

Griffith JF, Yeung DK, Tsang PH, Choi KC, Kwok TC, Ahuja AT, Leung KS, Leung PC (2008) Compromised bone marrow perfusion in osteoporosis. J Bone Miner Res 23:1068–1075

Griffith JF, Yeung DK, Chow SK, Leung JC, Leung PC (2009) Reproducibility of MR perfusion and (1)H spectroscopy of bone marrow. J Magn Reson Imaging 29:1438–1442

Griffith JF, Engelke K, Genant HK (2010) Looking beyond bone mineral density: Imaging assessment of bone quality. Ann N Y Acad Sci 1192:45–56

Griffith JF, Yeung DKW, Ma HT, Leung JSC, Kwok TCY, Leung PC (2012) Bone marrow fat content in the elderly: a reversal of trend seen in younger subjects J Magn Reson Imaging (In press)

Hamerman D (2005) Osteoporosis and atherosclerosis: biological linkages and the emergence of dual-purpose therapies. QJM 98:467–484

Hannan MT, Felson DT, Dawson-Hughes B, Tucker KL, Cupples LA, Wilson PW, Kiel DP (2000) Risk factors for longitudinal bone loss in elderly men and women: the Framingham Osteoporosis Study. J Bone Miner Res 15:710–720

Hartsock RJ, Smith EB, Petty CS (1965) Normal variations with aging of the amount of hematopoetic tissue in bone marrow from the anterior iliac crest. A study made from 177 cases of sudden death examined by necropsy. Am J Clin Pathol 43:326–331

Hatipoglu HG, Selvi A, Ciliz D, Yuksel E (2007) Quantitative and diffusion MR imaging as a new method to assess osteoporosis. Am J Neuroradiol 28:1934–1937

Herneth AM, Philipp MO, Naude J, Funovics M, Beichel RR, Bammer R, Imhof H (2002) Vertebral metastases: assessment with apparent diffusion coefficient. Radiology 225:889–894

Hillengass J, Stieltjes B, Bäuerle T, McClanahan F, Heiss C, Hielscher T, Wagner-Gund B, Habetler V, Goldschmidt H, Schlemmer HP, Delorme S, Zechmann CM (2011) Dynamic contrast-enhanced magnetic resonance imaging (DCE-MRI) and diffusion-weighted imaging of bone marrow in healthy individuals. Acta Radiol 1(52):324–330

Hwang S, Panicek DM (2007) Magnetic resonance imaging of bone marrow in oncology, Part 1. Skeletal Radiol 36:913–920

Ishijima H, Ishizaka H, Horikoshi H, Sakurai M (1996) Water fraction of lumbar vertebral bone marrow estimated from chemical shift misregistration on MR imaging: normal variations with age and sex. AJR Am J Roentgenol 167:355–358

Jung CM, Kugel H, Schulte O, Heindel W (2000) Proton-MR spectroscopy of the spinal bone marrow. An analysis of physiological signal behavior. Radiologe 40:694–699

Kahn D, Weiner GJ, Ben-Haim S, Ponto LL, Madsen MT, Bushnell DL, Watkins GL, Argenyi EA, Hichwa RD (1994) Positron emission tomographic measurement of bone marrow blood flow to the pelvis and lumbar vertebrae in young normal adults. Blood 15(83):958–963

Kha HT, Basseri B, Shouhed D, Richardson J, Tetradis S, Hahn TJ, Parhami F (2004) Oxysterols regulate differentiation of mesenchymal stem cells: pro-bone and anti-fat. J Bone Miner Res 19:830–840

Khan F, Green FC, Forsyth JS, Greene SA, Morris AD, Belch JJ (2003) Impaired microvascular function in normal children: effects of adiposity and poor glucose handling. J Physiol 551:705–711

Khoo MM, Tyler PA, Saifuddin A, Padhani AR (2011) Diffusion-weighted imaging (DWI) in musculoskeletal MRI: a critical review. Skeletal Radiol 40:665–681

Kugel H, Jung C, Schulte O, Heindel W (2001) Age- and sex-specific differences in the 1H-spectrum of vertebral bone marrow. J Magn Reson Imaging 13:263–268

Laroche M, Ludot I, Thiechart M, Arlet J, Pieraggi M, Chiron P, Moulinier L, Cantagrel A, Puget J, Utheza G et al (1995) Study of the intraosseous vessels of the femoral head in patients with fractures of the femoral neck or osteoarthritis of the hip. Osteoporos Int 5:213–217

Lau EM, Leung PC, Kwok T, Woo J, Lynn H, Orwoll E, Cummings S, Cauley J (2006) The determinants of bone mineral density in Chinese men—results from Mr. Os (Hong Kong), the first cohort study on osteoporosis in Asian men. Osteoporos Int 17:297–303

Lecka-Czernik B, Moerman EJ, Grant DF, Lehmann JM, Manolagas SC, Jilka RL (2002) Divergent effects of selective peroxisome proliferator-activated receptor-gamma 2 ligands on adipocyte versus osteoblast differentiation. Endocrinology 143:2376–2384

Lehnert A, Machann J, Helms G, Claussen CD, Schick F (2004) Diffusion characteristics of large molecules assessed by proton MRS on a whole-body MR system. Magn Reson Imaging 22:39–46

Letechipia JE, Alessi A, Rodriguez G, Asbun J (2010) Would increased interstitial fluid flow through in situ mechanical stimulation enhance bone remodeling? Med Hypotheses 75:196–198

Lichtman MA (1981) The ultrastructure of the hemopoietic environment of the marrow: a review. Exp Hematol 9:391–410

Liney GP, Bernard CP, Manton DJ, Turnbull LW, Langton CM (2007) Age, gender, and skeletal variation in bone marrow composition: a preliminary study at 3.0 Tesla. J Magn Reson Imaging 26:787–793

Link TM (2012) Osteoporosis imaging: state of the art and advanced imaging. Radiology 263:3–17

Liu Y, Tang GY, Tang RB, Peng YF, Li W (2010) Assessment of bone marrow changes in postmenopausal women with varying bone densities: magnetic resonance spectroscopy and diffusion magnetic resonance imaging. Chin Med J (Engl) 123:1524–1527

Maeda M, Sakuma H, Maier SE, Takeda K (2003) Quantitative assessment of diffusion abnormalities in benign and malignant vertebral compression fractures by line scan diffusion-weighted imaging. AJR Am J Roentgenol 181:1203–1209

Manolagas SC, Almeida M (2007) Gone with the Wnts: beta-catenin, T-cell factor, forkhead box O, and oxidative stress in age-dependent diseases of bone, lipid, and glucose metabolism. Mol Endocrinol 21:2605–2614

Marcovitz PA, Tran HH, Franklin BA, O'Neill WW, Yerkey M, Boura J, Kleerekoper M, Dickinson CZ (2005) Usefulness of bone mineral density to predict significant coronary artery disease. Am J Cardiol 96:1059–1063

McCarthy ID (2005) Fluid shifts due to microgravity and their effects on bone: a review of current knowledge. Ann Biomed Eng 33:95–103

McCarthy EF (2011) Perspective: skeletal complications of space flight. Skeletal Radiol 40:661–663

Mills R (1973) Self-diffusion in normal and heavy water in the range 1–45 deg. J Phy Chem 77:685–688

Montazel JL, Divine M, Lepage E, Kobeiter H, Breil S, Rahmouni A (2003) Normal spinal bone marrow in adults: dynamic gadolinium-enhanced MR imaging. Radiology 229:703–709

Müller R, Van Campenhout H, Van Damme B, Van Der Perre G, Dequeker J, Hildebrand T, Rüegsegger P (1998) Morphometric analysis of human bone biopsies: a quantitative structural comparison of histological sections and micro-computed tomography. Bone 23:59–66

Nonomura Y, Yasumoto M, Yoshimura R, Haraguchi K, Ito S, Akashi T, Ohashi I (2001) Relationship between bone marrow cellularity and apparent diffusion coefficient. J Magn Reson Imaging 13:757–760

Nordström A, Eriksson M, Stegmayr B, Gustafson Y, Nordström P (2010) Low bone mineral density is an independent risk factor for stroke and death. Cerebrovasc Dis. 29:130–136

Parfitt AM (2002) Misconceptions (2): turnover is always higher in cancellous than in cortical bone. Bone 30:807–809

Pfitzner J (1976) Poiseuille and his law. Anaesthesia 31:273–275

Piert M, Machulla HJ, Jahn M, Stahlschmidt A, Becker GA, Zittel TT (2002) Coupling of porcine bone blood flow and metabolism in high-turnover bone disease measured by [(15)O]H(2)O and [(18)F]fluoride ion positron emission tomography. Eur J Nucl Med Mol Imaging 29:907–914

Poulsen RC, Wolber FM, Moughan PJ, Kruger MC (2008) Long chain polyunsaturated fatty acids alter membrane-bound RANK-L expression and osteoprotegerin secretion by MC3T3-E1 osteoblast-like cells. Prostaglandins Other Lipid Mediat 85:42–48

Poulton TB, Murphy WD, Duerk JL, Chapek CC, Feiglin DH (1993) Bone marrow reconversion in adults who are smokers: MR Imaging findings. Am J Roentgenol 161:1217–1221

Prisby RD, Ramsey MW, Behnke BJ, Dominguez JM 2nd, Donato AJ, Allen MR, Delp MD (2007) Aging reduces skeletal blood flow, endothelium-dependent vasodilation, and NO bioavailability in rats. J Bone Miner Res 22:1280–1288

Ratcliffe JF (1986) Arterial changes in the human vertebral body associated with aging. The ratios of peripheral to central arteries and arterial coiling. Spine 11:235–240

Rosen CJ, Klibanski A (2009) Bone, fat, and body composition: evolving concepts in the pathogenesis of osteoporosis. Am J Med 122:409–414

Samuels A, Perry MJ, Gibson RL, Colley S, Tobias JH (2001) Role of endothelial nitric oxide synthase in estrogen-induced osteogenesis. Bone 29:24–29

Sanada M, Taguchi A, Higashi Y, Tsuda M, Kodama I, Yoshizumi M, Ohama K (2004) Forearm endothelial function and bone mineral loss in postmenopausal women. Atherosclerosis 176:387–392

Savvopoulou V, Maris TG, Vlahos L, Moulopoulos LA (2008) Differences in perfusion parameters between upper and lower lumbar vertebral segments with dynamic contrast-enhanced MRI (DCE MRI). Eur Radiol 18:1876–1883

Schellinger D, Lin SC, Fertikh D et al (2000) Normal lumbar vertebrae: anatomic, age, and sex variance in subjects at proton MR spectroscopy-initial experience. Radiology 215:910–916

Shen W, Chen J, Punyanitya M, Shapses S, Heshka S, Heymsfield SB (2007) MRI-measured bone marrow adipose tissue is inversely related to DXA-measured bone mineral in Caucasian women. Osteoporos Int 18:641–647

Shih TT, Chang CJ, Hsu CY, Wei SY, Su KC, Chung HW (2004) Correlation of bone marrow lipid water content with bone mineral density on the lumbar spine. Spine (Phila Pa 1976) 15(29):2844–2850

Shouhed D, Kha HT, Richardson JA, Amantea CM, Hahn TJ, Parhami F (2005) Osteogenic oxysterols inhibit the adverse effects of oxidative stress on osteogenic differentiation of marrow stromal cells. J Cell Biochem 95:1276–1283

Sorenson JA (1990) Effects of nonmineral tissues on measurement of bone mineral content by dual-photon absorptiometry. Med Phys 17:905–912

Steiner RM, Mitchell DG, Rao VM, Schweitzer ME (1993) Magnetic resonance imaging of diffuse bone marrow disease. Radiol Clin North Am 31:383–409

Sumino H, Ichikawa S, Kasama S, Takahashi T, Sakamoto H, Kumakura H, Takayama Y, Kanda T, Murakami M, Kurabayashi M (2007) Relationship between brachial arterial endothelial function and lumbar spine bone mineral density in postmenopausal women. Circ J 71:1555–1559

Tang G, Liu Y, Li W, Yao J, Li B, Li P (2007) Optimization of b value in diffusion-weighted MRI for the differential diagnosis of benign and malignant vertebral fractures. Skeletal Radiol 36:1035–1041

Tang GY, Lv ZW, Tang RB, Liu Y, Peng YF, Li W, Cheng YS (2010) Evaluation of MR spectroscopy and diffusion-weighted MRI in detecting bone marrow changes in postmenopausal women with osteoporosis. Clin Radiol 65:377–381

Thawait SK, Marcus MA, Morrison WB, Klufas RA, Eng J, Carrino J (2011) Research synthesis: what is the diagnostic performance of MRI to discriminate benign from malignant vertebral compression fractures? Systematic review and meta-analysis. Spine (Phila Pa 1976) [Epub ahead of print]

Toth MJ, Tchernof A, Sites CK, Poehlman ET (2000) Menopause-related changes in body fat distribution. Ann N Y Acad Sci 904:502–506

Travlos GS (2006) Normal structure, function, and histology of the bone marrow. Toxicol Pathol 34:548–565

Van Dyke D, Parker H, Anger HO, McRae J, Dobson EL, Yano Y, Naets JP, Linfoot J (1971) Markedly increased bone blood flow in myelofibrosis. J Nucl Med 12:506–512

Wang YX, Griffith JF (2010) Effect of menopause on lumbar disk degeneration: potential etiology. Radiology 257:318–320

Wang YX, Griffith JF, Kwok AW, Leung JC, Yeung DK, Ahuja AT, Leung PC (2009) Reduced bone perfusion in proximal femur of subjects with decreased bone mineral density preferentially affects the femoral neck. Bone 45:711–715

Ward R, Caruthers S, Yablon C, Blake M, DiMasi M, Eustace S (2000) Analysis of diffusion changes in posttraumatic bone marrow using navigator-corrected diffusion gradients. Am J Roentgenol 174:731–734

Wehrli FW, Hopkins JA, Hwang SN, Song HK, Snyder PJ, Haddad JG (2000) Cross-sectional study of osteopenia with quantitative MR imaging and bone densitometry. Radiology 217:527–538

Wimalawansa SJ (2010) Nitric oxide and bone. Ann N Y Acad Sci 1192:391–403

Yeung DK, Wong SY, Griffith JF, Lau EM (2004) Bone marrow diffusion in osteoporosis: evaluation with quantitative MR diffusion imaging. J Magn Reson Imaging 19:222

Yeung DK, Griffith JF, Antonio GE, Lee FK, Woo J, Leung PC (2005) Osteoporosis is associated with increased marrow fat content and decreased marrow fat unsaturation: a proton MR spectroscopy study. J Magn Reson Imaging 22:279–285

Yeung DK, Lam SL, Griffith JF, Chan AB, Chen Z, Tsang PH, Leung PC (2008) Analysis of bone marrow fatty acid composition using high-resolution proton NMR spectroscopy. Chem Phys Lipids 151:103–109

Zampa V, Cosottini M, Michelassi C, Ortori S, Bruschini L, Bartolozzi C (2002) Value of opposed-phase gradient-echo technique in distinguishing between benign and malignant vertebral lesions. Eur Radiol 12:1811–1818

Zhou XJ, Leeds NE, McKinnon GC, Kumar AJ (2002) Characterization of benign and metastatic vertebral compression fractures with quantitative diffusion MR imaging. Am J Neuroradiol 23:165–170

The Use of FRAX® in DXA Interpretation

S. M. Ploof, S. Wuertzer, and Leon Lenchik

Contents

Abstract

The World Health Organization (WHO) recently developed a fracture risk algorithm (FRAX®) that has fundamentally changed how clinical Dual X-ray Absorptiometry (DXA) scans are interpreted. The impact of FRAX on the community of clinicians who diagnose and treat patients with osteoporosis almost rivals the introduction of the T-score two decades ago. We review the clinical utility of FRAX in this chapter and show how our practice of DXA interpretation and reporting has changed with its introduction.

1   Introduction

Many effective pharmacologic treatments are available to significantly decrease the risk of fracture in men and women with decreased bone mineral density (BMD) and/or elevated fracture risk. Determining which patients to treat for low BMD is a common clinical dilemma. In particular, there is concern that many patients who have low-trauma fractures do not have osteoporosis based on DXA-measured BMD (Pasco et al. 2006; Sanders et al. 2006; Wainwright et al. 2005). Recently, a validated, computer-based tool has become widely available that can help to determine an individual's risk of fracture. Based on 10 clinical risk factors and BMD of the femoral neck measured by DXA, FRAX is designed to identify individuals at high risk for osteoporotic fracture. In many countries, clinical practice guidelines incorporate FRAX to help identify men and women who may benefit from pharmacologic therapy.

2   Overview of FRAX

FRAX is a widely used clinical tool that has caused a paradigm shift in the interpretation of DXA examinations. For the first time, a quantitative measure of fracture risk can be

S. M. Ploof · S. Wuertzer · L. Lenchik (✉)
Department of Radiology, Wake Forest University
School of Medicine, Winston-Salem, NC, USA
e-mail: llenchik@wakehealth.edu

G. Guglielmi (ed.), *Osteoporosis and Bone Densitometry Measurements*, Medical Radiology. Diagnostic Imaging,
DOI: 10.1007/174_2012_652, © Springer-Verlag Berlin Heidelberg 2013

obtained, thereby helping target pharmacologic therapy more effectively, to those patients who have the highest risk of fracture. FRAX is a free, internet-based computer algorithm that can be accessed on its website (http://www.shef.ac.uk/FRAX). Recently, FRAX has been incorporated into the DXA scanner software so that FRAX results are displayed on the same DXA printout as the BMD results (Fig. 1). Smartphone applications are also available. Since its release in 2008, fracture risk has been calculated in over six million individuals (FRAX website accessed 3/2012).

A screenshot of the FRAX website is shown in Fig. 2. First, the user selects the country where the patient lives. This data is important because fracture rates and life expectancy vary significantly in different countries (Kanis et al. 2002). The current version of FRAX is available for 39 countries including China, Japan, Philippines, South Korea, Singapore, Taiwan, Austria, Belgium, Czech Republic, Denmark, Finland, France, Germany, Hungary, Italy, Malta, Netherlands, Norway, Poland, Romania, Russia, Slovakia, Sri Lanka, Spain, Sweden, Switzerland, Turkey, United Kingdom, Jordan, Lebanon, Tunisia, Canada, United Sates, Argentina, Columbia, Ecuador, Mexico, Australia, and New Zealand. If a particular country is not included in FRAX, a similar country should be selected for the analysis. In the United States, the user then selects one of the four subgroups: Caucasian, Black, Hispanic, or Asian.

The user then answers the following questions about the patient: age, gender, weight, height, previous fracture, parental hip fracture, current smoking, use of glucocorticoids, rheumatoid arthritis (RA), secondary osteoporosis, and alcohol intake of 3 units or more daily.

Finally, the user enters the femoral neck BMD in g/cm^2 and selects the manufacturer of the DXA device used to measure the BMD. In settings where BMD measurement is not available, FRAX may be used to calculate fracture risk without BMD input.

Based on the provided data, FRAX calculates a 10-year probability of experiencing a hip fracture and a 10-year probability of experiencing what it terms, "major osteoporotic fracture." Major osteoporotic fracture includes fractures involving the proximal femur, spine, proximal humerus, or distal radius.

3   Risk Factors Included in FRAX

Although BMD is an important factor in the assessment of osteoporotic fracture risk; it is not the only factor. In fact, nearly half of low-trauma fractures occur in non-osteoporotic individuals (Wainwright et al. 2005). Many clinical factors have been recognized as increasing the risk for fracture, independent of BMD. FRAX incorporates many of these risk

factors in its algorithm, and it accounts for interactions between various risk factors (Kanis et al. 2007). FRAX, however, does not utilize every risk factor. For example, uncommon risk factors are excluded. Additionally, some common risk factors such as high bone turnover do not have sufficient data to be included in fracture prediction models. Some risk factors such as frailty and high frequency of falls are not easily measured. Some risk factors do not contribute to fracture risk independent of BMD. FRAX uses only those risk factors that are common, easily measurable, and have been proven in large epidemiological trials to predict fracture risk, independent of BMD.

3.1   Age

FRAX includes a question about the patient's date of birth. It is well established that age and BMD are not only the two most powerful predictors of fracture risk, but are also partially independent predictors of that risk (Siris et al. 2006).

3.2   Gender

FRAX includes a question about the patient's gender. It is well established that gender is an important determinate of fracture risk (Baron et al. 1996). The lifetime risk of a 50-year-old woman developing an osteoporotic fracture is approximately 50 %. The risk for the same age man is 20–30 %. It is important to recognize that despite the higher risk of fractures in women, nearly one-third of hip fractures occur in men (Eastell et al. 1998).

3.3   Height and Weight

The FRAX questionnaire includes the patient's height and weight. Individuals with low body mass index (BMI) are at an increased risk of fracture (De Laet et al. 2005; Felson et al. 1993). Importantly, decreasing BMI over time may contribute more to fracture risk than low BMI at a given time point (Cummings et al. 1995). In the Study of Osteoporotic Fractures, women who lost 10 % of their body weight since age 25 had a hip fracture rate of 15 per 1,000 patient-years, while those who gained more than 50 % of their body weight had a rate of 1.1 per 1,000 patient-years (Cummings et al. 1995).

3.4   Previous Fracture

FRAX includes a yes or no question about the patient's history of prior fracture. A previous fracture is defined as a spontaneous fracture in adult life or a traumatic fracture that would not normally occur in a healthy individual.

Sex: Female	Height: 59.3 in
Ethnicity: White	Weight: 159.6 lb
Menopause Age: 49	Age: 67

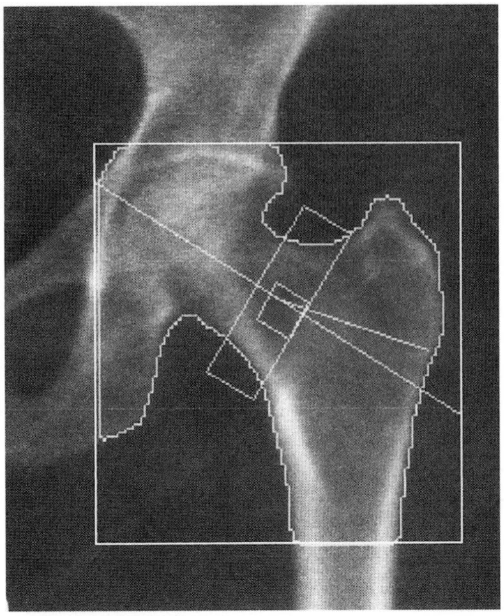

Scan Information:

Scan Date: February 29, 2012   ID: A02291206
Scan Type: a Left Hip
Analysis: February 29, 2012 14:17 Version 13.3:3
            Hip
Operator: SH
Model: Discovery A (S/N 70314)
Comment: FV3-

DXA Results Summary:

Region	Area (cm²)	BMC (g)	BMD (g/cm²)	T-score	PR (%)	Z-score	AM (%)
Neck	5.02	3.00	0.596	-2.3	70	-0.6	90
Troch	9.72	6.03	0.621	-0.8	88	0.4	107
Inter	17.14	18.18	1.061	-0.3	96	0.9	114
Total	31.88	27.21	0.854	-0.7	91	0.6	110

Total BMD CV 1.0%, ACF = 1.025, BCF = 1.008, TH = 6.208
WHO Classification: Osteopenia

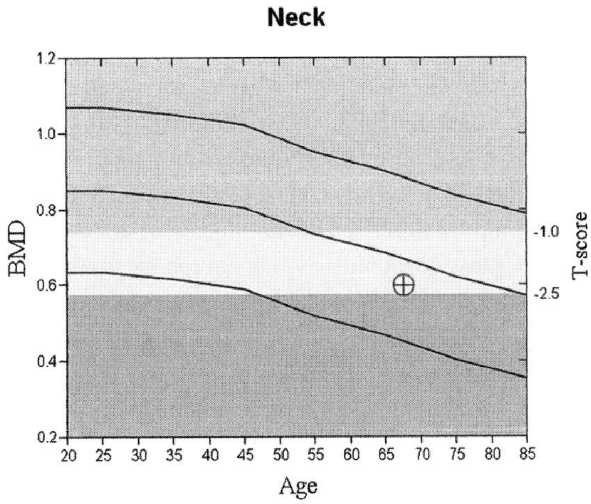

FRAX®   WHO Fracture Risk Assessment Tool

10-year Fracture Risk[1]

Major Osteoporotic Fracture	**19%**
Hip Fracture	**3.6%**

Reported Risk Factors:
US (Caucasian), T-score(WHO)=-2.2, BMI=31.9, previous fracture

[1] FRAX® Version 3.01. Fracture probability calculated for an untreated patient. Fracture probability may be lower if the patient has received treatment.

Image not for diagnostic use
k = 1.149, d0 = 46.8
94 x 100
NECK: 49 x 15

Neck

Comment:

All treatment decisions require clinical judgment and consideration of individual patient factors, including patient preferences, comorbidities, previous drug use and risk factors not captured in the FRAX model (e.g. frailty, falls, vitamin D deficiency, increased bone turnover, interval significant decline in BMD).

Fig. 1 DXA scan results at the hip in a 67-year-old woman with a history of proximal humerus fracture. The femoral neck T-score is −2.3. The FRAX results are shown on the DXA printout just below the BMD results. Ten-year fracture risk is 3.6 % for hip fracture and 19 % for major osteoporotic fracture

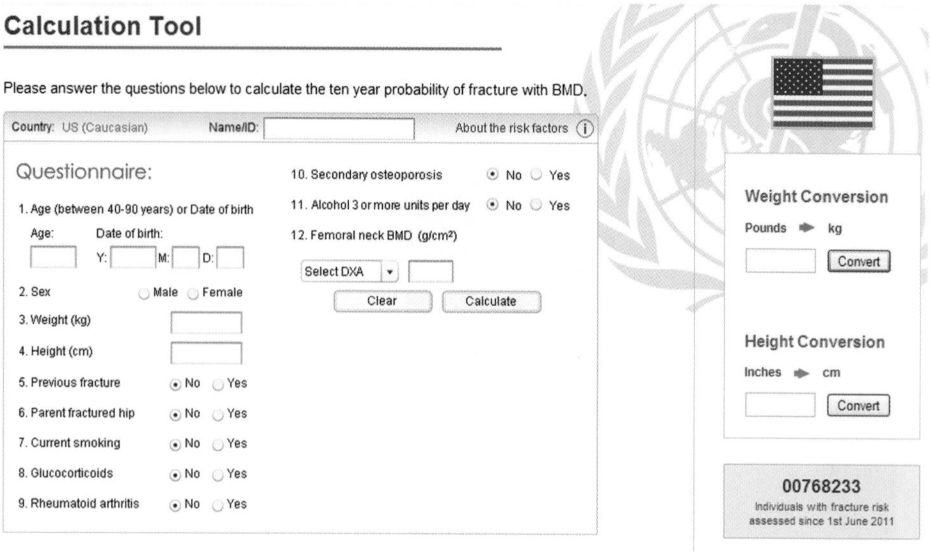

Fig. 2 FRAX Calculation tool
website. The United States
database is selected. The
questionnaire includes: age,
gender, weight, height, previous
fracture, parental hip fracture,
current smoking, use of
glucocorticoids, rheumatoid
arthritis, secondary osteoporosis,
alcohol intake, femoral neck
BMD

Importantly, radiographic or clinical vertebral fractures may be used when answering this question.

There is abundant evidence that prior fracture is a risk factor for future fractures, independent of BMD (Center et al. 2007; Ettinger et al. 2003; Lindsay et al. 2001; Kanis et al. 2004a, b, c; Klotzbuecher et al. 2000; Schousboe et al. 2006). In a meta-analysis of peri- and postmenopausal women, fracture risk was doubled in women who had a prior fracture compared to those who had no prior fracture (Klotzbuecher et al. 2000).

3.5 Parental Hip Fracture

FRAX asks if the patient's parent had a history of hip fracture. The question requires a yes or no response. There is evidence that fractures in parents increase the risk of fractures in the offspring. In the Study of Osteoporotic Fractures, women with a maternal history of hip fracture had twice the fracture risk compared to women without maternal history (Cummings et al. 1995). In a large meta-analysis Kanis et al. (2004a, b, c) reported that men and women with a parental history of fracture had an increased risk of any fracture (relative risk = 1.17), osteoporotic fracture (relative risk = 1.18), and hip fracture (relative risk = 1.49).

3.6 Smoking

FRAX includes a yes or no question about the patient's current tobacco smoking. There is evidence that smoking increases fracture risk (Cornuz et al. 1999; Høidrup et al.

2000; Law and Hackshaw 1997; Kanis et al. 2005a, b, c; Vestergaard and Mosekilde 2003; Ward and Klesges 2001).

3.7 Glucocorticoids

FRAX includes a yes or no question about patient's use of glucocorticoids. The question should be answered yes if there is present or past oral glucocorticoid therapy for more than three months and equivalent to at least 5 mg of prednisone per day.

Glucocorticoids are associated with an increased risk of fracture (van Staa et al. 2002, 2003; Weinstein 2011). In a study of 244,235 oral corticosteroid users and 244,235 controls, relative rates of non-vertebral fractures during treatment were 1.33 and hip fractures 1.61 (van Staa et al. 2000a, b).

The use of glucocorticoids as risk factor for fracture is inversely related to the patient's age. In a meta-analysis, Kanis et al. (2004a, b, c) reported that in 50-year olds, the relative risk of osteoporotic fractures was 2.63 and hip fractures was 4.42. In the same meta-analysis, in 80-year olds, the relative risk of osteoporotic fractures was 1.71 and hip fractures was 2.48. Importantly, the effect of glucocorticoids is independent of BMD.

3.8 Rheumatoid Arthritis

FRAX includes a yes or no question about RA. The etiology of fractures in patients with RA is multifactorial, resulting from chronic inflammation, inactivity, increased fall risk, and use of glucocorticoids (Broy and Tanner 2011). However, the increased fracture risk appears to be independent of the use of glucocorticoids.

3.9 Secondary Osteoporosis

FRAX asks if the patient has secondary osteoporosis. The question requires a yes or no response. Conditions associated with secondary osteoporosis include Type I diabetes, untreated long-standing hyperthyroidism, overtreated hypothyroidism, hypogonadism, premature menopause (<45 years), anorexia nervosa, certain breast cancer chemotherapeutic agents, hypopituitarism, inflammatory bowel disease, organ transplantation, COPD, chronic liver disease, chronic malnutrition, osteogenesis imperfecta, or prolonged immobility in conditions such as spinal cord injury, Parkinson's disease, stroke, or muscular dystrophy (Kanis et al. 2008a, b, c).

Although most of these conditions are associated with low BMD, the association with fractures risk is less certain. It is important to recognize that in FRAX there is no increased fracture risk attributed to secondary osteoporosis if the BMD value is entered. The only exception is RA, which is a separate question in FRAX.

3.10 Alcohol Use

FRAX asks if the patient drinks three or more units of alcohol per day. The question requires a yes or no response.

The association between alcohol use and risk of fracture has not been consistent across studies (Berg et al. 2008; Høidrup et al. 1999; Kanis et al. 2005a, b, c; Mukamal et al. 2007). In one large study (Kanis et al. 2005a, b, c) intake above two units daily was associated with an increased relative risk of any fracture (RR = 1.23), osteoporotic fracture (RR = 1.38), and hip fracture (RR = 1.68). Importantly, this elevated fracture risk was independent of BMD.

3.11 Bone Mineral Density

When available, femoral neck BMD measured by DXA should be included in FRAX. The association between low BMD and an increased risk of fracture has been well established (Cranney et al. 2007; Cummings et al. 1993; Marshall et al. 1996). Importantly, the combination of BMD with clinical factors has been shown to improve risk prediction, compared to BMD or clinical risk factors alone (Kanis et al. 2007, 2012). This combination is what makes FRAX such a powerful clinical tool.

4 Various Ways to Use FRAX

In 1994, when the World Health Organization (WHO) first used BMD to define osteoporosis, the definition was intended mainly as a research tool for epidemiologists. Soon after,

T-scores emerged and revolutionized the care of patients being evaluated for osteoporosis. In contrast, the introduction of FRAX by the WHO in 2008 was intended for clinical use rather than research. For this reason, various professional organizations developed guidelines for the use of FRAX in managing patients. What emerged is an approach to FRAX that is somewhat different in different countries. In particular, clinicians in the United States and the United Kingdom have chosen distinct approaches to the use of FRAX.

4.1 Indications for FRAX

In the United States, the National Osteoporosis Foundation (NOF) recommends using FRAX in postmenopausal women and in men age 50 and older. The NOF does not recommend FRAX in patients who are receiving pharmacologic therapy (NOF 2010).

In the United Kingdom, the National Osteoporosis Guideline Group (NOGG) recommends using FRAX in postmenopausal women and men over 50 years of age. However, unlike the NOF, the NOGG recommends initial use of FRAX *without* BMD. So in fact, FRAX results are used to determine what patients are candidates for BMD measurement using DXA. Based on age-specific thresholds of FRAX-derived risk of major osteoporotic fracture, patients are divided into three categories: (1) high risk–consider treatment, (2) intermediate risk–measure BMD, and (3) low risk–no treatment (NOGG 2010). The individuals that fall into the second group (intermediate risk) have their BMD measured and have a second FRAX calculation, this time *with* BMD. Based on FRAX-derived risk of major osteoporotic fracture, these patients are divided into two categories: (1) high risk–consider treatment, (2) low risk–no treatment (NOGG 2010).

In summary, in the UK, FRAX is used to select patients for DXA. In other words, every patient with DXA will have FRAX first. In contrast, in the US, DXA is used to select patients for FRAX. Based on the recommendations of the NOF and the International Society for Clinical Densitometry (ISCD), only patients with osteopenic BMD (T-score between −1.0 and −2.5) by DXA should have a FRAX calculation.

Importantly, FRAX does not provide treatment guidelines. As the indications for FRAX differ among individual countries, treatment recommendations based on FRAX are also different in various countries.

4.2 Treatment Recommendations Based on FRAX

FRAX has changed how men and women suspected of having osteoporosis are selected for pharmacologic therapy. Prior to FRAX, many guidelines relied on BMD results

(*T*-score) for treatment recommendations. After FRAX became available, these guidelines were revised to recommend therapy in individuals who are at high risk for fracture based on FRAX. Thresholds for therapy vary by country.

In the United Sates, the NOF recommends pharmacologic intervention in men and women with osteopenia (*T*-score between −1.0 and −2.5 at the femoral neck or spine) and a 10-year probability of a hip fracture ≥3 % or a 10-year probability of a major osteoporosis-related fracture ≥20 % (NOF 2010). The NOF also recommends treatment in individuals with osteoporosis (*T*-score ≤−2.5 at the femoral neck or spine) and in individuals with a hip or vertebral (clinical or radiologic) fracture (NOF 2010).

Prior to FRAX, a 70-year-old Caucasian woman in the United States with a BMI of 19, a *T*-score of −1.4, and a maternal history of hip fracture would not qualify for treatment. Using FRAX, the same woman has a 10 % probability of a hip fracture and 22 % probability of a major osteoporotic fracture and would qualify for therapy based on NOF guidelines.

In the United Kingdom, the NOGG algorithm stratifies patients into low, intermediate, and high risk categories based on FRAX *without* BMD. High risk individuals can be considered for treatment without BMD testing. Intermediate risk individuals have DXA with FRAX. Intervention thresholds are set by age and are equivalent to the risk associated with a prior fracture for a person of that age (NOGG 2010). Like the NOF, the NOGG recommends that women with a prior fragility fracture should be considered for treatment, without the need for BMD testing.

In summary, the FRAX treatment thresholds in the UK vary by age, whereas in the US the FRAX treatment thresholds of 3 and 20 % are used for all postmenopausal women and men age 50 and older. The economic modeling that underlies these two approaches is also quite different.

4.3 Economic Modeling

FRAX-based treatment thresholds vary by country. Treatment thresholds are determined in part by country-specific economic analysis which includes costs associated with fractures and costs associated with pharmacologic therapy (Borgström et al. 2006; Burge et al. 2007; Kanis et al. 2008a, b, c).

In the United States, a cost-benefit analysis with the following assumptions was used: bisphosphonate therapy for 5 years ($600/year), yearly doctor visit ($49/year), BMD in year 2 ($82), fracture risk reduction of 35 %, and willingness-to-pay threshold of $60,000 per quality-adjusted-life-year (QUALY) gained (Tosteson et al. 2008). Osteoporosis treatment was cost-effective when 10-year hip fracture rates reached 3 %.

In the United Kingdom, a cost-benefit analysis with a different set of assumptions was used (Kanis et al. 2008a, b, c, 2009). The intervention threshold was set to coincide with the fracture probability of someone with a prior osteoporotic fracture. The cost of generic aldendronate was set at £95 a year. Unlike the NOF thresholds, the NOGG thresholds vary by age. For example, in a 50-year-old, a 7.5 % probability of major fracture is used; in an 80-year-old, a 30 % probability is used.

In the future, the treatment thresholds based on FRAX are expected to change based on changing drug costs, drug effectiveness, and health economics within a given country.

5 How We Use FRAX

We include FRAX in our DXA reports only in patients with DXA measured *T*-score between −1 and −2.5, who are older than age 50, and who are not currently being treated for osteoporosis. We do not include FRAX in our DXA reports in patients with normal or osteoporotic BMD, in non-steroid-treated patients younger than age 50, or in patients undergoing pharmacotherapy. As such, our practice is consistent with the recommendations of the NOF and ISCD.

To understand how we use FRAX, it is important to review how we use DXA (Dasher et al. 2010). Figure 3 shows our DXA report template. In the vast majority of our patients, we use our DXA interpretation to help answer three clinical questions: (1) what is the patient's diagnosis based on BMD, (2) what is the patient's prognosis or risk of fracture, (3) could the patient benefit from pharmacologic therapy.

The second question was always the most problematic because there are different ways to express fracture risk. For example, we could state *qualitatively* that the risk is increased or we could state *quantitatively* that the risk has a certain number. Quantitative risk, in turn, could be expressed as relative risk or absolute risk. While relative risk compares two groups, absolute risk evaluates just one group, typically over 1 year, 5 years, or 10 years. In that sense, FRAX provides an absolute risk of fracture over 10 years. Thus, when combined with DXA-measured BMD, FRAX has proven to be extremely valuable for determining a patient's prognosis.

FRAX can also address the third clinical question by helping to select osteopenic patients for pharmacologic therapy.

In order to further emphasize the utility of FRAX in the interpretation of clinical DXA examinations, we contrast our current approach with our approach before FRAX became available.

Fig. 3 Our DXA report
template. Note that the report is
organized into sections including
clinical history, BMD Results,
Conclusions, and additional
information. The conclusion
section includes statements about
diagnosis, fracture risk,
monitoring, treatment
recommendations, and follow-up.
When appropriate, we include
FRAX results in the fracture risk
portion of our conclusion

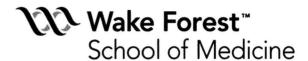

DXA REPORT

CLINICAL HISTORY:
Age: _____
Race: _____
Gender: _____
Menopausal Status: _____
Osteoporosis Therapy: _____
Prior DXA Exam: _____
Risk Factors: _____

BMD RESULTS:

PA Lumbar Spine:
BMD measured in _____region of interest is _____ g/cm².
T-score: _____Z-score: _____
Comments: _____

Proximal Femur:
BMD measured in _____region of interest is _____ g/cm².
T-score: _____Z-score: _____
Comments: _____

CONCLUSIONS:
- Diagnosis:_____
- Fracture Risk:_____
- BMD Monitoring:_____
- Treatment Recommendations:_____
- Follow up DXA:_____

ADDITIONAL INFORMATION:

World Health Organization Classification:
Osteoporosis:	T-score = -2.5 or below.
Osteopenia (low bone mass):	T-score between -1.0 and -2.5.
Normal:	T-score = -1.0 or above.

National Osteoporosis Foundation recommends pharmacologic therapy in postmenopausal women and men > 50 y/o with:
- Hip or vertebral (clinical or morphometric) fractures
- T-score ≤ -2.5 at the femoral neck, total hip, or spine
- T-score between -1 and -2.5 with FRAX 10-year fracture risk:
  ≥ 3% for hip fracture or ≥ 20% for major osteoporotic fracture

---

5.1 DXA Interpretation Before FRAX

Figure 4 shows one of our typical DXA reports prior to the use of FRAX. This was a 64-year-old woman with a history of distal radius fracture. Because her BMD was in the osteopenic range (femoral neck T-score $= -1.7$) the fracture risk in our DXA report was expressed qualitatively as "increased." Although at one time we used a quantitative expression of relative risk in our DXA reports, this practice was not standardized. Statements such as, "this patient's risk

Fig. 4 Our DXA report prior to the use of FRAX. This is a 64-year-old woman with previous distal radius fracture. L1–L4 T-score of −1.1 and femoral neck T-score of −1.7. Note that the risk is expressed in qualitative terms as "increased"

DXA REPORT

CLINICAL HISTORY:

Age: <u>64</u>

Race: <u>Caucasian</u>

Gender: <u>Woman</u>

Menopausal Status: <u>Postmenopausal</u>

Osteoporosis Therapy: <u>None</u>

Prior DXA Exam: <u>No priors</u>

Risk Factors: <u>Previous distal radius fracture</u>

BMD RESULTS:

PA Lumbar Spine:

BMD measured in <u>L1-L4</u> region of interest is <u>0.799</u> g/cm^2.

T-score: <u>-1.1</u> Z-score: <u>0.4</u>

Comments: <u>No artifacts.</u>

Proximal Femur:

BMD measured in <u>left femoral neck</u> region of interest is <u>0.678</u> g/cm^2.

T-score: <u>-1.7</u> Z-score: <u>-0.2</u>

Comments: <u>Scan is technically valid.</u>

CONCLUSIONS:

Diagnosis: <u>Osteopenia (low bone mass).</u>

Fracture Risk: <u>Increased.</u>

BMD Monitoring: <u>No prior studies.</u>

Treatment Recommendations: <u>According to NOF, therapy should be considered.</u>

Follow up DXA: <u>Two years.</u>

ADDITIONAL INFORMATION:

World Health Organization Classification:

Osteoporosis:	T-score = -2.5 or below.
Osteopenia (low bone mass):	T-score between -1.0 and -2.5.
Normal:	T-score = -1.0 or above.

National Osteoporosis Foundation recommends pharmacologic therapy in postmenopausal women with:
- Hip or vertebral fractures
- T-score ≤ -2.0 without risk factors
- T-score ≤ -1.5 with clinical risk factors

Fig. 4 Our DXA report prior to the use of FRAX. This is a 64-year-old woman with previous distal radius fracture. L1–L4 T-score of −1.1 and femoral neck T-score of −1.7. Note that the risk is expressed in qualitative terms as "increased"

is increased four-fold" were found to be confusing to many of our referring clinicians and thus were consequently abanoned. Prior to FRAX, there was no accepted way to express absolute fracture risk in DXA reports. Before FRAX, the NOF recommended therapy in patients with T-scores below −1.5 if they had clinical risk factors. Because the patient in Fig. 4 met the above NOF criteria, our DXA report included a statement, "Therapy should be considered."

5.2 Current DXA Interpretation

Figure 5 shows one of our typical DXA reports with the use of FRAX. Note that this 66-year-old woman with prior history of distal radius fracture and a femoral neck T-score of −1.5 is similar to the patient in Fig. 4. Because the patient has osteopenic BMD, the fracture risk was calculated using FRAX. However, unlike the patient in Fig. 4,

a

Sex: Female	Height: 63.7 in
Ethnicity: White	Weight: 191.4 lb
Menopause Age: 48	Age: 66

b

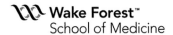

DXA REPORT

Scan Information:

Scan Date: January 09, 2012   ID: A0109120B
Scan Type: a Left Hip
Analysis: January 09, 2012 14:10 Version 13.3:3
            Hip
Operator: SH
Model: Discovery A (S/N 70314)
Comment: FV3-

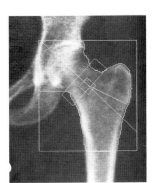

Image not for diagnostic use
k = 1.142, d0 = 45.6
91 x 100
NECK: 46 x 15

CLINICAL HISTORY:
Age: 66
Race: Caucasian
Gender: Woman
Menopausal Status: Postmenopausal
Osteoporosis Therapy: None
Prior DXA Exam: No priors
Risk Factors: Previous distal radius fracture

BMD RESULTS:

PA Lumbar Spine:
BMD measured in L1-L4 region of interest is 0.958 g/cm².
T-score: -0.8 Z-score: 0.7
Comments: There are mild degenerative changes.

Proximal Femur:
BMD measured in left femoral neck region of interest is 0.680 g/cm².
T-score: -1.5 Z-score: 0.0
Comments: The scan is technically valid.

DXA Results Summary:

Region	Area (cm²)	BMC (g)	BMD (g/cm²)	T-score	PR (%)	Z-score	AM (%)
Neck	4.98	3.39	0.680	-1.5	80	0.0	101
Troch	9.40	6.13	0.652	-0.5	93	0.6	111
Inter	18.79	17.34	0.922	-1.1	84	-0.1	98
Total	33.18	26.85	0.809	-1.1	86	0.2	103

Total BMD CV 1.0%, ACF = 1.026, BCF = 1.010, TH = 6.922
WHO Classification: Osteopenia

FRAX®   WHO Fracture Risk Assessment Tool

10-year Fracture Risk¹

| Major Osteoporotic Fracture | 14% |
| Hip Fracture | 1.5% |

Reported Risk Factors:
US (Caucasian), T-score(WHO)=-1.5, BMI=33.2, previous fracture

¹ FRAX® Version 3.01. Fracture probability calculated for an untreated patient. Fracture probability may be lower if the patient has received treatment.

CONCLUSIONS:
Diagnosis: Osteopenia (low bone mass).
Fracture Risk: According to FRAX, 1.5% risk of hip fracture and 14% risk of major osteoporotic fracture.
BMD Monitoring: No prior studies.
Treatment Recommendations: Does not meet the NOF guidelines for therapy.
Follow up DXA: Two years.

ADDITIONAL INFORMATION:

World Health Organization Classification:
Osteoporosis: T-score = -2.5 or below.
Osteopenia (low bone mass): T-score between -1.0 and -2.5.
Normal: T-score = -1.0 or above.

National Osteoporosis Foundation recommends pharmacologic therapy in postmenopausal women and men > 50 y/o with:
• Hip or vertebral (clinical or morphometric) fractures
• T-score ≤ -2.5 at the femoral neck, total hip, or spine
• T-score between -1 and -2.5 with FRAX 10-year fracture risk:
  ≥ 3% for hip fracture or ≥ 20% for major osteoporotic fracture

Neck

(graph: BMD vs Age, T-score axis -1.0, -2.5)

Comment:
All treatment decisions require clinical judgment and consideration of individual patient factors, including patient preferences, comorbidities, previous drug use and risk factors not captured in the FRAX model (e.g. frailty, falls, vitamin D deficiency, increased bone turnover, interval significant decline in BMD).

Fig. 5 a Hip DXA printout in a 66-year-old woman with previous distal radius fracture. L1–L4 T-score (*not shown*) is −0.8. Femoral neck T-score is −1.5. Note that the FRAX results are shown because the patient is osteopenic. **b** DXA report in the same patient. Note that the risk is expressed in quantitative terms based on FRAX: 10-year fracture risk is 1.5 % for hip fracture and 14 % for major osteoportic fracture. Because the patient does not meet the NOF criteria for therapy, therapy was not recommended

this patient did not qualify for pharmacologic therapy. With a 10-year risk of hip fracture of 1.5 % and major osteoporotic fracture of 14 %, the patient did not meet the post-FRAX criteria for therapy from the NOF.

Figure 6 shows our use of FRAX in a DXA report of another patient, a 78-year-old woman with a history of low-trauma tibia fracture. Like the patient in Fig. 5, this patient has osteopenic BMD (femoral neck T-score is −2.0). Unlike the patient in Fig. 5, this patient met the post-FRAX criteria for pharmacologic therapy from the NOF. The 10-year risk was 5.1 % for hip fracture and 21 % for major osteoporotic fracture.

How do we express risk in patients with normal or osteoporotic BMD? The same way we did before FRAX. Figure 7 shows our DXA printouts in patients who have normal BMD, osteoporotic BMD, prior spine or hip fracture, or are undergoing therapy for osteoporosis. In these patients, our DXA reports make no mention of FRAX. If the BMD is in the normal range, we report the fracture risk as "normal." If the BMD is in the osteoporotic range or the patient is on therapy, we report the risk as "increased." How do we recommend therapy in patients with osteoporosis (T-score below −2.5),

or history of spine or hip fracture? The same way we did before FRAX; we report "therapy should be considered."

Outside of the radiology setting, another benefit of FRAX is its use as an educational tool for patients. FRAX results are often used by clinicians to explain to patients why some are candidates for therapy while others are not. By manipulating FRAX results in front of a given patient, clinicians are able to show the benefit of lifestyle modifications such as smoking cessation or excessive alcohol intake.

6   Controversies

Despite the obvious clinical utility of FRAX, its use has attracted controversy (Ensrud et al. 2009; Giangregorio et al. 2012; Hillier et al. 2011; Joop et al. 2010; Kanis et al. 2011; Leslie et al. 2012; Lewiecki et al. 2011; Roux and Thomas 2009; Silverman and Calderon 2010; Tremollieres et al. 2010). To help organize the controversial aspects of FRAX, we first review some key aspects in its development and then attempt to answer two questions: (1) Does FRAX

a

Sex: Female	Height: 61.9 in
Ethnicity: White	Weight: 165.0 lb
Menopause Age: 41	Age: 78

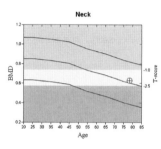

Image not for diagnostic use
k = 1.139, d0 = 49.0
98 x 99
NECK: 49 x 15

Scan Information:

Scan Date: February 08, 2012   ID: A02081207
Scan Type: a Left Hip
Analysis: February 08, 2012 11:08 Version 13.3:3
    Hip
Operator: SH
Model: Discovery A (S/N 70314)
Comment: FV3-

DXA Results Summary:

Region	Area (cm²)	BMC (g)	BMD (g/cm²)	T-score	PR (%)	Z-score	AM (%)
Neck	4.81	3.02	0.628	-2.0	74	0.2	104
Troch	9.64	5.63	0.584	-1.2	83	0.5	110
Inter	17.21	15.29	0.889	-1.4	81	0.4	107
Total	31.66	23.94	0.756	-1.5	80	0.4	108

Total BMD CV 1.0%, ACF = 1.026, BCF = 1.010, TH = 6.069
WHO Classification: Osteopenia

FRAX®   WHO Fracture Risk Assessment Tool

10-year Fracture Risk¹

| Major Osteoporotic Fracture | 21% |
| Hip Fracture | 5.1% |

Reported Risk Factors:
US (Caucasian), T-score(WHO)=-1.9, BMI=30.3, previous fracture

¹ FRAX® Version 3.01. Fracture probability calculated for an untreated patient.
Fracture probability may be lower if the patient has received treatment.

Comment:

All treatment decisions require clinical judgment and consideration of
individual patient factors, including patient preferences, comorbidities,
previous drug use and risk factors not captured in the FRAX model
(e.g. frailty, falls, vitamin D deficiency, increased bone turnover,
interval significant decline in BMD).

Neck

Graph: BMD vs Age, with T-score axis

b

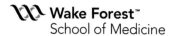

DXA REPORT

CLINICAL HISTORY:
Age: 78
Race: Caucasian
Gender: Woman
Menopausal Status: Postmenopausal
Osteoporosis Therapy: None
Prior DXA Exam: No priors
Risk Factors: Previous proximal tibia fracture

BMD RESULTS:

PA Lumbar Spine:
BMD measured in L1-L4 region of interest is 0.805 g/cm².
T-score: -2.2 Z-score: 0.3
Comments: No significant artifacts.

Proximal Femur:
BMD measured in left femoral neck region of interest is 0.628 g/cm².
T-score: -2.0 Z-score: 0.2
Comments: Scan acquisition is technically valid.

CONCLUSIONS:
Diagnosis: Osteopenia (low bone mass).
Fracture Risk: According to FRAX, 5.1% risk of hip fracture and 21% risk of major osteoporotic fracture.
BMD Monitoring: No prior studies.
Treatment Recommendations: According to NOF, therapy should be considered.
Follow up DXA: Two years.

ADDITIONAL INFORMATION:

World Health Organization Classification:
Osteoporosis: T-score = -2.5 or below.
Osteopenia (low bone mass):   T-score between -1.0 and -2.5.
Normal: T-score = -1.0 or above.

National Osteoporosis Foundation recommends pharmacologic therapy in postmenopausal women and men > 50 y/o with:
 • Hip or vertebral (clinical or morphometric) fractures
 • T-score ≤ -2.5 at the femoral neck, total hip, or spine
 • T-score between -1 and -2.5 with FRAX 10-year fracture risk:
    ≥ 3% for hip fracture or ≥ 20% for major osteoporotic fracture

Fig. 6 **a** Hip DXA printout in a 78-year-old woman with previous low-trauma tibia fracture. L1–L4 T-score (*not shown*) is −2.2. Femoral neck T-score is −2.0. Note that the FRAX results are shown because the patient is osteopenic. **b** DXA report in the same patient. Note that the risk is expressed in quantitative terms based on FRAX: 10-year fracture risk is 5.1 % for hip fracture and 21 % for major osteoportic fracture. Because the patient meets the NOF criteria for therapy, therapy was recommended

work? (2) Can it work better? In answering these questions we glimpse into the future of how this tool may be used to help improve patient care.

6.1   Development of FRAX

FRAX was developed using country-specific epidemiologic data. Risk factors for fracture were chosen from multiple meta-analyses using 60,000 men and women, with approximately 250,000 patient years (McCloskey et al. 2009). The results have been confirmed in 11 independent cohorts from around the world, with over a million patient years (Kanis et al. 2007).

Unlike other absolute fracture risk tools, FRAX accounts for competing mortality (Kanis et al. 2003). The mortality modifier is used because the average life expectancies vary substantially in different countries. The closer someone is to their life-expectant age, the higher their probability of dying before they sustain an osteoporotic fracture. For this reason, future versions of FRAX will have to take into account not only changing fracture rates but also changing mortality rates.

It is important to realize that FRAX provides probability of fracture over a 10-year period instead of a lifetime. From a clinical standpoint, lifetime risk is not as important as a short-term risk. For example, a 50-year-old individual has a much higher lifetime risk of fracture compared to an 85-year-old simply because they will live longer. But the 85-year old is much more likely to fracture in the next 10 years than a 50-year old.

Ten-year risk is also used because the prognostic value of some clinical risk factors may diminish with time (Lewiecki 2010). For example, the fracture risk after an osteoporotic fracture decreases as the time from that fracture increases (Schousboe et al. 2006). Excess risk for hip fracture (after adjusting for BMD and age) in individuals with prevalent vertebral fractures was 110 % in the first 5 years, 75 % at 5–10 years, and 41 % more than 10 years after the baseline examination (Schousboe et al. 2006).

Although FRAX has undergone multiple updates with new epidemiologic data (Watts et al. 2009), many osteoporosis experts still wonder if FRAX can be further improved. This question revolves around two issues: (1) Clinical risk factors and (2) Measurement of BMD.

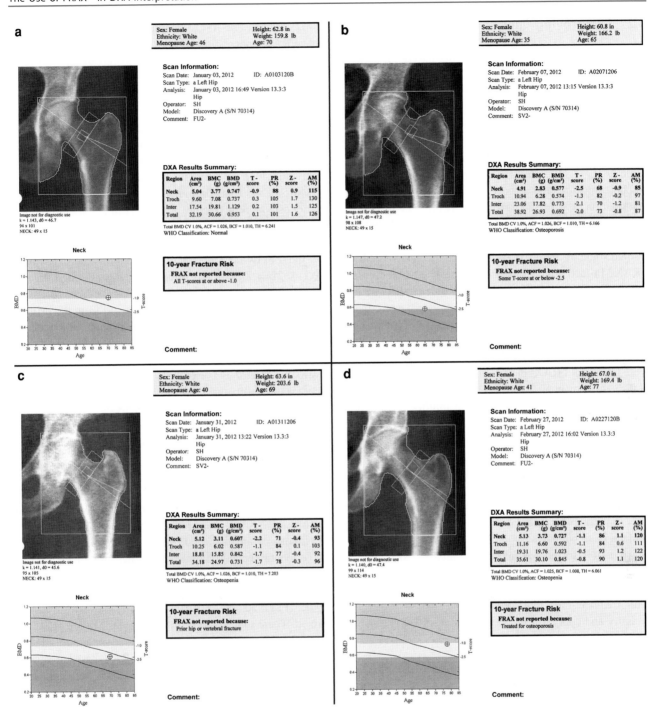

Fig. 7 **a** Hip DXA printout in a 70-year-old woman with a 43-year history of cigarette smoking. L1–L4 T-score (*not shown*) is 0.2. Femoral neck T-score is −0.9. Note that the FRAX results are not reported because the T-scores are within normal range (above −1.0). **b** Hip DXA printout in a 65-year-old woman with a maternal history of hip fracture. L1–L4 T-score (*not shown*) is −1.7. Femoral neck T-score is −2.5. Note that the FRAX results are not reported because some of the T-scores are within osteoporotic range. **c** Hip DXA printout in a 69-year-old woman with a history of T8 vertebral body fracture. L1–L4 T-score (*not shown*) is -1.2. Femoral neck T-score is −2.2. Note that the FRAX results are not reported because the patient has a history of a low-trauma spine fracture. **d** Hip DXA printout in a 77-year-old woman on bisphosphonate therapy for the past 3 years. L1–L4 T-score (*not shown*) is −1.7. Femoral neck T-score is −1.1. Note that the FRAX results are not reported because the patient is being treated for osteoporosis

6.2   Improving Clinical Risk Factors in FRAX

There has been controversy surrounding the use of dichotomous (Yes or No) variables in FRAX (Blank 2011; Dimai and Chandran 2011; Leib et al. 2011). Previous fracture, smoking, glucocorticoids use, and alcohol use are all dichotomous variables. Yet there is evidence that increased *number* of prior fractures and increased *severity* of prior vertebral fractures substantially increases future risk of fracture (Black et al. 1999; Lindsay et al. 2001; Puisto et al. 2012). Similarly, the use of alcohol, smoking, and glucocorticoids has a dose-dependent contribution to increased fracture risk (Cornuz et al. 1999; de Vries et al. 2007; Høidrup et al. 1999; van Staa et al. 2000a, b; Ward and Klesges 2001; Weatherall et al. 2008). Is it possible to treat some of these risk factors as continuous variables in FRAX? In fact, a recent meeting of the International Osteoporosis Foundation (IOF) and ISCD considered that question. They decided that FRAX may underestimate fracture risk in patients with multiple fractures, severe vertebral fractures, and doses of oral glucocorticoids >7.5 mg/day (Hans et al. 2011).

Controversy also exists about the clinical risk factors that were left out of FRAX; in particular, falls and frailty (Masud et al. 2011; Roy et al. 2002). In the elderly, 40–60 % of falls result in an injury; 5–10 % of these injuries are fractures (Masud and Morris 2001). According to the Study of Osteoporotic Fractures, a woman has a 30 % increase in 10-year fracture probability with each fall compared to her counterpart without any falls. The most important risk factors for falling include previous falls, decreased muscle strength, instability, dizziness, visual impairment, depression, cognitive impairment, urinary incontinence, chronic musculoskeletal pain, woman sex, and age >80 (Masud et al. 2011). Is it possible to include falls and frailty as risk factors in FRAX? A recent IOF–ISCD Position Statement on FRAX acknowledges evidence for increased fracture risk in patients with frequent falls but states that the risk is difficult to quantify and apply to FRAX (Hans et al. 2011).

6.3   Improving BMD Measurement in FRAX

There has been some controversy about the choice of BMD measurement site in FRAX. Because some of the epidemiologic trials used in FRAX meta-analyses did not include total hip BMD or spine BMD, femoral neck BMD was chosen. There are other reasons for using only femoral BMD: (1) Femoral BMD predicts hip fractures better than other BMD measurement sites; (2) Frequent age-related degenerative changes in the lumbar spine, coupled with the absence of a standardized approach for excluding artifacts, limits use of lumbar spine BMD.

In clinical patients there is significant inter-site variability (discordance) in BMD between spine and hip (Leslie et al.

2007). Recent IOF–ISCD Position Statement acknowledges that FRAX underestimates fracture risk in individuals with significantly lower spine BMD compared to femoral neck BMD (Hans et al. 2011).

Leslie et al. (2011) derived a correction factor for FRAX to account for spine-hip discordance based on the Manitoba BMD database. The FRAX estimate was increased or decreased by one-tenth for each rounded T-score difference between the femoral neck and lumbar spine. For example, an individual with a T-score of -1.9 at the femoral neck and a T-score of -3.8 at the lumbar spine has a FRAX-derived major osteoporotic fracture probability of 22 %. A difference of 1.9 exists between the BMD at the spine and hip (-3.8 minus -1.9). This number is rounded to 2.0. One-tenth of the FRAX-derived fracture probability is determined ($0.1 \times 22 = 2.2$). This value is then multiplied by the rounded difference between the sites ($2.0 \times 2.2 = 4.4$). The resultant number is added to or subtracted from the original FRAX fracture probability to derive a modified FRAX fracture probability. In this example, the modified FRAX fracture probability is 26.4 % ($22 + 4.4 = 26.4$ %). Although, this correction factor is currently not being applied to FRAX, there is possibility that some similar correction factor may be included in the future versions of FRAX.

7   Conclusion

By providing a country-specific 10-year risk of fracture that takes into account not just BMD but 10 other clinical risk factors, FRAX has changed the way patients with suspected osteoporoses are managed. Using FRAX, many clinicians have recommended pharmacologic therapy to patients who have not yet reached osteoporotic BMD. The use of FRAX in clinical practice will certainly be refined in the future. Other risk factors or BMD measurement sites may be added. There may even be further standardization on its use in different countries. In our practice, including FRAX-derived fracture risk and applying FRAX-based treatment algorithms in our DXA interpretation has fundamentally changed the way these examinations are reported. The purpose of this chapter was to share our perspective on this important tool.

References

Baron JA, Karagas M, Barrett J (1996) Basic epidemiology of fractures of the upper and lower limb among Americans over 65 years of age. Epidemiology 7(6):612–618

Berg KM, Kunins HV, Jackson JL, Nahvi S, Chaudhry A, Harris KA Jr, Malik R, Arnsten JH (2008) Association between alcohol consumption and both osteoporotic fracture and bone density. Am J Med 121(5):406–418

Black DM, Arden NK, Palermo L, Pearson J, Cummings SR (1999) Prevalent vertebral deformities predict hip fractures and new vertebral fractures, but not wrist fractures. J Bone Miner Res 14:821–828

Blank RD (2011) Official positions for FRAX® clinical regarding prior fractures from joint official positions development conference of the international society for clinical densitometry and international osteoporosis foundation on FRAX®. J Clin Densitom 14(3):205–211

Borgström F, Johnell O, Kanis JA, Jönsson B, Rehnberg C (2006) At what hip fracture risk is it cost-effective to treat? International Intervention thresholds for the treatment of osteoporosis. Osteoporos Int 17:1459–1471

Broy SB, Tanner SB (2011) Official positions for FRAX® clinical regarding rheumatoid arthritis. J Clin Densitom 14(3):184–189

Burge R, Dawson-Hughes B, Solomon DH, Wong JB, King A, Tosteson A (2007) Incidence and economic burden of osteoporosis-related fractures in the United States, 2005–2025. J Bone Miner Res 22:465–475

Center JR, Bliuc D, Nguyen TV, Eisman JA (2007) Risk of subsequent fracture after low-trauma fracture in men and women. J Am Med Assoc 297(4):387–394

Cornuz J, Feskanich D, Willett WC, Colditz GA (1999) Smoking, smoking cessation, and risk of hip fracture in women. AJM 106(3):311–314

Cranney A, Jamal SA, Tsang JF, Josse RG, Leslie WD (2007) Low bone mineral density and fracture burden in postmenopausal women. CMAJ 177(6):575–580

Cummings SR, Black DM, Nevitt MC et al (1993) Bone density at various sites for the prediction of hip fractures. Lancet 341:72–75

Cummings SR, Nevitt MC, Browner WS, Stone K, Fox KM, Ensrud KE et al (1995) Risk factors for hip fracture in white women. Study of osteoporotic fractures research group. N Engl J Med 332(12):767–773

Dasher LG, Newton CD, Lenchik L (2010) Dual X-ray absorptiometry in today's clinical practice. Radiol Clin North Am 48:541–560

De Laet C, Kanis JA, Oden A, Johanson H, Johnell O, Delmas P et al (2005) Body mass index as a predictor of fracture risk: a meta-analysis. Osteoporos Int 16(11):1330–1338

de Vries F, Pouwels S, Lammers JW et al (2007) Use of inhaled and oral glucocorticoids, severity of inflammatory disease and risk of hip/femur fracture: a population-based case-control study. J Intern Med 261(2):170–177

Dimai HP, Chandran M (2011) Official positions for FRAX® clinical regarding smoking. J Clin Densitom 14(3):190–193

Ensrud KE, Lui LY, Taylor BC, Schousboe JT, Donaldson MG, Fink HA, Cauley JA, Hillier TA, Browner WS, Cummings SR (2009) A comparison of prediction models for fractures in older women: is more better? Arch Intern Med 169(22):2087–2094

Eastell R, Boyle IT, Compston J et al (1998) Management of male osteoporosis: report of the UK consensus group. Q J Med 91:71

Ettinger B, Ray GT, Pressman AR et al (2003) Limb fractures in elderly men as indicators of subsequent osteoporotic fractures. Arch Intern Med 163(22):2741–2747

Felson DT, Zhang Y, Hannan MT, Anderson JJ (1993) Effects of weight and body mass index on bone mineral density in men and women: the Framingham study. J Bone Miner Res 8(5):567–573

Giangregorio LM, Leslie WD, Lix LM, Johansson H, Oden A, McCloskey E, Kanis JA (2012) FRAX underestimates fracture risk in patients with diabetes. J Bone Miner Res 27(2):301–308

Hans DB, Kanis JA, Baim S, Bilenzikian JP, Binkley N et al (2011) Joint official positions of the international society for clinical densitometry and international osteoporosis foundation on FRAX. J Clin Densitom 14(3):171–180

Hillier TA, Cauley JA, Rizzo JH, Pedula KL, Ensrud KE, Bauer DC, Lui L, Vesco KK, Black DM, Donaldson MG, LeBlanc ES,

Cummings SR (2011) WHO absolute fracture risk models (FRAX): do clinical risk factors improve fracture prediction in older women without osteoporosis? J Bone Miner Res 26(8):1774–1782

Høidrup S, Gronbaek M, Gottschau A, Lauritzen JB, Schroll M (1999) Alcohol intake, beverage preference, and risk of hip fracture in men and women. Am J Epidemiol 149(11):993–1001

Høidrup S, Prescott E, Sørensen TIA, Gottschau A, Lauritzen JB, Schroll M, Grønbaek M (2000) Tobacco smoking and risk of hip fracture in men and women. Int J Epidemiol 29(2):253–259

Joop PW, van den Bergh Tineke ACM, van Geel Lems WF, Geusens PP (2010) Assessment of individual fracture risk: FRAX and beyond. Curr Osteoporos Rep 8:131–137

Kanis JA, Johnell O, De Laet C et al (2002) International variations in hip fracture probabilities: implications for risk assessment. J Bone Miner Res 17:1237–1244

Kanis JA, Oden A, Johnell O et al (2003) The components of excess mortality after hip fracture. Bone 32:468

Kanis JA, Johansson H, Oden A et al (2004a) A family history of fracture and fracture risk: a meta-analysis. Bone 35:1029–1037

Kanis JA, Johansson H, Oden A et al (2004b) A meta-analysis of prior corticosteroid use and fracture risk. J Bone Miner Res 19:893–899

Kanis JA, Johnell O, De Laet C et al (2004c) A meta-analysis of previous fracture and subsequent fracture risk. Bone 35:375–382

Kanis JA, Borgstrom F, De Laet C, Johansson H, Johnell O, Jonsson B (2005a) Assessment of fracture risk. Osteoporos Int 16:581–589

Kanis JA, Johansson H, Johnell O, Oden A, De Laet C, Eisman JA, Pols H, Tenenhouse A (2005b) Alcohol intake as a risk factor for fracture. Osteoporos Int 16(7):737–742

Kanis JA, Johnell O, Oden A et al (2005c) Smoking and fracture risk: a meta-analysis. Osteoporos Int 16:155–162

Kanis JA, Oden A, Johnell O et al (2007) The use of clinical risk factors enhances the performance of BMD in the prediction of hip and osteoporotic fractures in men and women. Osteoporos Int 18:1033–1046

Kanis JA, Burlet N, Cooper C, Delmas PD, Reginster JY, Borgstrom F et al (2008a) European guidance for the diagnosis and management of osteoporosis in postmenopausal women. Osteoporos Int 19(4):399–428

Kanis JA, McCloskey EV, Johansson H, Oden A, Melton LJ, Khaltaev N (2008b) A reference standard for the description of osteoporosis. Bone 42:467–475

Kanis JA, McCloskey EV, Johansson H, Strom O, Borgstrom F, Oden A (2008c) Case finding for the management of osteoporosis with FRAX®—assessment and intervention thresholds for the UK. Osteoporos Int 19:1395–1408

Kanis J, Oden A, Johansson H, Borgström F, Ström O, McCloskey E (2009) FRAX® and its applications to clinical practice. Bone 44:734–743

Kanis JA, Johansson H, Oden A et al (2011) Guidance for the adjustment of FRAX according to the dose of glucocorticoids. Osteoporos Int 22:809–816

Kanis JA, McCloskey E, Johansson H, Oden A, Leslie WD (2012) FRAX with and without BMD. Calcif Tissue Int 90:1–13

Klotzbuecher CM, Ross PD, Landsman PB, Abbott TA III, Berger M (2000) Patients with prior fractures have an increased risk of future fractures: a summary of the literature and statistical synthesis. J Bone Miner Res 15(4):721–739

Law MR, Hackshaw AK (1997) A meta-analysis of cigarette smoking, bone mineral density and risk of hip fracture: recognition of major effects. BMJ 315(7112):841–846

Leib ES, Saag KG, Adachi JD et al (2011) Official positions for FRAX® clinical regarding glucocorticoids: the impact of the use of glucocorticoids on the estimate by FRAX® of the 10 year risk of fracture. J Clin Densitom 14(3):212–219

Leslie WD, Lix LM, Tsang JF, Caetano PA (2007) Single-site vs multisite bone density measurement for fracture prediction. Arch Intern Med 167(15):1641–1647

Leslie WD, Lix LM, Johansson H, Oden A, McCloskey E, Kanis JA (2011) Spine-hip discordance and fracture risk assessment: a physician-friendly FRAX enhancement. Osteoporos Int 22: 839–847

Leslie WD, Majumdar SR, Lix LM, Johansson H, Oden A, McCloskey E, Kanis JA (2012) High fracture probability with FRAX® usually indicates densitometric osteoporosis: implications for clinical practice. Osteoporos Int 23:391–397

Lewiecki EM (2010) Fracture risk assessment in clinical practice: T-scores, FRAX, and beyond. Clinic Rev Bone Miner Metab 8: 101–112

Lewiecki EM, Compston JE, Miller PD, Adachi JD et al (2011) Official positions for FRAX® bone mineral density and FRAX® simplification. J Clin Densitom 14(3):226–236

Lindsay R, Silverman SL, Cooper C, Hanley DA, Barton I, Broy SB et al (2001) Risk of new vertebral fracture in the year following a fracture. J Am Med Assoc 285:320–323

Marshall D, Johnell O, Wedel H (1996) Meta-analysis of how well measures of bone mineral density predict occurrence of osteoporotic fractures. Br Med J 312:1254–1259

Masud T, Morris RO (2001) Epidemiology of falls. Age Ageing 30(4):S9–S16

Masud T, Binkly N, Boonen S, Hannan MT (2011) Official positions for FRAX® clinical regarding falls and frailty: can falls and frailty be used in FRAX®? J Clin Densitom 14(3):194–204

McCloskey EV, Johansson H, Oden A, Kanis JA (2009) From relative risk to absolute fracture risk calculation: the FRAX algorithm. Curr Osteoporos Rep 7:77–83

Mukamal KJ, Robbins JA, Cauley JA, Kern LM, Siscovick DS (2007) Alcohol consumption, bone density, and hip fracture among older adults: the cardiovascular health study. Osteoporos Int 18(5):593–602

National Osteoporosis Guideline Group (2010) Osteoporosis: clinical guideline for prevention and treatment

National Osteoporosis Foundation (2010) Clinician's guide to prevention and treatment of osteoporosis

Pasco JA, Seeman E, Henry MJ, Merriman EN, Nicholson GC, Kotowicz MA (2006) The population burden of fractures originates in women with osteopenia, not osteoporosis. Osteoporos Int 17(9):1404–1409

Puisto V, Heliövaara M, Jalanko T, Kröger H, Knekt P, Aromaa A, Rissanen H, Helenius I (2012) Severity of vertebral fracture and risk of hip fracture: a nested case-control study. Osteoporos Int 22:63–69

Roux C, Thomas T (2009) Optimal use of FRAX®. Joint Bone Spine 76:1–3

Roy DK, Pye SR, Lunt M et al (2002) Falls explain between center differences in the incidence of limb fracture across Europe. Bone 31:712–717

Sanders KM, Nicholson GC, Watts JJ, Pasco JA, Henry MJ, Kotowicz MA et al (2006) Half the burden of fragility fractures in the community

occur in women without osteoporosis: When is fracture prevention cost effective? Bone 38(5):694–700

Schousboe JT, Fink HA, Lui LY, Taylor BC, Ensrud KE (2006) Association between prior non-spine non-hip fractures or prevalent radiographic vertebral deformities known to be at least 10 years old and incident hip fracture. J Bone Miner Res 21(10):1557–1564

Silverman SL, Calderon AD (2010) The utility and limitations of FRAX: a US perspective. Curr Osteoporos Rep 8:192–197

Siris ES, Brenneman SK, Barrett-Connor E, Miller PD, Saijan S, Berger ML, Chen YT (2006) The effect of age and bone mineral density on the absolute, excess, and relative risk of fracture in postmenopausal women aged 50–99: results from the National Osteoporosis Risk Assessment (NORA). Osteoporos Int 17: 565–574

Tosteson AN, Melton LJ III, Dawson-Hughes B, Baim S, Favus MJ, Khosla S et al (2008) Cost-effective osteoporosis treatment thresholds: the United States perspective. Osteoporos Int 19(4):437–447

Tremollieres FA, Pouille JM, Drewniak N, Laparra J, Ribot C, Dargent-Molina P (2010) Fracture risk prediction using BMD and clinical risk factors in early postmenopausal women: sensitivity of the WHO FRAX tool. J Bone Miner Res 25(5):1002–1009

van Staa TP, Leufkens HGM, Abenhaim L, Zhang B, Cooper C (2000a) Use of oral corticosteroids and risk of fractures. J Bone Miner Res 15:993–1000

van Staa TP, Leufkens HGM, Abenhaim L, Zhang B, Cooper C (2000b) Oral corticosteroids and fracture risk: relationship to daily and cumulative dosing. Rheumatology 39:1383–1389

van Staa TP, Leufkens HG, Cooper C (2002) The epidemiology of corticosteroid-induced osteoporosis: a meta-analysis. Osteoporos Int 13(10):777–787

van Staa TP, Laan RF, Barton IP, Cohen S, Reid DM, Cooper C (2003) Bone density threshold and other predictors of vertebral fracture in patients receiving oral glucocorticoid therapy. Arthritis Rheum 48:3224–3229

Vestergaard P, Mosekilde L (2003) Fracture risk associated with smoking: a meta-analysis. J Intern Med 254(6):572–583

Wainwright SA, Marshall LM, Ensrud KE et al (2005) Hip fracture in women without osteoporosis. J Clin Endocrinol Metab 90(5): 2787–2793

Ward KD, Klesges RC (2001) A meta-analysis of the effects of cigarette smoking on mineral density. Calcif Tissue Int 68:259–270

Watts NB, Ettinger B, LeBoff MS (2009) FRAX Facts. J Bone Miner Res 24(6):975–979

Weinstein RS (2011) Glucocorticoid-induced bone disease. NEJM 365:62–70

Weatherall M, James K, Clay J et al (2008) Dose response relationship for risk of non-vertebral fracture with inhaled corticosteroids. Clin Exp Allergy 38(9):1451–1458

Dual-Energy X-Ray Absorptiometry

J. E. Adams

Contents

Abstract

Dual-energy X-ray absorptiometry (DXA) is the most widely available and utilised quantitative method for diagnosis of osteoporosis and assessment of fracture risk. The strengths of DXA are low radiation dose (1–6μSv) and rapid scanning (1–2min); it provides an 'areal' bone mineral density (BMD; g/cm^2) of integral (cortical and trabecular) bone. A limitation is that the measures are size dependent, a particular problem in growing children. A number of methods have been suggested to correct for this size dependency but there is no consensus yet on which is ideal. Diagnosis of osteoporosis in made by DXA in the hip, lumbar spine and distal 1/3 radius using a T score of ≤ 2.5. Introduction of the WHO FRAX® 10-year fracture risk assessment tool will improve clinical use of DXA and the cost effectiveness of therapeutic interventions for osteoporosis. An important clinical development in DXA is vertebral fracture assessment (VFA) which is being increasingly applied. Whole body DXA provides total and regional BMD, lean and fat mass measurements and recently android/gynoid ratio and visceral adipose tissue (VAT) results have become available. Extended research applications include hip strength analysis (HAS) and trabecular bone score (TBS), but their role in clinical practice is still to be determined.

1   Introduction

Osteoporosis is the most common metabolic bone disease, and is characterised by reduced bone mass, altered bone architecture and the clinical consequence of easy fracture with little or no trauma (low-trauma insufficiency fractures). These fractures tend to occur most commonly in sites of the skeleton that are rich in trabecular bone: the wrist, spine and hip (Cummings and Melton 2002). The latter have the greatest morbidity and mortality, but all osteoporotic

J. E. Adams (✉)
Manchester Academic Health Science Centre and Radiology Department, Manchester Royal Infirmary, Central Manchester Universities NHS Foundation Trust, Oxford Road, Manchester, M13 9WL, UK
e-mail: judith.adams@manchester.ac.uk

G. Guglielmi (ed.), *Osteoporosis and Bone Densitometry Measurements*, Medical Radiology. Diagnostic Imaging,
DOI: 10.1007/174_2012_789, © Springer-Verlag Berlin Heidelberg 2013

fractures result in pain and suffering for affected patients and have considerable socio-economic impact on healthcare systems and society generally (Compston 2010a). Over the past two decades there has been considerable improvement in the therapeutic interventions that can be made to increase bone mineral density (BMD) and, more importantly, reduce future fracture risk. Such therapies include bisphosphonates (etidronate, alendronate, risedronate, ibandronate, zoledronate), selective oestrogen modulator regulators (SERMs; raloxifene), strontium ranelate, denusomab and teriparatide, a recombinant form of parathyroid hormone (Rachner et al. 2011). These developments in therapeutic options have made it even more relevant to identify accurately those patients at risk of osteoporosis, and to do so before they suffer a fracture.

The diagnosis of osteoporosis can be made from radiographs when multiple fractures are present, or if structural abnormalities characteristic of osteoporosis are evident. These include reduction in both bone density (osteopenia) and the number of trabeculae, thinned cortices, prominent vertical trabeculae in the vertebrae with preferential loss of horizontal trabeculae giving a striated appearance (Anil et al. 2010). However, judging bone density on a radiograph can be imprecise, as technical aspects such as patient size, exposure and processing factors influence how radio-dense the bones appear. Although whether a patient suffers a fracture depends on a number of factors, including the propensity to fall and the nature of, and the response to, a fall, about 60–70 % of bone strength is related to BMD (Ammann and Rizzoli 2003). These factors lead to the importance of having available accurate and reproducible methods to quantitate the BMD of the skeleton in order to:
1. Diagnose osteoporosis
2. Predict fracture risk
3. Determine appropriate therapeutic intervention
4. Monitor response to therapy, or change with time, which are the diagnostic and management roles of bone densitometry.

2   Historical Aspects

Quantitative measurements of bone mineral content (BMC) of the skeleton first became available in 1963, with the introduction of single photon absorptiometry (SPA) for peripheral bone densitometry (Cameron and Sorenson 1963). For application to central sites (lumbar spine and proximal femur), a dual photon source (DPA) was required to correct for the overlying soft tissues (Dunn et al. 1980). These techniques used radionuclide sources for the production of the photons; the sources decayed and needed regular replacement, and scanning took a considerable length of time (15–30 min) because the photon flux was low. Thus, the patient might move during the scan causing artefact, and the image quality was relatively poor due to limited spatial resolution; both these factors adversely affected reproducibility (precision). However, a large amount of useful clinical data was collected using these methods. In the mid-1980s the radionuclide sources of these scanners were replaced with low-dose X-ray tubes. These had a higher photon flux and so allowed faster scanning and improved spatial resolution providing better image quality (Kelly et al. 1988; Cullum et al. 1989; Mazess 1990). This heralded the introduction of single- and dual-energy X-ray absorptiometry (SXA, DXA), with improved precision, which could be applied to peripheral and central skeletal sites respectively.

3   Technical Aspects

The first DXA scanners were introduced in the late 1980s, and DXA is now the most widely used and available method amongst the techniques applied for quantitative assessment of the skeleton (Blake and Fogelman 2007; Dasher et al. 2010; Guglielmi et al. 2011; Chun 2011), although its availability varies in different countries. The dual-energy X-ray beams are required to correct bone density measurements for overlying soft tissue, and are produced by a variety of techniques by different manufacturers (energy switching; k-edge filtration) (Blake and Fogelman 1997). The energies used are selected to optimise the separation of the mineralised calcium hydroxyapatite component of bone and adjacent soft tissue of the skeletal site scanned. Scanners manufactured by Hologic (Bedford, Mass., USA) use an energy-switching system in which the X-ray tube potential is switched rapidly from 70 to 140 kVp, alternating 60 times per second. The problems in quantitative applications of beam hardening that are usually associated with the polychromatic beam produced by an X-ray tube are overcome by simultaneous calibration and correction using a disc of reference bone and soft tissue equivalents which rotates synchronously with the X-ray pulses. The scanners manufactured by General Electric/Lunar (Madison, Wisconsin, USA) use a constant potential X-ray source, combined with a rare-earth filter with energy-specific absorption characteristics due to the k-edge of the atomic structure of the element (k-edge filtration). The k-edge filter separates the X-ray distribution into two separate components of "high-energy" and "low-energy" photons (70 and 40 keV using cerium; 45 and 80 keV using a samarium filter) (Blake et al. 1999). Edge detection software is used to find the bone outline, and the pixels inside the bone edges are summed to find the bone area (BA) in cm^2. The BMD result reported on the scan printout is the average BMD measurement within the bone area. Finally, BMD is multiplied by BA to find the bone mineral content (BMC; g), equal to the total mass of hydroxyapatite within the bone region of interest (Blake et al. 2012). DXA therefore provides an areal (BMD), rather than a volumetric, density in g/cm^2. There is a depth of bone which cannot be taken into account from two-dimensional (2D) DXA images, which leads to DXA being size-dependent, a particular problem in growing children.

If a single-energy photon beam is used, which is only applicable to scanning of peripheral skeletal sites using dedicated peripheral scanners, then the site has to be placed in a water bath to allow correction for the overlying soft tissues.

3.1 Technical Developments

The original DXA scanners used a pencil X-ray beam and a single detector, and scanned in a rectilinear fashion across the anatomical site being examined. Scanning time was approximately 10–15 min per single site, and up to 30–40 min for whole-body scanning in a large patient. Technical developments in DXA have taken place over recent years. These include fan-beam X-ray sources and a bank of detectors. This allows faster scanning (approximately 1–2 min per site; similar times for whole-body scans) with improved image quality and spatial resolution (Eiken et al. 1994). The spatial resolution of DPA was 3 mm; that of third-generation DXA scanners is approximately 0.5–0.7 mm (Felsenberg et al. 1995; Kastl et al. 2002) and with current modern scanners spatial resolution is between 0.5 and 0.35 mm. With fan-beam scanners there is some magnification (approximately 7 %) in the horizontal plane, but not in the cranio-caudal plane. This magnification does not affect BMD, but there are significant differences in BMC, bone area and parameters of hip geometry. This can be corrected by performing two scans at different distances from the X-ray tube (Griffiths et al. 1997).

Lateral scanning for BMD in the lumbar spine is feasible, with the patient repositioned in the lateral decubitus position on scanners with fixed arms, and on scanners which have a "C" arm which rotates though 90° the patient can remain in the supine position. Such lateral spinal BMD is not often performed in clinical practice, because of the additional time required for repositioning and as L1 is often superimposed by rib and L4 by iliac crest, leaving only one or two vertebrae for assessment (Blake et al. 1996).

Postero-anterior and lateral scanning of the whole spine also became available for Vertebral Fracture Assessment (VFA) (Genant et al. 2000; Rea et al. 1998, 2000, 2001), and will be described in more detail in a later section.

3.2 Sites of Application and Measures Provided by DXA

DXA can be applied to sites of the skeleton where osteoporotic fractures occur; in the central skeleton this includes the lumbar spine (L1–4) (Fig. 1a, b) and proximal femur (total hip, femoral neck, trochanter and Ward's area) (Fig. 2a–c). Interpretation is currently made only from femoral neck and total hip. The spine and hip are chosen for interpretation because the hip is the most reliable measurement site for predicting hip fracture risk (Cummings et al. 1993; Marshall et al. 1996), femoral neck T-score is used in the WHO FRAX 10-year fracture risk calculator (World Health Organisation FRAX® 2010), the spine BMD is optimum for monitoring treatment (Faulkner 1998), and there is consensus that osteoporosis can be diagnosed in postmenopausal women in terms of DXA from spine and hip measurements using the WHO T-score definitions of osteoporosis and osteopenia (International Society for Clinical Densitometry 2007; National Osteoporosis Foundation 2010).

DXA can also be applied to peripheral skeletal sites (forearm and calcaneus), using either full-sized body (Fig. 3a–c), or dedicated peripheral, DXA scanners, although the latter are diminishing in availability and utilisation. Central DXA measures are currently used as the "gold standard" for the clinical diagnosis of osteoporosis by bone densitometry.

The measurements provided by DXA are BMC in grams, projected area of the measured site in cm^2 and BMD in g/cm^2. As the DXA image is a two-dimensional image of a three-dimensional object, this is an "areal", rather than a true volumetric, density; there is the depth of the bones, which cannot be taken into account with a single postero-anterior (PA) projection. This results in one of the limitations of DXA, as the measurement is size-dependent. This is a particular problem in children, in whom the bones change markedly in size during growth, especially during puberty, and in patients whose disease might result in their being small in stature or having slender, small bones (e.g. chronic illness, growth hormone deficiency, Turner's syndrome) (Gilsanz 1998; Blake et al. 2012; Adams 2013). To overcome this limitation to some extent, bone mineral apparent density (BMAD) can be calculated (Katzman et al. 1991). In the spine BMAD can be calculated assuming that the vertebra is a cube (Carter et al. 1992) or a cylinder (Kröger et al. 1993) and in the femoral neck assuming this is a cylinder (Lu et al. 1996).

If hyperparathyroidism (primary or secondary) is suspected a distal 1/3 radius measurement is relevant, a site at which cortical bone predominates (95 %), since cortical bone can be lost preferentially from this site in

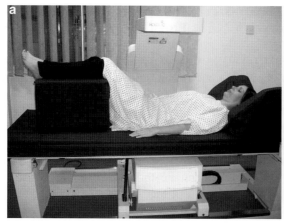
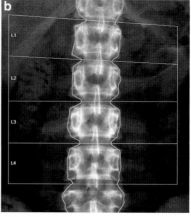

Fig. 1 *DXA of the lumbar spine.* **a** Patient positioned on DXA scanner (with fixed over-couch arm) for postero-anterior (PA – the X-ray source is below the table and the detectors in the scanning arm) for scanning of the lumbar spine. The legs are flexed at the hip and knee, and rest on a foam pad, to eliminate the natural lumbar lordosis so the spine is flat on the table. **b** DXA of normal lumbar spine L1–4. Measurements of BMC (g) and area (cm^2) are provided for each vertebra L1–4. Results are expressed as a mean "areal" density (g/cm^2) for all four vertebrae. For interpretation an appropriate race- and gender-matched reference database must be available (usually provided by the manufacturer of the scanner) and expressed as a standard deviation score (SD) from the mean of either mean peak bone mass PBM (T-score) or age-matched BMD (Z-score)

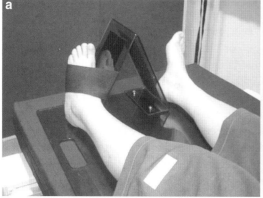
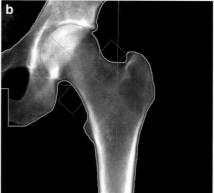
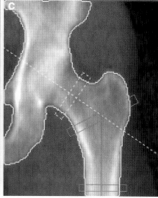

Fig. 2 *DXA of left hip.* **a** The leg is well positioned, being a little abducted and internally rotated, to bring the femoral neck parallel to the table, and with the foot secured on a positioner which is provided by the scanner manufacturer This position prevents foreshortening of the femoral neck (the lesser trochanter should not be prominently seen) which would cause falsely higher BMD. **b** Scan of left hip. Although "areal" bone mineral density (g/cm2) is provided in a number of different sites (femoral neck, *oblong box*; Ward's area, *small box*; trochanter and total hip), for clinical diagnosis femoral neck and total hip are used. The morphometric measure of the hip — hip axis length (HAL) is the length of the line drawn parallel and between the cortical margins of the femoral neck and extending from the inner margin of the bony pelvis to the lateral margin of the femur. An increase in this length has been found to be predictive of hip fracture. **c** Hip strength analysis (HAS), calculated from the distribution of bone mineral around a central axis in sites in the femoral neck, inter-trochanteric and proximal femoral shaft regions, can be measured. Biomechanical properties of stress strain index and moment of inertia can be derived automatically. DXA scans of the hip are not recommended in children as the femoral shape has not yet acquired the shape of that in an adult

hyperparathyroidism (Fig. 3c) (Wishart et al. 1990; Silverberg et al. 2009). The forearm scan is also a useful alternative site to scan when it is not possible to obtain a valid DXA measurement at the spine or hip. This occurs in patients with bilateral hip replacement, elderly patients with severe degenerative disease in the lumbar spine and patients whose weight exceeds the safety limit of the scanner.

With appropriate software whole-body scanning can also be performed, from which can be extracted whole-body and regional bone mineral content (BMC; gm) and body composition of lean muscle and fat mass (Fig. 4) (Pietrobelli et al. 1996; Tothill and Hannan 2000; Albanese et al. 2003; Schoeller et al. 2005; Chun 2011). Whole-body DXA (less head) is advocated in children with a growing skeleton in whom the adult hip scan may not be appropriate (Gordon et al. 2008; Lewiecki et al. 2008). There have recently been significant improvements in body composition measurements with the availability of the National Health and

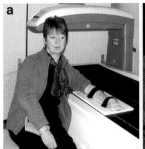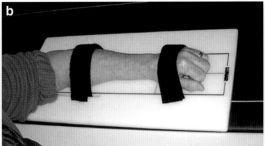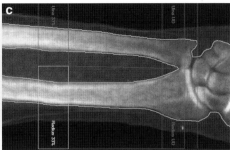

Fig. 3 *Peripheral DXA*. Can be obtained on dedicated peripheral DXA scanners, but are increasing being performed on central DXA scanners. **a** Positioning of patient and **b** arm pronated on the table. **c** DXA of the non-dominant forearm. The anatomical sites measured vary between scanners, but are generally the ultra-distal and distal 1/3.

The latter is 95 % cortical, is particularly pertinent in patients with hyperparathyroidism (primary and secondary), has good precision (CV = 1 %) and can be used if there are factors which preclude DXA at central sites (excessive weight)

Nutrition Examination Survey (NHANES) USA reference data which extends from 8 to 85 years. Additionally, measurements for android and gynoid region of interest can be extracted, and visceral adipose tissue estimated (Fig. 4) (Kelly et al. 2009; Micklesfield et al 2012).

3.3 Precision and Accuracy

Precision measures the reproducibility of a bone densitometry technique, and is usually expressed as a coefficient of variation (CV) or standardised CV, which takes into account the range of measurements of the particular method (Gluer et al. 1995). To be clinically useful the precision needs ideally to be in the region of 1 %, and certainly better than 3 %. The precision for total hip and lumbar spine is approximately 1 %; for femoral neck and trochanter CV it is 2.5 % and for Ward's area it is 2.5–5 %. In peripheral sites precision is 1 % in the distal radius, 2.5 % in the ultra-distal radius and 1.4 % in the calcaneus (Grampp et al. 1993; Pacheco et al. 2002; Shepherd et al. 2006). The measurement sites generally used in clinical diagnosis, in contrast to research studies, are therefore lumbar spine (L1–4), femoral neck and total hip (Kanis and Gluer 2000). Precision can be measured in either phantoms, normal individuals or in patients with osteoporosis. Precision is optimum in phantoms, and will be less good in patients with osteoporosis than in normal people, because positioning is more problematic in the former. Precision can be calculated by making repeat BMD measurements in the same individual after repositioning (usually a minimum of 10, but preferably 20 individuals or patients), although the International Society for Clinical Densitometry recommends 100 repeat scans (ISCD Position Development Conference—Writing Group 2004). Departments performing bone densitometry should ideally calculate their own precision but this is not always feasible. Precision is optimised by using

the minimum number of expert and highly motivated and well trained technical staff; it is not ideal to have a large number of staff who rotate through different departments and perform bone density scanning only infrequently.

Accuracy is how close the BMD measured by densitometry is to the actual calcium content of the bone (ash weight). The accuracy of DXA lies between 3 % and 8 %. The inaccuracies are related to marrow fat and DXA taking soft tissue as a reference (Tothill and Pye 1992; Blake et al. 1999; Blake et al. 2009). Although DXA measurements are affected by accuracy errors similar inaccuracies are present when other basic clinical measurements are made of blood pressure and body temperature (Blake et al. 2012).

Specificity is the ability of the measurement to discriminate between patients with and without fractures, and to measure small changes with time and/or treatment. A statistically significant change in BMD is calculated from the precision of the measurement technique. To reach a statistically significant change, the BMD has to increase or decrease by at least 2.77 times the precision error. This is termed the least significant change (LSC) and implies that changes in BMD of 3–4.5 % in the lumbar spine and total hip, and of 6–7.5 % in the femoral neck BMD (Gluer 1999; Bonnick et al. 2001) have to be present for change in BMD to be significant. Changes in bone density are generally small; even in the early post-menopausal period in women, when bone loss is greatest, bone density decrements may only be in the region of 1–2 % per annum. Therefore, when performing follow-up BMD measures in an individual patient it is essential to leave an adequate time interval between measures, usually 18–24 months (Gluer 1999), unless particularly large changes in BMD are expected, for example after large doses of oral glucocorticoids (International Society for Clinical Densitometry 2007).

Since whether a patient develops a fracture depends on factors in addition to BMD (whether the patient falls, the nature of the fall, the patient's age and response to the fall),

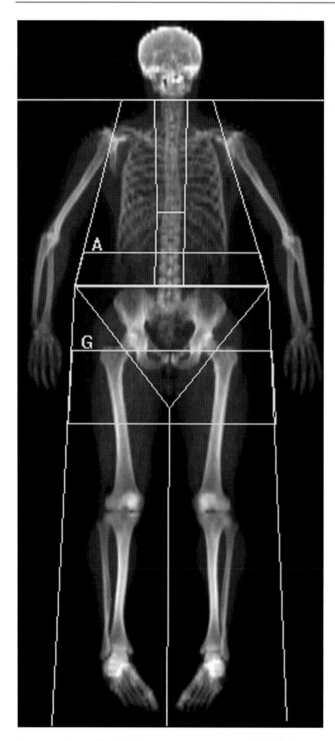

Fig. 4 *Whole-body DXA scan*: these can be acquired rapidly 1–2 min on fan beam DXA scanners, depending on patient size, and provides information on total and regional bone mineral content (BMC, g), area (cm²), bone mineral density (BMD; g/cm²) and body composition of lean muscle and fat mass. Sub-regional analyses are now available for body composition of the android (*rectangular box* below A) and gynoid (*rectangular box* below G) regions, and additionally visceral adipose tissue (VAT), which is found to correlate well with the measures made from cross-sectional CT

it is impossible for BMD techniques to completely discriminate between those with and without fractures (Stone et al. 2003). However, approximately 60–70 % of bone strength depends on BMD (Ammann and Rizzoli 2003), the lower the BMD the more at risk the patient is of suffering a fracture and fracture prediction is optimum from the site-specific DXA BMD measurement (Marshall et al. 1996).

3.4 Correlations

DXA provides an "areal" density (g/cm²) of integral (cortical and trabecular) bone. The cortical/trabecular ratios vary in different sites (Eastell et al. 1989; Faulkner et al. 1991), being approximately:

- 50/50 in the PA lumbar spine
- 10/90 in the lateral lumbar spine scan
- 60/40 in total hip
- 80/20 in total body
- 5/95 in calcaneus
- 95/5 in distal 1/3 radius
- 40/60 in ultra-distal radius (depending on site of region of interest).

As a result of the different composition of bones and rates of change in these various skeletal sites, it is not surprising that measurements in different sites in the same individual will not give the same results (Eastell et al. 1989). The correlations between the BMD measurements made in the same patient vary between $r = 0.4$ and $r = 0.9$; it is not possible to predict from a DXA BMD measurement made in one site, what the BMD will be in another site using DXA or other bone densitometry methods (Grampp et al. 1997). In research studies, BMD measurements in different anatomical sites and by various bone density methods (DXA, QCT, QUS) may be complementary.

3.5 Radiation Dose

These quantitative photon absorptiometric techniques involve very low radiation doses, which are similar to those of natural background radiation (NBR; 2400 μSv per annum; about 7 μSv per day) (Kalender 1992; Huda and Morin 1996; Blake et al. 2006; Damilakis et al. 2010) (Table 1). For the first-generation pencil-beam scanners the dose per site scanned was about 1 μSv, but the dose may be up to 6 μSv for the hip scan in pre-menopausal women, when the ovaries are included in the scan field (Lewis et al. 1994). The doses are a little higher for the fan-beam scanners (generally 3–9 μSv), but were up to 62 μSv with some scanners (Lunar Expert, which is no longer manufactured)

Table 1 Approximate ionising radiation doses of fan beam DXA and some comparable investigations used in osteoporosis

Examination	Site	Effective dose (µSv)	NBR	FC
DXA	Spine	13	2 day	<1 in few million
	Femur	9	1 day	<1 in few million
	Total body	5	17 h	<1 in few million
Vertebral fracture assessment (DXA VFA)	Spine: Single energy	12	2 days	1 in 1 million
	Dual energy	42	6 days	1 in 1 million
Radiographs	Hand	<1	<1 h	<1 in few million
	Chest Lumbar spine	20 700–1000	3 days 7 months	1 in 1 million 1 in 200,000
Return flight UK/USA		80	12 days	
Background radiation		7–20 per day (2400–7300 per year)		

NBR natural background radiation; FC fatal cancer risk. Doses will be higher in children. Data drawn from reference Damilakis et al. 2010

(Eiken et al. 1994; Njeh et al. 1996). Radiation doses for forearm and calcaneus scans are extremely low (0.5 and 0.03 µSv respectively). These DXA doses are less than one-quarter of the dose of a chest radiograph (20 µSv), and considerably lower than doses involved in other radiographic examinations carried out to confirm the diagnosis of osteoporosis in patients at risk; lateral spinal radiographs involve doses in the region of 300–700 µSv per projection, depending on patient size and exposure factors (Damilakis et al. 2010).

4 Indications, Including WHO FRAX®

There has been much debate concerning the appropriate use of bone densitometry, particularly in population screening in women at menopause (Melton et al. 1990), and the cost-effectiveness of such a programme has not been established. However, there is now consensus that DXA bone densitometry is the quantitative method of choice for the diagnosis of osteoporosis before fractures occur (Compston et al. 1995; Kanis et al. 1997, 2009; Adams 2013). DXA

Table 2 Factors used in the WHO FRAX® 10 year fracture calculator

- Country or geographic region
- Ethnic origin (US only)
- Age
- Gender
- Weight (kg) and height (cm) (BMI)
- Previous low trauma fracture in adult life
- Parental hip fracture
- Current smoking
- Current or past oral glucocorticoid therapy (≥5mg for >3 months)
- Rheumatoid arthritis
- Secondary osteoporosis*
- Alcohol intake ≥3 units daily

+/- DXA femoral neck BMD (scanner manufacturer specified)
  BMI body mass index; BMD bone mineral density
*Secondary causes of osteoporosis: type I (insulin dependent) diabetes, osteogenesis imperfecta in adults, untreated long-standing hyperthyroidism, hypogonadism or premature menopause (<45 years), chronic malnutrition, or malabsorption and chronic liver disease

bone densitometry has high specificity but low sensitivity. Selection of patients who would most appropriately be referred for DXA bone densitometry was in the past based on a case-finding strategy in those who have had an insufficiency (low trauma) fracture or have other strong risk factors (Royal College of Physicians 1999), and there were national differences in such referral guidelines.

A new approach for appropriate DXA scan referral and interpretation was introduced by the World Health Organisation (WHO) in 2010. This tool is based on using clinical risk factors (Table 2), with or without femoral neck BMD, to estimate a patient's 10-year probability of a fracture at the hip or one of the major osteoporotic sites (Johnell et al. 2005; Kanis et al. 2007; Compston 2009a). The latter are defined as the hip, spine, forearm and humerus. The FRAX WHO fracture risk assessment tool is accessed using the web site http://www.shef.ac.uk/FRAX (World Health Organisation 2010), is applicable in women and men aged 40–90 years, is currently available for use in 30 different countries and has been incorporated into manufacturers' DXA scan reports (Fig. 5a, b). The FRAX algorithm was developed from data based on meta-analyses from nine different international (North America, Europe and Asia) fracture studies. These included 46,000 men and women with 190,000 person-years of follow-up, and 850 cases of hip fracture and 3,300 other osteoporotic fractures (Kanis et al. 2007; Blake et al. 2012). FRAX is increasingly being incorporated into guidelines on the appropriate referral for DXA and treatment of osteoporosis, but these vary between nations. In the United States the National Osteoporosis Foundation (NOF) has added FRAX to the criteria for

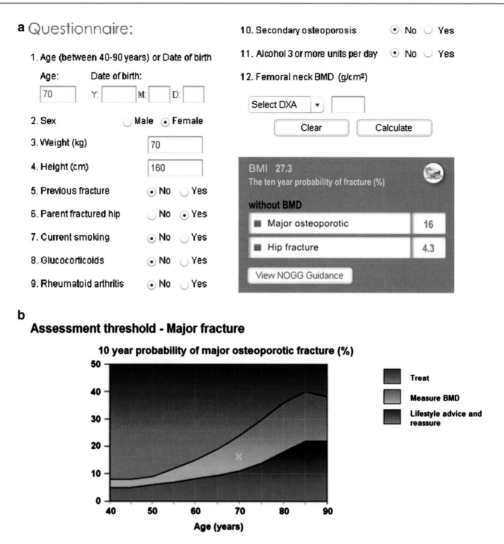

a Questionnaire:

1. Age (between 40-90 years) or Date of birth

Age: 70   Date of birth: Y: ___ M: ___ D: ___

2. Sex   Male ⦿ Female

3. Weight (kg)   70

4. Height (cm)   160

5. Previous fracture   ⦿ No   ○ Yes

6. Parent fractured hip   ○ No   ⦿ Yes

7. Current smoking   ⦿ No   ○ Yes

8. Glucocorticoids   ⦿ No   ○ Yes

9. Rheumatoid arthritis   ⦿ No   ○ Yes

10. Secondary osteoporosis   ⦿ No   ○ Yes

11. Alcohol 3 or more units per day   ⦿ No   ○ Yes

12. Femoral neck BMD (g/cm²)

Select DXA ▾   ___

[Clear]   [Calculate]

BMI 27.3
The ten year probability of fracture (%)

without BMD

Major osteoporotic	16
Hip fracture	4.3

View NOGG Guidance

b
Assessment threshold - Major fracture

10 year probability of major osteoporotic fracture (%)

Treat

Measure BMD

Lifestyle advice and reassure

Fig. 5 WHO FRAX® 10 year fracture risk calculator: **a** this can be accessed at http://www.shef.ac.uk/FRAX and the fracture risk for patients aged between 40–90 years can be calculated using clinical risk factors alone, or with the addition of femoral neck BMD, with knowledge of the DXA scanner manufacturer. The risk for major osteoporotic fractures, (defined as the hip, spine, forearm or humerus) and hip fracture are calculated and guidelines determine appropriate management interventions. These may vary between nations. The National Osteoporosis Foundation (NOF) in the USA has criteria for treating patients using therapeutic threshold fracture risk levels of 3 % for hip fracture and 20 % for a major osteoporotic fracture (National Osteoporosis Foundation 2010). **b** The tool can be used with just clinical risk factors and guidelines (National Osteoporosis Guidelines group NOGG in UK) will indicate if DXA scan should be performed. Consequently FRAX should lead to a more appropriate utilization of DXA scanning and results, and more cost effective intervention strategies

treating patients using therapeutic threshold fracture risk levels of 3 % for hip fracture and 20 % for a major osteoporotic fracture (National Osteoporosis Foundation 2010). In the United Kingdom a different treatment algorithm was produced by the National Osteoporosis Guidelines Group (NOGG), which recommended that FRAX is used to select the patients who would most appropriately be referred for a DXA scan (Kanis et al. 2008; Compston et al. 2009) (Fig. 5a, b). FRAX should lead to a more appropriate utilisation of DXA scanning and results, and more cost-effective intervention strategies (Johansson et al. 2012). Whether other clinical risk factors and additional quantitative skeletal assessments can be added to the FRAX calculator is being explored (Binkley and Lewiecki 2010; Lewiecki et al. 2011).

5   Positioning, Artefacts and Errors

5.1   Patient Positioning

For measurement of the lumbar spine the patient is positioned supine on the scanner table with the legs flexed at the hips and knees and the calves resting on a square pad

(Fig. 1a). This removes the natural lumbar lordosis, so that the lumbar spine lies flat on the scanner table. For scanning of the proximal femur the leg is slightly abducted and internally rotated and fixed to a shaped block provided by the scanner manufacturer (Fig. 2a). This ensures that the femoral neck is parallel to the table to avoid foreshortening. Any foreshortening will result in false elevation of BMD (same amount of calcium in reduced area) (Fig. 6d), and poor positioning of the femur can result in errors in BMD of the femoral neck of 0.95–4.5 % (Wilson et al. 1991; Goh et al. 1995). For whole-body DXA, the technician must ensure that all parts of the body, including arms and hands, are positioned inside the marker line on the scanner table.

For scanning of the forearm on a central DXA scanner the hand is pronated and the arm and hand are positioned flat on the scanner table (Fig. 3a and b). In dedicated peripheral scanners the forearm is scanned in a vertical position with the hand gripping a short vertical pole to ensure reproducible positioning. The non-dominant forearm is generally scanned unless there are contraindications to this, such as a previous fracture or metal artefact, when the dominant forearm is scanned. For measurements of the calcaneus on a dedicated peripheral DXA scanner the foot is positioned in a foot well, as prescribed by the manufacturer of the equipment; on a central DXA scanner the patient is placed in the lateral decubitus position on the side of the calcaneus to be examined so that a lateral calcaneus scan can be obtained.

5.2 Artefacts

Imaging artefacts can cause inaccuracies in DXA measurements (Fig. 6a–d). They are most common in the lumbar spine, particularly in more elderly patients (Table 3). All the calcium in the path of the X-ray beam will contribute to the BMD measured. If there is heavy aortic calcification, degenerative disc disease (osteophytes, osteoarthritis and hyperostosis of the facet joints) or a vertebral fracture (in which the same amount of calcium as was present before the fracture occurred is contained in the vertebra which is reduced in area following fracture) present, then the BMD will be falsely elevated (Orwoll et al. 1990, Frohn et al. 1991, Laskey et al. 1993, Franck et al. 1995, Jaovisidha et al. 1997). Other aetiologies can also cause false elevation or underestimation of BMD measured by DXA (Table 3) (Fig. 6a–c). It is therefore essential that all DXA images be scrutinised for such artefacts. The vertebra affected significantly by artefact should be excluded from analysis, but there must be a minimum of two vertebrae assessable for interpretation. Anomalies in spinal segmentation may be quite frequent (16.5 %), and may cause the vertebral bodies to be misidentified (Peel et al. 1993). Approximately 50 % of the increment in BMD with

Table 3 DXA artefacts causing errors in estimation of BMD

Artefacts causing overestimation of BMD:
Spinal degeneration and hyperostosis (osteophytes)
Vertebral fracture
Extraneous calcification (lymph nodes, aortic calcification)
Sclerotic metastases
Overlying metal (clips, coins, navel rings, surgical rods)
Overlying objects (wallets, buttons)
Vertebral haemangioma
Ankylosing spondylitis with paravertebral ossification
Strontium ranelate therapy
Vertebroplasty/kyphoplasty
Poor positioning of femoral neck (inadequate internal rotation)
Artefacts causing underestimation of BMD:
Laminectomy
Lytic metastases
Barium contrast medium in bowel
Recent radionuclide investigation

strontium ranelate treatment will be artifactual due to the high atomic number strontium being taken up in the bone, and effects may differ between different manufacturer's scanners (Blake et al. 2007; Liao et al. 2010). Laminectomy will cause DXA BMD to be falsely reduced and affected vertebrae must be excluded. DXA will also not differentiate low BMD being due to osteoporosis or osteomalacia.

To overcome the problems of degenerative disc disease and hyperostosis in PA DXA of the spine, lateral DXA has been developed (Fig. 7c). On scanners with "C" arms lateral scanning can be performed with the patient remaining in the supine position; otherwise the patient has to be repositioned in the lateral decubitus position, which limits its clinical practicality and precision ($CV = 2.8$–5.9 % in lateral decubitus position, 1.6 %–2 % in the supine position). L3 may be the only vertebra in which lateral DXA can be measured, as there may be superimposition of ribs over L1 and L2 and the iliac crest over L4. So although lateral DXA may be a more sensitive predictor of vertebral fracture than PA spinal DXA as it is principally measuring trabecular BMD and is less affected by degenerative spine changes than is the PA scan projection, the limited precision and impracticality has resulted in lateral DXA BMD not often performed in clinical practice (Guglielmi et al. 1994; Del Rio et al. 1995; Jergas et al. 1995; Blake et al 1996).

Because of these artefacts on PA DXA scans of the lumbar spine, it has been suggested that in the more elderly population (over 65 years) only the proximal femur (femoral neck, total hip) should be scanned (Kanis and Gluer 2000). However, monitoring change is performed optimally in the lumbar spine, if there are no artefacts present.

Fig. 6 *Artefacts on DXA*: lumbar spine. **a** Degenerative disc disease and marginal osteophytes on the right: falsely elevated BMD at L2/3 and L3/4. **b** Vertebral fracture of L1. BMD at this level will be falsely elevated (same BMC as non-fractured vertebra, but in a smaller projected area, giving higher apparent BMD). **c** Laminectomy L4. The removal of the laminae and spinous process will falsely reduce the BMD of this vertebra. The DXA images must always be carefully scrutinised for such artefacts, and the affected vertebra excluded from analysis. There must be a minimum of at least two vertebrae for diagnosis; interpretation should not be made on a single vertebra. If a vertebral fracture has occurred between sequential DXA measurements, then the results from that vertebra must be excluded from all scans to calculate longitudinal change in BMD. **d** Proximal femur: the lesser trochanter is prominent, indicating inadequate internal rotation of the femur. This external rotation of the leg will cause foreshortening of the femoral neck and hence overestimation of BMD (same BMC as well-positioned femoral neck, in a smaller projected area)

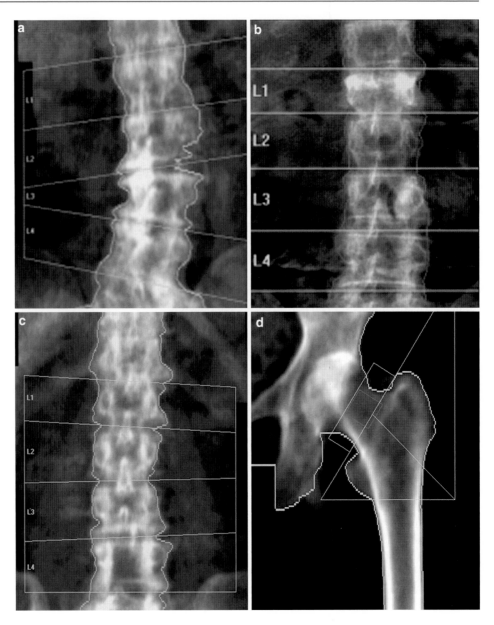

As DXA makes some assumptions about the composition of soft tissue adjacent to the skeletal site in which BMD is being measured inaccuracies may occur when excessive obesity, or underweight in patients with anorexia, are present. Excessive weight changes between DXA scans performed for monitoring BMD will also introduce inaccuracies and affect precision; but how such inaccuracies should be corrected for is not yet established.

5.3 Sources of Error

Spinal scoliosis may make DXA scans of the spine difficult to analyse, and it may prove impossible to perform DXA if the patient is not able to lie flat (e.g. if the patient is in cardiac failure or has severe chronic obstructive airways disease or thoracic kyphosis), or if pain or deformity makes positioning problematic.

As DXA uses the soft tissues as a reference, errors in BMD can arise if the patient is excessively under- or overweight. Some manufacturers (GE/Lunar) used to apply a weight correction to the results provided (Z score), but such weight correction should not now be applied. Precision errors increase in obese patients (Knapp et al. 2012).

6 Interpretation of Results

When a BMD measurement has been made in a patient, this has to be interpreted as normal or abnormal and a report formulated that will be of assistance to the referring clinician (Miller et al. 1996). For this it is essential that age-, sex- and racially matched reference data are available. The scanner manufacturer supplies such normal reference databases. These databases are predominantly, but not exclusively, drawn from a white, Caucasian, American-based population. There is a paucity of appropriate reference ranges for children and certain ethnic minorities (e.g. Asians; Afro-Caribbean). A patient's results can be interpreted in terms of the standard deviations (SD) from the mean of either sex-matched peak bone mass (PBM) (T-score) or age-matched BMD (Z-score) (Parfitt 1990). Alternative methods of interpretation are as a percentage or percentile of expected PBM, either gender- and age-matched or just gender-matched.

The WHO has defined osteoporosis in terms of bone densitometry. A T-score of less than −2.5 defines osteoporosis (World Health Organisation 1994). This was arbitrarily defined as the level of BMD in post-menopausal women that identified approximately 30 % of that population as having osteoporosis in their lifetime (this is thought to be the percentage of post-menopausal women who will suffer a vertebral fracture in their lifetime). The definition applied to DXA measurements made in the lumbar spine, the proximal femur and the forearm. The definition does not apply to other techniques (e.g. QCT, QUS) or other anatomical sites (e.g. calcaneus) (Grampp et al. 1997; Faulkner et al. 1999; Miller 2000), nor is it yet confirmed to be applicable to younger women and men.

T-scores are calculated by taking the difference between a patient's measured BMD and the mean BMD in healthy young adults matched for gender and ethnicity, and expressing the difference relative to the young adult population SD:

$$\text{T-score} = \frac{\text{Measured BMD} - \text{Young adult mean BMD}}{\text{Young adult population SD}}$$

A T-score measurement of less than, or equal to, −2.5 at the spine, distal 1/3 radius, femoral neck or total hip sites is taken to indicate osteoporosis. Measurements between −2.5 and −1.0 are interpreted as indicating osteopenia, while measurements greater than −1.0 at all three sites are classified as normal (World health Organisation 1994). A limitation of this T-score method for making decisions about patient therapies is that factors such as age and a history of previous insufficiency fracture are independent risk factors that are as important as BMD in determining the 10-year risk of fracture. In the FRAX fracture risk calculator a selected list of clinical risk factors (Table 2) is used together with femoral neck BMD to improve fracture risk prediction.

Z-scores compare the patient's BMD with the mean BMD for a healthy subject matched for age, gender and ethnicity (International Society for Clinical Densitometry 2007; Chun 2011).

$$\text{Z-score} = \frac{\text{Measured BMD} - \text{Age matched mean BMD}}{\text{Age matched population SD}}$$

Until PBM has been reached (i.e. in children and young adults up to approximately 19 years) interpretation can be made only by comparison to the age-matched mean (Z-score) (Faulkner et al. 1993b; Gordon et al. 2008).

BMD measurements in the whole skeleton can be performed using total body scans (Nuti and Martini 1992). These are usually interpreted after excluding the head from the scan analysis, particularly in children (Lewiecki et al. 2008; Ward et al. 2007).

Variations in the mean and standard deviation of reference ranges may alter the number of patients identified as osteoporotic (Ahmed et al. 1997); in DXA of the hip, use of the NHANES reference database is preferred for white Caucasians (Looker et al. 1998).

In calculating change over time, the absolute BMD values (g/cm^2) have to be used. To be statistically significant the change in BMD has to be 2.77 times greater than the precision to reach the least significant change (LSC); in longitudinal studies in individual patients one needs to leave an intervening period of at least 18–24 months between measures to ensure significant change in individual patients (Gluer 1999).

7 Applications

7.1 Clinical

7.1.1 Diagnosis of Osteoporosis

Osteoporosis is defined as "a condition characterised by reduced bone mass and deterioration of bone structure". It is the most common of the metabolic bone diseases, affecting 1 in 3 women and 1 in 12 men during their lifetime. DXA is currently the most widely available bone densitometric technique for the diagnosis of osteoporosis, although its availability in different countries varies (Chun 2011; Guglielmi et al. 2011; Adams 2013). Central DXA scanners cost approximately 80,000 EUR to 120,000 EUR, depending on the sophistication and versatility of scan functions; dedicated peripheral DXA scanners are less expensive (approximately 30,000 EUR), smaller and portable, with the potential for use in a community rather than a hospital setting. For clinical diagnosis the lumbar spine and proximal femur are scanned; forearm scanning can be performed on either central or dedicated peripheral scanners. Although the ionising radiation from these DXA scanners is low, ionising radiation regulations apply to their installation and operation. Dedicated and highly motivated technical staff with appropriate training will ensure high quality of positioning of the patient and good precision of the results.

Table 4 Relative risk (RR) of fracture per 1 SD decrease in BMD (measured by photon absorptiometry) below age-adjusted mean (Marshall et al. 1996)

BMD site	Forearm	Hip	Vertebral	All
Radius, distal	1.8	2.1	2.2	1.5
Radius, ultradistal	1.7	1.8	1.7	1.4
Hip	1.4	2.6	1.8	1.6
Lumbar spine	1.5	1.6	2.3	1.5
Calcaneum	1.6	2.0	2.4	1.5
All	1.6	2.0	2.1	1.5

Different manufacturers use different edge detection algorithms and analyse different ROIs for analysis in the hip. For this reason, results from different scanners are not interchangeable. In longitudinal studies it is vital to use the same scanner and software program. With technical developments it may become necessary to replace a scanner. In order to cross-calibrate between the old and the new scanner, scanning patients (approximately 100, with a spread of BMD from high to low) and phantoms (manufacturers or European Spine Phantom) will generally allow the required calculations to be made (Genant et al. 1994; Kalender et al. 1995; Hui et al. 1997; International Society for Clinical Densitometry 2004).

7.1.2 Prediction of Fracture

DXA BMD measurements made in any skeletal site (central and peripheral) are predictive of fracture (Marshall et al. 1996), with the risk of fracture increased in individuals with the lower BMD, but it is impossible to define a specific fracture threshold (Siris et al. 2004). The relative risk of fracture in various skeletal sites for every 1SD reduction in age-adjusted mean BMD were published in a meta-analysis study and are given in (Table 4) (Marshall et al. 1996). This reduction in BMD in predicting fracture is as good as a rise of 1SD in blood pressure is in predicting stroke, and a 1SD rise in cholesterol is in predicting myocardial infarction. Site-specific measurements are best in predicting fracture in that particular anatomical place.

7.1.3 Decisions for Treatment

Although there is consensus on the definition of osteoporosis (T-score at, or below, –2.5), there is as yet no consensus on levels of BMD which justify therapeutic intervention. This is perhaps not surprising, since it is the individual patient that is being treated, not the bone density result. Other risk factors including age, gender, parental history of osteoporosis, history of insufficiency fractures, oral glucocorticoid therapy, cigarette smoking, alcohol consumption, associated diseases that cause secondary osteoporosis will influence fracture risk and appropriate

management. These clinical risk factors are used in the WHO FRAX 10-year fracture risk calculator which therefore makes referral for DXA bone densitometry and therapeutic intervention more appropriate through various international national guidelines (Compston et al. 2009; National Osteoporosis Foundation 2010) (Fig. 5b).

Other guidelines have been published as to the appropriate use and interpretation of DXA in glucocorticoid therapy (Compston 2010b), and when aromatase inhibitors are used in patients with breast cancer (Reid et al. 2008), which may have different T-score intervention thresholds recommended: T-scores: glucocorticoids below −1.5; breast cancer on aromatase inhibitors below −2.0.

7.1.4 Monitoring Change with Time and Treatment

There is controversy as to whether DXA should be used to monitor change in BMD to assess efficacy of therapeutic interventions such as bisphosphonates, in which response of bone turnover markers will confirm effect in 3-4 months, whereas a significant change in BMD may take 18–24 months (Compston 2009b; Lewiecki et al. 2010). Despite this debate DXA is widely used to monitor the change in BMD to access disease progression and the efficacy of therapy in clinical practice (Bonnick et al. 2001; Bell et al. 2009). As the rate of change in BMD, under most circumstances, is relatively slow, it is essential that an adequate interval of time exists between BMD assessments (Gluer 1999). A statistically significant change in BMD has to be greater than 2.77 times the precision of the technique. The rate of change will vary at different skeletal sites, and will be influenced by the ratio of cortical to trabecular bone, as trabecular bone is some eightfold more metabolically active than cortical bone (Eastell et al. 1989). As the distal forearm is predominantly cortical bone, this is not a sensitive site for monitoring change in BMD (Bouxsein et al. 1999); however, bone may be lost preferentially from this site in parathyroid overactivity (Wishart et al. 1990; Silverberg et al. 2009). DXA of the lumbar spine and total hip (precision 1 %) are generally used for monitoring change, and an interval of approximately 2 years should be left between measurements, unless rapid loss of bone is suspected. Excessive changes in weight between measurements may account for apparent changes in BMD (Patel et al. 1997).

7.1.5 Vertebral Fracture Assessment and Aortic Calcification Scoring

Lateral views of the thoracic and lumbar spine (T4–L4) can be obtained with fan-beam scanners, using dual- or single-energy scanning, and with the patient either in the supine ("C" arm scanners) or lateral decubitus position (Fig. 7a, b, d). Single (SE) and dual energy (DE) images can be acquired, but differently between scanner manufacturers; simultaneously in

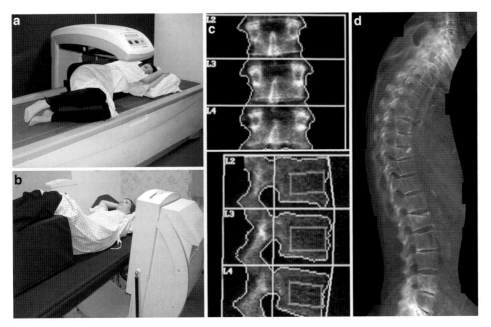

Fig. 7 *Lateral DXA of the spine for BMD measurement, vertebral fracture assessment (VFA) and abdominal aortic calcification (AAC) scoring.* **a** With a scanner with a fixed arm the patient has to be repositioned in the lateral decubitus position to enable lateral scanning to be performed. This repositioning takes additional time, and may be problematic in patients with osteoporosis. **b** On scanners with a "C" arm this can be rotated (as illustrated) to allow lateral scanning of the patient in the supine position without repositioning. **c** Bone densitometry, PA (*upper* image) and lateral (*lower* image) projections. From such scanning in two planes some calculations can be made to calculate true volumetric BMD (g/cm3). The lateral DXA gives a measurement that is predominantly trabecular bone (*oblong box*) and is therefore is not so affected by degenerative spinal changes as is the PA measurement. However, the ribs may overlie L1 and L2, and the iliac crest may overlie L4, leaving only one vertebra (L3) for analysis. The precision of BMD measurement from lateral spinal DXA is also poorer than for PA DXA, so that it is not often used in clinical

practice. **d** *Vertebral fracture assessment*: grade 2 moderate vertebral fractures at T 9 and L1, grade 1 mild endplate fractures of T6 and T8 and spindylosis evident at l4/5 and L5/S1. With the introduction of fan-beam DXA the spatial resolution of the images has improved (approximately 0.35–0.5 mm) and scan times are shorter. It is possible to obtain a lateral view of the vertebrae from approximately T4 to L4 with single- and dual-energy images. A visual assessment can be made for vertebral fracture, or vertebral shape can be defined by morphometric assessment with 6 point placements on the anterior, mid and posterior edges of the upper and lower vertebral endplates. *Abdominal aortic calcification (AAC) scoring*: calcification is present anterior to the lumbar vertebrae L1-4; this can be scored by either the 8 or 24 point scale. AAC has been found to be independently associated with incident myocardial infarction or stroke in women and so offers an opportunity to capture this cardiovascular risk factor in postmenopausal women undergoing bone densitometry, at very little additional cost

a single pass with General Electric Lunar (Madison, WI, USA) scanners and separately with scanners manufactured by Hologic (Bedford, MA, USA). DE images are superior to SE images to visualise vertebrae in the thoracic spine. The identification of vertebral fractures, which may be clinically silent, is important as it is a relevant entry into the FRAX tool (previous fracture), and there is enhanced prediction of fracture risk when combining vertebral fracture status and BMD (Siris et al. 2007).

The advantages of VFA are that the entire spine is visualised on a single lateral image (in contrast to spinal radiographs in which two separate images are acquired in the thoracic and lumbar spine with appropriate overlap at the thoraco-lumbar junction to enable vertebral levels to be counted). From these vertebral fracture assessment (VFA) images a visual assessment can be made as to whether or not vertebral fractures are present, and the images have the potential for morphometric assessment of vertebral shape

(Genant et al. 2000; Rea et al. 1998, 2000, 2001; Guglielmi et al. 2008). The latter is currently time-consuming, with the requirement of considerable operator interaction, and so is not often used in clinical practice. Such morphometric analysis has the potential for automation by the application of computer analysis techniques (active shape models; active appearance models) that may make them more practical for use in a clinical setting (Smyth et al. 1999; Roberts et al. 2007; Roberts et al. 2010). DXA VFA is being increasingly applied to identify vertebral fracture in clinical practice (Link et al. 2005; Diacinti et al. 2012) and research studies (Fuerst et al. 2009), although VFA under-performed in the identification of mild grade 1 vertebral fractures when compared to spinal radiographs (Fuerst et al. 2009). However, spatial resolution has improved in recent years with improvement in vertebral fracture diagnosis by VFA (Diacinti et al. 2012). VFA has several advantages over conventional radiography, including exposing the patient to a lower dose of ionising radiation (approximately 40 μSv compared to around 700 μSv per projection for spinal radiographs) (Damilakis et al. 2010) and avoiding the problems resulting from the divergent X-ray beam of radiography that can distort vertebral shape ('bean can' effect), causing apparent bi-concavity of the endplates (Lewis and Blake 1995). DXA uses a lateral scan projection method, with simultaneous movement of the X-ray source and detectors along the spine, so the projection is always parallel to the vertebral endplates. The ISCD has issued guidelines as to the appropriate use of VFA (Vokes et al. 2006; Schousboe et al. 2008a). The method has been shown to be satisfactory for excluding the presence of vertebral fractures (Rea et al. 2000). However, more scientific studies are required to establish the exact clinical role of this alternative technology to conventional spinal radiography for the identification of vertebral fractures (Blake et al. 2012).

Abdominal aortic calcification scoring: an additional measurement which can be made from DXA images is abdominal aortic calcification (AAC) scoring (Fig. 7d) (Schousboe et al. 2006; Bazzocchi et al. 2012). AAC from VFA images has been found to be independently associated with incident myocardial infarction or stroke in women and so offers an opportunity to capture this cardiovascular risk factor in postmenopausal women undergoing bone densitometry, at very little additional cost (Schousboe et al. 2008b). There has also been found to be good agreement in AAC scoring made from VFA images and digital radiographs with areas under receiver operating characteristics (ROC) curves for VFA to detect those with a radiographic 24-point AAC score of greater than, or equal to' 5 were 0.86 (95 % C.I. 0.77–0.94) using the 24-point scale method and 0.84 (95 % C.I. 0.76–0.92) using the AAC-8 scale methods (Schousboe et al. 2007).

8 Research; Extended Use of DXA

There are other scanning options on central DXA scanners, which currently remain as research applications, as their role in clinical practice has not been established (Adams 2013). These include *whole-body DXA* in adults for total and regional BMC, lean and fat mass (Pietrobelli et al. 1996; Tothill and Hannan 2000) (Fig. 4a). In children whole-body DXA less head is advocated in routine clinical practice (Gordon et al. 2008). Software programs are available for measuring BMD around prostheses following hip and knee arthroplasty (Soininvaara et al. 2000; Wilkinson et al. 2001), but have not been widely applied. There is an increasing demand for dedicated software programs for DXA in bone specimens and small experimental animals in which scanning is now feasible (Griffin et al. 1993, Kastl et al. 2002); however, high resolution QCT is applied more

widely to these applications now. Applications of DXA to other established and novel anatomical sites (hand, mandible) have been described (Horner et al. 1996). Although there may be no specific commercial software program available for scanning such sites, programs available for scanning conventional sites (e.g. forearm) can be used, with analysis being performed by hand-placed ROIs; these would not be as precise as automated ROIs.

Hip axis length (HAL) is the length of the line which runs parallel to the cortices of the femoral neck and from the inner pelvic margin to the lateral margin of the femoral shaft below the greater trochanter (Fig. 2c). HAL was measured in women in the study of osteoporotic fracture (SOF) and for each SD increase in HAL there was almost a doubling of the risk of hip fracture with odds ratio = 1.8; 95 % CI 1.3, 2.5) (Faulkner et al. 1993a). Using the automated method of measurement now available on scanners the mean HAL in women was 10.5 cm; an HAL of 11.0 cm was associated with a twofold increase in hip fracture risk and one of 11.6 cm increased hip fracture risk by a factor of 4 (Faulkner et al. 1994). There will be some magnification of the hip geometry with fan-beam scanners, so that corrections have to be applied (Young et al. 2000).

Hip strength analysis (HSA) makes certain assumptions from DXA images about the distribution of mineral (cortical, mg) in the proximal femur in the neck, inter-trochanteric and proximal femoral shaft regions, providing cross-sectional area (CSA) from which a biomechanical parameter (cross-sectional moment of inertia [CSMI]) is extracted (Fig. 2b) (Beck 2007). These parameters measured from HSA compared favourably with those derived from volumetric QCT, supporting the validity of these DXA-derived geometrical properties of the proximal hip (Prevrhal et al. 2008). Advantages of HSA are that bone geometry and BMD, both of which contribute to bone strength, are taken into account, it can be applied retrospectively to DXA hip scans previously acquired and analysis is automated. However, HSA is limited to evaluating bending strength in the 2D plane of the DXA image, so precision is sensitive to consistent femur positioning (Beck 2007; Bouxsein and Karasik 2006). Body-size scaling is critically important when interpreting bone geometry, and the application of HSA to the hip DXA scans in young children, in whom the shape of the proximal femur does not yet resemble that in the adult, may provide results which are of questionable validity.

Femoral neck angle or Neck Shaft Angle (NSA) (Fig. 2c) can be measured but few data have investigated its application and in one study it was found not to be useful in prediction of hip fracture (Tuck et al. 2011). With the application of modern computer vision techniques (active appearance models [AAM] and active shape models [ASM]) studies have found that adding proximal femoral shape to hip DXA BMD improved hip fracture prediction from 82 to 90 % (Gregory et al. 2004; Gregory et al. 2005). However, whether such additional factors extracted from DXA scans will be applied widely in clinical practice for diagnosis of osteoporosis is still to be established.

Trabecular Bone Score (TBS) has recently been introduced to extract further information from PA DXA scans of the lumbar spine. The technique uses a greyscale, texture-based computer analysis which it is claimed is related to trabecular structure. The method was validated in a study in which 30 cadaver vertebrae were imaged by micro-computed tomography (isotropic resolution 92 μm) (Hans et al. 2011a). TBS was found to correlate with the various 3D parameters of bone micro-architecture (positively with connectivity and trabecular number; negatively with trabecular spacing and solid volume fraction [Bone volume/total volume] in combination with trabecular thickness), independent of any correlation between TBS and BMD. TBS was applied retrospectively to the Manitoba Study; both TBS and BMD were significantly lower in patients with major osteoporotic, spine and hip fractures, and TBS and BMD predicted fractures equally well (Hans et al. 2011b). TBS shows potential for fracture prediction from rapid and retrospective analysis of DXA spine images, after relevant calibration of the DXA scanner from which the images have been acquired. However, there are limitations, such as the effect of spondylosis, and for spatial resolution and technical reasons, the TBS correlates with, but does not measure, bone microarchitecture (Bousson et al. 2012). Data are sparse and further studies are required to determine the clinical and research applications and relevance of the technique (Bousson et al. 2012).

Research studies may involve different scanners in multiple centres. To make the results comparable it is necessary to cross-calibrate between scanners with phantoms such as the European Spine Phantom or others (Kalender et al. 1995). To combine results from different scanners, standardised bone mineral density (sBMD) is provided by most manufacturers or can be calculated (Nord 1992; Genant et al. 1994; Kalender et al. 1995; Hui et al. 1997). In bone densitometry generally, and in research studies in particular, quality assurance programmes must be rigorous (Faulkner and McClung 1995; Damilakis and Guglielmi 2010; Guglielmi et al. 2012).

9 Peripheral DXA

An increasing number of small, portable DXA scanners did become available for application to peripheral sites, generally the forearm and the calcaneus. The peripheral DXA (pDXA) scanners had several advantages over central DXA scanners in that they were smaller, portable and lower in costs and ionising radiation doses. BMD measurements in these sites are as predictive of fractures in all sites, and equally as strongly related to clinical risk fractures, as the more conventional DXA measurements in central sites (Table 4) (Patel et al. 2007). The forearm measurements are particularly predictive of wrist fractures; the calcaneus measurements are particularly predictive of spine fractures, even in the elderly, in whom spinal DXA is confounded by degenerative disease (Cheng et al. 1997; Marshall et al. 1996; National Osteoporosis Society 2001). For monitoring change in BMD, the forearm site, being predominantly cortical bone, is not a sensitive site; the calcaneus, being 95 % trabecular bone, offers more potential for this purpose.

Although the WHO criterion for the diagnosis of osteoporosis (T-scores less than −2.5) is applicable to the forearm, it is not to the calcaneus. T-scores between −1.0 and −1.5 for BMD in the calcaneus have been suggested as more appropriate in this site, but the definitive threshold for diagnosis is yet to be determined (Pacheco et al. 2002). A method for determining site-specific thresholds for pDXA have been reported (Blake et al. 2005). In recent years the use and manufacture of pDXA scanners have diminished and peripheral sites are increasingly scanned on central DXA scanners.

10 DXA in Children

Children are difficult to study with DXA as the bones both grow in size and increase in density during childhood development (Kalkwarf et al. 2010) Fractures are also frequent; by the end of the teenage years, up to half of all boys and a third of girls will have sustained a fracture (Jones et al. 2002; Cooper et al. 2004). Consequently, a single fracture in an otherwise healthy child should not therefore require investigation of skeletal health. The measurement of bone size or bone mineral density in children needs to provide data which are relevant to skeleton health and management. DXA is the most widely used quantitative bone imaging technique in paediatric practice, but many aspects of its use, and the interpretation of the results obtained, remain controversial (Fewtrell et al. 2003; van Rijn et al. 2003; Mughal et al. 2004; Bachrach 2005; Blake et al. 2012).

Indications: DXA is generally appropriate in children who are at increased risk of fracture. These include children with primary bone (osteogenesis imperfecta; idiopathic juvenile osteoporosis) or endocrine (Cushing's disease; anorexia nervosa) diseases, chronic immobilisation (cerebral palsy; Duchenne muscular dystrophy), inflammatory conditions (Crohn's disease, cystic fibrosis; juvenile idiopathic arthritis), following chemotherapy or organ transplantation or with a history of recurrent fractures (Bishop et al. 2008).

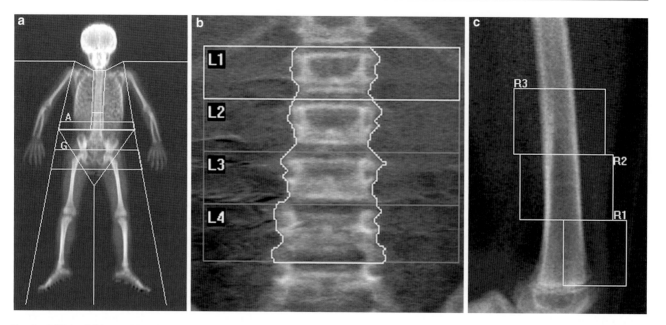

Fig. 8 *DXA in children*: **a** Total body less head (TBLH) and **b** lumbar spine L1-4 is recommended in children; hip scans are generally not. This is because in young children (particularly under 10 years) the proximal femur has not attained the adult shape. There are various techniques of adjusting for the size dependency of DXA, which is a particular problem in growing children, in whom the bones are changing in shape, size and density, but there is not yet consensus on the optimum method to implement. **c** Lateral DXA of the distal femur, with the regions where BMC and BMD are measured indicated. This has been proposed in children in whom the use of DXA in the normal measurement sites is precluded by deformity and contracture which prohibit ideal positioning (e.g. cerebral palsy, Duchenne muscular dystrophy) and for which reference data are available

Measurements and sites of application: the advantages of using DXA in children are short scan time, low radiation dose, good precision and widespread availability in most of the countries of the Western world. The measurement sites for DXA in children are typically the lumbar spine (L1-4) and total body less head (TBLH) (Fig. 8a and b), where precision (CV = 1.0 %) is similar to that achieved in adults (Gordon et al. 2008; Bishop et al. 2008). The mean time interval (MTI) for monitoring least significant change in children in these sites is approximately 12 months (Shepherd et al. 2011). As the proximal femur in young children has not developed into the shape of that in adults, and the precision is less good, scanning of this site is generally not advocated, particularly in children aged less than 10 years. However, the proximal femur and forearm have been used in some studies, as has the lateral distal femur where deformity and contracture preclude the use of DXA in the normal measurement sites. In children in whom the use of DXA in the normal measurement sites is precluded by deformity and contracture prohibiting ideal positioning (e.g. in cerebral palsy, Duchenne muscular dystrophy) lateral DXA of the distal femur has been proposed (Fig. 8c) and for which reference data are available (Zemel et al. 2009). Normal reference data are available for spine, femoral neck, total body and lateral distal femur (Ward et al. 2007; Kalkwarf et al. 2007; Zemel et al. 2009).

There are some limitations of the technique, including an initial paucity of appropriate reference data and the size dependency of DXA (Gilsanz 1998; van Kuijk 2010). Originally there were reference data only for the spine, but most of these were based on chronological age and did not take into account the pubertal staging of the child, which is crucial to changes in size and density of the developing skeleton (Faulkner et al. 1993b). However, there have been improvements made in this over recent years and normal reference data are available for spine, femoral neck and total body (Ward et al. 2007; Kalkwarf et al. 2007; Zemel et al. 2011), although significant discrepancies in BMD Z-scores exist between various references ranges as there are other differences in children's bone mass, shape, strength and body size that are not detected by DXA (Kocks et al. 2010).

Some correction for the size dependency of DXA can be made in the spine by calculating bone mineral apparent density (BMAD) (Katzman et al. 1991), either assuming that the vertebral bodies are cubes (Carter et al. 1992) or cylinders (Kröger et al. 1993), and in the femoral neck assuming a cylindrical shape (Lu et al. 1996). Alternative methods adjust BMC of whole body for various parameters including bone area ('are bones under-mineralised?'), bone area for height ('are bones narrow?') and height for age ('are bones short?') (Mølgaard et al. 1997). Alternatively, BMC can be related to lean muscle mass, since loading of the skeleton by muscular activity is a strong determinant of

BMC (Crabtree et al. 2004). However, to date, there is no consensus as to which of the methods should be applied, although some reference data with size adjustments are available (Ward et al. 2007; Zemel et al. 2011).

Fracture prediction: the relationship between DXA BMD and fracture prediction in children is less strong and well understood than that in adults, and there are racial disparities similar to those in adults, with white Caucasian children being at higher risk of fracture (Goulding 2007; Rauch et al. 2008; Wren et al. 2012). DXA measures of BMD in healthy children are predictive of fracture risk both at the measurement site (in the forearm) and elsewhere; in a prospective cohort study at age 9.9 years total body BMD less head (Fig. 8a), adjusted for weight, height and bone area, was found to be most strongly associated with fracture risk over the following two years (Clark et al. 2006). However, there are no data for the predictive value of DXA at other ages in apparently healthy children, and no similar data for children with bone disease.

Interpretation: measurements are reported in relation to reference data drawn from normal children matched for gender, age and ethnicity (Kalkwarf et al. 2007; Zemel et al. 2011). Interpretation of the scan results depends on the clinical context, and T-scores must not be used in children who have not yet reached peak bone mass. A diagnosis of osteoporosis should not be made in children and management must not be based on the BMD measurement in isolation (Lewiecki et al. 2008). Terminology such as 'low bone density for chronological age' may be used if the Z-score is below -2.0 (International Society for Clinical Densitometry. ISCD 2007).

DXA in children should probably still be regarded predominantly as a research tool rather than an established clinical service. Those referring children for bone densitometry, and those performing the measurements and providing interpretation of the results, need to have experience in the field and be aware of the limitations of the technique. Nonetheless, the method is being increasingly applied to the investigation of bone in children, including neonates (Salle et al. 1992; Koo 2000).

Quantitative CT has some important advantages in children, as it provides separate measurements of cortical and trabecular bone, and true volumetric density (mg/cm^3), so it is not size-dependent. Quantitative CT is therefore an important tool in assessing BMD in the developing skeleton, and is applied to the central (T12–L3) and peripheral (usually forearm, but also tibia) skeleton (Adams 2009; Bachrach 2005; Gordon 2005). A limitation of central QCT in its application to children is that it involves significantly larger doses of ionising radiation (Damilakis et al. 2010).

11 Conclusions

DXA offers a precise and reasonably accurate technique for measuring BMD in both central and peripheral sites, using very small doses of radiation (in the region of natural background radiation). DXA is currently regarded as the "gold standard" for BMD measurements, but there are some important limitations ["areal" density, size dependency, measurement of integral (cortical and trabecular) bone], of which users and operators need to be aware. Good precision is dependent on scanners being operated by skilled and appropriately trained staff, and quality assurance protocols being in place. DXA can be used to diagnose osteoporosis using the WHO threshold, to predict fractures, to contribute to the decision on patient management and therapeutic intervention, and to monitor change in BMD. Introduction of the World Health Organisation (WHO) 10-year fracture risk assessment tool (FRAX^{TM}) will improve clinical use of DXA and cost-effectiveness of therapeutic intervention. VFA is used increasingly for the identification of vertebral fractures, an important element in defining the most appropriate management of patients with osteoporosis. There are increasing, and varied, applications of DXA which extend its role in research studies (hip strength analysis [HAS], hip axis length [HAL], trabecular bone score [TBS], android/gynoid body composition and visceral adipose tissue from whole-body scans) but the role of which is yet to be established in clinical practice.

References

Adams JE (2009) Quantitative computed tomography. Eur J Radiol 71(3):415–424

Adams J (2013) Advances in bone imaging for osteoporosis. Nat Endocrinol 9(1):28–42

Ahmed AIH, Blake GM, Rymer JM, Fogelman I (1997) Screening for osteoporosis and osteopenia: do the accepted normal ranges lead to overdiagnosis? Osteoporos Int 7:432–438

Albanese CV, Diessel E, Genant HK (2003) Clinical applications of body composition measurements using DXA. J Clin Densitom 6(2):75–85

Ammann P, Rizzoli R (2003) Bone strength and its determinants. Osteoporos Int14(Suppl 3):S13–S18

Anil G, Guglielmi G, Peh WC (2010) Radiology of osteoporosis. Radiol Clin North Am 48(3):497–518

Bachrach LK (2005) Osteoporosis and measurement of bone mass in children and adolescents. Endocrinol Metab Clin North Am 34(3):521–535

Bazzocchi A, Ciccarese F, Diano D, Spinnato P, Albisinni U, Rossi C, Guglielmi G (2012) Dual-energy X-ray absorptiometry in the evaluation of abdominal aortic calcifications. J Clin Densitom 15(2):198–204

Beck TJ (2007) Extending DXA beyond bone mineral density: understanding hip structure analysis. Curr Osteoporos Rep 5(2):49–55

Bell KJ, Hayen A, Macaskill P, Irwig L, Craig JC, Ensrud K, Bauer DC (2009) Value of routine monitoring of bone mineral density after starting bisphosphonate treatment: secondary analysis of trial data. BMJ 23(338):b2266

Binkley N, Lewiecki EM (2010) The evolution of fracture risk estimation. J Bone Miner Res 25(10):2098–2100

Bishop N, Braillon P, Burnham J, Cimaz R, Davies J, Fewtrell M, Hogler W, Kennedy K, Mäkitie O, Mughal Z, Shaw N, Vogiatzi M, Ward K, Bianchi ML (2008) Dual-energy X-ray aborptiometry assessment in children and adolescents with diseases that may affect the skeleton: the 2007 ISCD Pediatric Official Positions. J Clin Densitom 11(1):29–42

Blake GM, Herd RJ, Fogelman I (1996) A longitudinal study of supine lateral DXA of the lumbar spine: a comparison with postero-anterior spine, hip and total-body DXA. Osteoporos Int 6(6):462–470

Blake GM, Fogelman I (1997) Technical principles of dual energy X-ray absorptiometry. Semin Nucl Med 27:210–228

Blake GM, Wahner HW, Fogelman I (1999) The evaluation of osteoporosis: dual energy x-ray absorptiometry and ultrasound in clinical practice. Martin Dunitz, London

Blake GM, Chinn DJ, Steel SA, Patel R, Panayiotou E, Thorpe J, Fordham JN (2005) National Osteoporosis Society Bone Densitometry Forum A list of device-specific thresholds for the clinical interpretation of peripheral x-ray absorptiometry examinations. Osteoporos Int 16(12):2149–2156

Blake GM, Naeem M, Boutros M (2006) Comparison of effective dose to children and adults from dual x-ray absorptiometry examinations. Bone 38(6):935–942

Blake GM, Lewiecki EM, Kendler DL, Fogelman I (2007) A review of strontium ranelate and its effect on DXA scans. J Clin Densitom 10(2):113–119

Blake GM, Fogelman I (2007) The role of DXA bone density scans in the diagnosis and treatment of osteoporosis. Postgrad Med J 83(982):509–517

Blake GM, Griffith JF, Yeung DK, Leung PC, Fogelman I (2009) Effect of increasing vertebral marrow fat content on BMD measurement, T-Score status and fracture risk prediction by DXA. Bone 44(3):495–501

Blake G, Adams J, Bishop N (2012) DXA in adults and children. In: Primer on the metabolic bone diseases and disorders of mineral metabolism Rosen C (ed) 8th edn. American Society of Bone and Mineral Research (ASBMR), Washington, USA. In press

Bonnick SL, Johnston CC Jr, Kleerekoper M, Lindsay R, Miller P, Sherwood L, Siris E (2001) Importance of precision in bone density measurements. J Clin Densitom 4(2):105–110

Bousson V, Bergot C, Sutter B, Levitz P, Cortet B (2012) Scientific committee of the groupe de recherche et d'Information sur les Ostéoporoses Trabecular bone score (TBS): available knowledge, clinical relevance, and future prospects. Osteoporos Int 23(5):1489–1501

Bouxsein ML, Parker RA, Greenspan SL (1999) Forearm bone mineral densitometry cannot be used to monitor response to alendronate. Osteoporos Int 10:505–509

Bouxsein ML, Karasik D (2006) Bone geometry and skeletal fragility. Curr Osteoporos Rep 4(2):49–56

Cameron JR, Sorenson J (1963) Measurement of bone mineral density in vivo: an improved method. Science 142:230–232

Carter DR, Bouxsein ML, Marcus R (1992) New approaches for interpreting projected bone densitometry data. J Bone Miner Res 7(2):137–145

Cheng S, Suominen H, Sakari-Rantala R, Laukkanen P, Avikainen V, Heikkinen E (1997) Calcaneal bone mineral density predicts fracture occurrence: a five-year follow-up study in elderly people. J Bone Miner Res 12:1075–1082

Chun KJ (2011) Bone densitometry. Semin Nucl Med 41(3):220–228

Clark EM, Ness AR, Bishop NJ, Tobias JH (2006) Association between bone mass and fractures in children: a prospective cohort study. J Bone Miner Res 21(9):1489–1495

Compston J (2009a) Recent advances in the management of osteoporosis. Clin Med 9(6):565–569

Compston J (2009b) Monitoring osteoporosis treatment. Best Pract Res Clin Rheumatol 23(6):781–788

Compston J (2010a) Osteoporosis: social and economic impact. Radiol Clin North Am 48(3):477–482

Compston J (2010b) Management of glucocorticoid-induced osteoporosis. Nat Rev Rheumatol 6(2):82–88

Compston JE, Cooper C, Kanis JA (1995) Bone densitometry in clinical practice. Br Med J 310:1507–1510

Compston J, Cooper A, Cooper C, Francis R, Kanis JA, Marsh D, McCloskey EV, Reid DM, Selby P, Wilkins M (2009) National Osteoporosis Guideline Group (NOGG) Guidelines for the diagnosis and management of osteoporosis in postmenopausal women and men from the age of 50 years in the UK. Maturitas 62(2):105–108

Cooper C, Dennison EM, Leufkens HG, Bishop N, van Staa TP (2004) Epidemiology of childhood fractures in Britain: a study using the general practice research database. J Bone Miner Res 19(12):1976–1981

Crabtree NJ, Kibirige MS, Fordham JN, Banks LM, Muntoni F, Chinn D, Boivin CM, Shaw NJ (2004) The relationship between lean body mass and bone mineral content in paediatric health and disease. Bone 35(4):965–972

Cummings SR, Black DM, Nevitt MC, Browner W, Cauley J, Ensrud K, Genant HK, Palermo L, Scott J, Vogt TM (1993) Bone density at various sites for prediction of hip fractures. Lancet 341(8837):72–75

Cummings SR, Melton LJ (2002) Epidemiology and outcomes of osteoporotic fractures. Lancet 359(9319):1761–1767

Cullum ID, Ell PJ, Ryder JP (1989) X-ray dual-photon absorptiometry: a new method for the measurement of bone density. Br J Radiol 62(739):587–592

Damilakis J, Guglielmi G (2010) Quality assurance and dosimetry in bone densitometry. Radiol Clin North Am 48(3):629–640

Damilakis J, Adams JE, Guglielmi G, Link TM (2010) Radiation exposure in X-ray-based imaging techniques used in osteoporosis. Eur Radiol 20(11):2707–2714

Dasher LG, Newton CD, Lenchik L (2010) Dual X-ray absorptiometry in today's clinical practice. Radiol Clin North Am 48(3):541–560

Del Rio L, Pons F, Huguet M, Setoain FJ (1995) Anteroposterior versus lateral bone mineral density of spine assessed by dual X-ray absorptiometry. Eur J Radiol 22:407–412

Diacinti D, Guglielmi G, Pisani D, Diacinti D, Argirò R, Serafini C, Romagnoli E, Minisola S, Catalano C, David V (2012) Vertebral morphometry by dual-energy X-ray absorptiometry (DXA) for osteoporotic vertebral fractures assessment (VFA). Radiol Med 117(8):1374–1385

Dunn WL, Wahner HW, Riggs BL (1980) Measurement of bone mineral content in human vertebrae and hip by dual photon absorptiometry. Radiology 136:485–487

Eastell R, Wahner HW, O"Fallon WM, Amadio PC, Melton LJ 3rd, Riggs BL (1989). Unequal decrease in bone density of the lumbar spine and ultradistal radius in Colles" and vertebral fracture syndromes. J Clin Invest 83:168–174

Eiken P, Kolthoff N, Barenholdt O, Hermansen F, Pors Nielsen S (1994) Switching from pencil-beam to fan-beam. II. Studies in vivo. Bone 15:671–676

Faulkner KG (1998) Bone densitometry: choosing the proper site to measure. J Clin Densitom 1(3):279–285

Faulkner KG, McClung MR (1995) Quality control of DXA instruments in multicentre trials. Osteoporos Int 5:218–227

Faulkner KG, Glüer CC, Majumdar S, Lang P, Engelke K, Genant HK (1991) Noninvasive measurements of bone mass, structure, and strength: current methods and experimental techniques. AJR Am J Roentgenol 157(6):1229–1237

Faulkner KG, Cummings SR, Black D, Palermo L, Glüer CC, Genant HK (1993a) Simple measurement of femoral geometry predicts hip fracture: the study of osteoporotic fractures. J Bone Miner Res 8(10):1211–1217

Faulkner KG, McClung M, Cummings SR (1994) Automated evaluation of hip axis length for predicting hip fracture. J Bone Miner Res 9:1065–1070

Faulkner KG, von Stetten E, Miller P (1999) Discordance in patient classification using T-score. J Clin Densitom 2:343–350

Faulkner RA, Bailey DA, Drinkwater DT, Wilkinson AA, Houston CS, McKay HA (1993b) Regional and total body bone mineral content, bone mineral density, and total body tissue composition in children 8–16 years of age. Calcif Tissue Int 3:7–12

Felsenberg D, Gowin W, Diessel E, Armbrust S, Mews J (1995) Recent developments in DXA. Quality of new DXA/MXA-devices for densitometry and morphometry. Eur J Radiol 20(3):179–184

Franck H, Munz M, Scherrer M (1995) Evaluation of dual-energy X-ray absorptiometry bone mineral measurement — comparison of a single-beam and fan beam design: the effect of osteophytic calcification on spine bone mineral density. Calcif Tissue Int 56:192–195

Fewtrell MS; British Paediatric & Adolescent Bone Group (2003) Bone densitometry in children assessed by dual x-ray absorptiometry: uses and pitfalls. Arch Dis Child 88(9):795–798

Frohn J, Wilken T, Falk S, Strutte HJ, Kollath J, Hor G (1991) Effect of aortic sclerosis on bone mineral measurements by dual-photon absorptimetry. J Nucl Med 32:259–262

Fuerst T, Wu C, Genant HK, von Ingersleben G, Chen Y, Johnston C, Econs MJ, Binkley N, Vokes TJ, Crans G, Mitlak BH (2009) Evaluation of vertebral fracture assessment by dual X-ray absorptiometry in a multicenter setting. Osteoporos Int 20(7):1199–1205

Genant HK, Grampp S, Glueer CC, Faulkner KG, Jergas M, Engelke K, Hagiwara S, van Kuijk C (1994) Universal standardisation for the dual X-ray absorptiometry: patient and phantom cross-calibration results. J Bone Miner Res 9:1503–1514

Genant HK, Li Y, Wu CY, Shepherd JA (2000) Vertebral fractures in osteoporosis: a new method for clinical assessment. J Clin Densitom 3:281–290

Gilsanz V (1998) Bone density in children: a review of the available techniques and indications. Eur J Radiol 26:177–182

Gluer CC (1999) Monitoring skeletal changes by radiological techniques. J Bone Miner Res 14:1952–1962

Gluer CC, Blake G, Blunt BA, Jergas M, Genant HK (1995) Accurate assessment of precision errors: how to measure the reproducibility of bone densitometry techniques. Osteoporos Int 5:262–270

Goh JC, Low SL, Bose K (1995) Effect of femoral rotation on bone mineral density measurements with dual energy X-ray absorptiometry. Calcif Tissue Int 57:340–343

Gordon CM (2005) Evaluation of bone density in children. Curr Opin Endocrinol Diabetes 12:444–451

Gordon CM, Bachrach LK, Carpenter TO, Crabtree N, El-Hajj Fuleihan G, Kutilek S, Lorenc RS, Tosi LL, Ward KA, Ward LM, Kalkwarf HJ (2008) Dual energy X-ray absorptiometry interpretation and reporting in children and adolescents: the 2007 ISCD pediatric official positions. J Clin Densitom 11(1):43–58

Goulding A (2007) Risk factors for fractures in normally active children and adolescents. Med Sport Sci 51:102–120

Grampp S, Jergas M, Glüer CC, Lang P, Brastow P, Genant HK (1993) Radiologic diagnosis of osteoporosis. Current methods and perspectives. Radiol Clin North Am 31(5):1133–1145

Grampp S, Genant HK, Mathur A, Lang P, Jergas M, Takada M, Gluer CC, Lu Y, Chavez M (1997) Comparisons of non-invasive bone mineral measurements in assessing age-related loss, fracture discrimination and diagnostic classification. J Bone Miner Res 12:697–711

Gregory JS, Testi D, Stewart A, Undrill PE, Reid DM, Aspden RM (2004) A method for assessment of the shape of the proximal femur and its relationship to osteoporotic hip fracture. Osteoporos Int 15(1):5–11

Gregory JS, Stewart A, Undrill PE, Reid DM, Aspden RM (2005) Bone shape, structure, and density as determinants of osteoporotic hip fracture: a pilot study investigating the combination of risk factors. Invest Radiol 40(9):591–597

Griffin MC, Kimble R, Hopfer W, Pacifici R (1993) Dual-energy X-ray absorptiometry of the rat: accuracy, precision and measurement of bone loss. J Bone Miner Res 8:795–800

Griffiths MR, Noakes KA, Pocock NA (1997) Correcting the magnification error of fan beam densitometers. J Bone Miner Res 12:119–123

Guglielmi G, Grimston SK, Fischer KC, Pacifici R (1994) Osteoporosis: diagnosis with lateral and posteroanterior dual X-ray absorptiometry compared with quantitative CT. Radiology 192:845–850

Guglielmi G, Diacinti D, van Kuijk C, Aparisi F, Krestan C, Adams JE, Link TM (2008) Vertebral morphometry: current methods and recent advances. Eur Radiol 18(7):1484–1496

Guglielmi G, Muscarella S, Bazzocchi A (2011) Integrated imaging approach to osteoporosis: state-of-the-art review and update. Radiographics 31(5):1343–1364

Guglielmi G, Damilakis J, Solomou G, Bazzocchi A (2012) Quality assurance of imaging techniques used in the clinical management of osteoporosis. Radiol Med (Epub ahead of print)

Hans D, Barthe N, Boutroy S, Pothuaud L, Winzenrieth R, Krieg MA (2011a) Correlations between trabecular bone score, measured using anteroposterior dual-energy X-ray absorptiometry acquisition, and 3-dimensional parameters of bone microarchitecture: an experimental study on human cadaver vertebrae. J Clin Densitom 14(3):302–312

Hans D, Goertzen AL, Krieg MA, Leslie WD (2011b) Bone microarchitecture assessed by TBS predicts osteoporotic fractures independent of bone density: the Manitoba study. J Bone Miner Res 26(11):2762–2769

Horner K, Devlin H, Alsop CW, Hodgkinson IM, Adams JE (1996) Mandibular bone mineral density as a predictor of skeletal osteoporosis. Br J Radiol 69:1019–1025

Huda W, Morin RL (1996) Patient doses in bone densitometry. Br J Radiol 69:422–425

Hui SL, Gao S, Zhou XH, Johston CC Jr, Lu Y, Gluer CC, Grampp S, Genant HK (1997) Universal standardisation of bone density measurements: a method with optimal properties for calibration among several instruments. J Bone Miner Res 12:1463–1470

ISCD Position Development Conference—Writing Group (2004) Technical standardization for dual-energy x-ray absorptiometry. J Clin Densitom 7(1):27–36

International Society for Clinical Densitometry. ISCD (2007) Official Positions & Pediatric Official Positions. West Hartford (CT): International Society for Clinical Densitometry; 2007 Oct. http://www.iscd.org

Jaovisidha S, Sartoris DJ, Martin EM, De Maeseneer M, Szollar SM, Deftos LJ (1997) Influence of spondylopathy on bone densitometry using dual energy X-ray absorptiometry. Calcif Tissue Int 60:424–429

Jergas M, Breitenseher M, Gluer CC, Black D, Grampp s LP, Engelke K, Genant HK (1995) Which vertebrae should be assessed using lateral dual-energy X-ray absorptiometry of the lumbar spine. Osteoporos Int 5:196–204

Johansson H, Kanis JA, Oden A, Compston J, McCloskey E (2012) A comparison of case-finding strategies in the UK for the management of hip fractures. Osteoporos Int 23(3):907–915

Johnell O, Kanis JA, Oden A, Johansson H, De Laet C, Delmas P, Eisman JA, Fujiwara S, Kroger H, Mellstrom D, Meunier PJ, Melton LJ 3rd, O'Neill T, Pols H, Reeve J, Silman A, Tenenhouse A (2005) Predictive value of BMD for hip and other fractures. J Bone Miner Res 20(7):1185–1194

Jones IE, Williams SM, Dow N, Goulding A (2002) How many children remain fracture-free during growth? A longitudinal study of children and adolescents participating in the Dunedin multidisciplinary health and development study. Osteoporos Int 13(12): 990–995

Kalkwarf HJ, Gilsanz V, Lappe JM, Oberfield S, Shepherd JA, Hangartner TN, Huang X, Frederick MM, Winer KK, Zemel BS (2010) Tracking of bone mass and density during childhood and adolescence. J Clin Endocrinol Metab 95(4):1690–1698

Kalender WA (1992) Effective dose values in bone mineral measurements by photon absorptiometry and computed tomography. Osteoporos Int 2:82–87

Kalender WA, Felsenberg D, Genant HK, Dequeker J, Reeve J (1995) The European Spine Phantom: a tool for standardisation and quality control in spinal bone mineral measurement by DXA and QCT. Eur J Radiol 20:83–92

Kalkwarf HJ, Zemel BS, Gilsanz V, Lappe JM, Horlick M, Oberfield S, Mahboubi S, Fan B, Frederick MM, Winer K, Shepherd JA (2007) The bone mineral density in childhood study: bone mineral content and density according to age, sex, and race. J Clin Endocrinol Metab 92(6):2087–2099

Kanis JA, Delmas P, Burckhardt P, Cooper C, Torgerson D (1997) Guidelines for diagnosis and management of osteoporosis: EFFO report. Osteoporos Int 7:390–406

Kanis JA, Gluer C (2000) The committee of the scientific advisors, international osteoporosis foundation. An update in the diagnosis and assessment of osteoporosis with densitometry. Osteoporos Int 11:192–202

Kanis JA, Oden A, Johnell O, Johansson H, De Laet C, Brown J, Burckhardt P, Cooper C, Christiansen C, Cummings S, Eisman JA, Fujiwara S, Glüer C, Goltzman D, Hans D, Krieg MA, La Croix A, McCloskey E, Mellstrom D, Melton LJ 3rd, Pols H, Reeve J, Sanders K, Schott AM, Silman A, Torgerson D, van Staa T, Watts NB, Yoshimura N (2007) The use of clinical risk factors enhances the performance of BMD in the prediction of osteoporotic fractures in men and women. Osteoporos Int 18(8): 1033–1046

Kanis JA, McCloskey EV, Johansson H, Strom O, Borgstrom F, Oden A (2008) Case finding for the management of osteoporosis with FRAX–assessment and intervention thresholds for the UK. Osteoporos Int 19(10):1395–1408

Kanis JA, Johansson H, Oden A, McCloskey EV (2009) Assessment of fracture risk. Eur J Radiol 71(3):392–397

Kastl S, Sommer T, Klein P, Hohenberger W, Engelke K (2002) Accuracy and precision of bone mineral density and bone mineral content in the excised rat humeri using fan beam dual-energy X-ray absorptiometry. Bone 30:243–246

Katzman DK, Bachrach LK, Carter DR, Marcus R (1991) Clinical and anthropometric correlates of bone mineral acquisition in healthy adolescent girls. J Clin Endocrinol Metab 73:1332–1339

Kelly TL, Slovik DM, Schoenfeld DA, Neer RM (1988) Quantitative digital radiography versus dual photon absorptiometry of the lumbar spine. J Clin Endocrinol Metab 67:839–844

Kelly TL, Wilson KE, Heymsfield SB (2009) Dual energy X-Ray absorptiometry body composition reference values from NHANES. PLoS ONE 4(9):e7038

Kocks J, Ward K, Mughal Z, Moncayo R, Adams J, Högler W (2010) Z-score comparability of bone mineral density reference databases for children. J Clin Endocrinol Metab 95(10):4652–4659

Koo WW (2000) Body composition measurements during infancy. Ann N Y Acad Sci 904:383–392

Knapp KM, Welsman JR, Hopkins SJ, Fogelman I, Blake GM (2012) Obesity increases precision errors in dual-energy X-ray absorptiometry measurements. J Clin Densitom 15(3):315–319

Kröger H, Kotaniemi A, Kröger L, Alhava E (1993) Development of bone mass and bone density of the spine and femoral neck: a prospective study of 65 children and adolescents. Bone Miner 23(3):171–182

Laskey MA, Crisp AJ, Compston JE, Khaw KT (1993) Heterogeneity of spine bone density. Br J Radiol 66:480–483

Lewiecki EM, Gordon CM, Baim S, Leonard MB, Bishop NJ, Bianchi ML, Kalkwarf HJ, Langman CB, Plotkin H, Rauch F, Zemel BS, Binkley N, Bilezikian JP, Kendler DL, Hans DB, Silverman S (2008) International society for clinical densitometry 2007 adult and pediatric official positions. Bone 43(6):1115–1121

Lewiecki EM (2010) Benefits and limitations of bone mineral density and bone turnover markers to monitor patients treated for osteoporosis. Curr Osteoporos Rep 8(1):15–22

Lewiecki EM, Compston JE, Miller PD, Adachi JD, Adams JE, Leslie WD, Kanis JA, Moayyeri A, Adler RA, Hans DB, Kendler DL, Diez-Perez A, Krieg MA, Masri BK, Lorenc RR, Bauer DC, Blake GM, Josse RG, Clark P, Khan AA (2011) FRAX® Position Development Conference Members (2011) Official Positions for FRAX® Bone Mineral Density and FRAX® simplification from Joint Official Positions Development Conference of the International Society for Clinical Densitometry and International Osteoporosis Foundation on FRAX®. J Clin Densitom 14(3):226–236

Lewis MK, Blake GM (1995) Patient dose in morphometric X-ray absorptiometry. Osteoporos Int 5:281–282

Lewis MK, Blake GM, Fogelman I (1994) Patient doses in dual X-ray absorptiometry. Osteoporos Int 4:11–15

Liao J, Blake GM, McGregor AH, Patel R (2010) The effect of bone strontium on BMD is different for different manufacturers' DXA systems. Bone 47(5):882–887

Link TM, Guglielmi G, van Kuijk C, Adams JE (2005) Radiologic assessment of osteoporotic vertebral fractures: diagnostic and prognostic implications. Eur Radiol 15(8):1521–1532

Looker AC, Wahner HW, Dunn WL, Calvo MS, Harris TB, Heyse SP, Johnston CC Jr, Lindsay R (1998) Updated data on proximal femur bone mineral levels of US adults. Osteoporos Int 8:468–489

Lu PW, Cowell CT, Lloyd-Jones SA, Briody JN, Howman-Giles R (1996) Volumetric bone mineral density in normal subjects, aged 5–27 years. J Clin Endocrinol Metab 81(4):1586–1590

Marshall D, Johnell O, Wedel H (1996) Meta-analysis of how well measures of bone density predict occurrence of osteoporotic fractures. Br Med J 312:1254–1259

Mazess RB (1990) Bone densitometry of the axial skeleton. Orthop Clin North Am 21(1):51–63

Melton LJ, Eddy DM, Johnson CC (1990) Screening for osteoporosis. Ann Intern Med 112:516–528

Micklesfield LK, Goedecke JH, Punyanitya M, Wilson KE, Kelly TL (2012) Dual-energy X-ray performs as well as clinical computed tomography for the measurement of visceral fat. Obesity (Silver Spring) 20(5):1109–1114

Miller P (2000) Controversies in bone mineral density diagnostic classification. Calcif Tissue Int 66:317–319

Miller P, Bonnick SL, Rosen CJ (1996) Consensus of an international panel on the clinical utility of bone mass measurements in the detection of low bone mass in the adult population. Calcif Tissue Int 58:207–214

Mølgaard C, Thomsen BL, Prentice A, Cole TJ, Michaelsen KF (1997) Whole body bone mineral content in healthy children and adolescents. Arch Dis Child 76(1):9–15

Mughal M, Ward K, Adams J (2004) Assessment of bone status in children by densitometric and quantitative ultrasound techniques. In: Carty H, Brunelle F, Stringer DA, Kao SC (eds) Imaging in children, vol 1. Elsevier Science, Edinburgh, pp 477–486

National Osteoporosis Foundation (2010) Clinician's Guide to Prevention and Treatment of Osteoporosis. National Osteoporosis Foundation, Washington (DC) http://www.nof.org/professionals/clinical-guidelines

National Osteoporosis Society (2001) Position statement on the use of peripheral X-ray absorptiometry in the management of osteoporosis. National Osteoporosis Society, Camerton, pp 1–15

Njeh CF, Apple K, Temperton DH, Boivin CM (1996) Radiological assessment of a new bone densitometer: the Lunar expert. Br J Radiol 69:335–340

Nord RH (1992) Work in progress: a cross-calibration study of four DXA instruments designed to culminate in inter-manufacturer standardization. Osteoporos Int 2:210–211

Nuti R, Martini G (1992) Measurements of bone mineral density by DXA total body absorptiometry in different skeletal sites in postmenopausal osteoporosis. Bone 13(2):173–178

Orwoll ES, Oviatt SK, Mann T (1990) The impact of osteophytic and vascular calcifications on vertebral mineral density measurements in men. J Clin Endocrinol Metab 70:1202–1207

Pacheco EM, Harrison EJ, Ward KA, Lunt M, Adams JE (2002) Detection of osteoporosis by dual energy X-ray absorptiometry (DXA) of the calcaneus: is the WHO criterion applicable? Calcif Tissue Int 70(6):475–482

Patel R, Blake GM, Herd RJM, Fogelman I (1997) The effect of weight change on DXA scans in a 2 year prospective clinical trial of cyclical etidronate therapy. Calcif Tissue Int 61:393–399

Patel R, Blake GM, Fogelman I (2007) Peripheral and central measurements of bone mineral density are equally strongly associated with clinical risk factors for osteoporosis. Calcif Tissue Int 80(2):89–96

Parfitt AM (1990) Interpretation of bone densitometry measurements: disadvantages of a percentage scale and a discussion of some alternatives. J Bone Miner Res 5:537–540

Peel N, Johnson A, Barrington NA, Smith TW, Eastell R (1993) Impact of anomalous vertebral segmentation on the measurements of bone mineral density. J Bone Miner Res 8:719–723

Prevrhal S, Shepherd JA, Faulkner KG, Gaither KW, Black DM, Lang TF (2008) Comparison of DXA hip structural analysis with volumetric QCT. J Clin Densitom 11(2):232–236

Pietrobelli A, Formica C, Wang Z, Heymsfield SB (1996) Dual-energy X-ray absorptiometry body composition model: review of physical concepts. Am J Physiol 271:E941–951

Rachner TD, Khosla S, Hofbauer LC (2011) Osteoporosis: now and the future. Lancet 377(9773):1276–1287

Rauch F, Plotkin H, DiMeglio L, Engelbert RH, Henderson RC, Munns C, Wenkert D, Zeitler P (2008) Fracture prediction and the definition of osteoporosis in children and adolescents: the ISCD 2007 pediatric official positions. J Clin Densitom 11(1):22–28

Rea JA, Steiger P, Blake GM, Fogelman I (1998) Optimizing data acquisition and analysis of morphometric X-ray absorptiometry. Osteoporos Int 8:177–183

Rea JA, Li J, Blake GM, Steiger P, Genant HK, Fogelman I (2000) Visual assessment of vertebral deformity by X-ray absorptiometry: a highly predictive method to exclude vertebral deformity. Osteoporos Int 11:660–668

Rea JA, Chen MB, Li J, Marsh E, Fan B, Blake GM, Steiger P, Smith IG, Genant HK, Fogelman I (2001) Vertebral morphometry: a comparison of long-term precision of morphometric X-ray absorptiometry and morphometric radiography in normal and osteoporotic subjects. Osteoporos Int 12:158–166

Reid DM, Doughty J, Eastell R, Heys SD, Howell A, McCloskey EV, Powles T, Selby P, Coleman RE (2008) Guidance for the management of breast cancer treatment-induced bone loss: a consensus position statement from a UK Expert Group. Cancer Treat Rev 34(Suppl 1):S3–18

Roberts M, Cootes T, Pacheco E, Adams J (2007) Quantitative vertebral fracture detection on DXA images using shape and appearance models. Acad Radiol 14(10):1166–1178

Roberts MG, Pacheco EM, Mohankumar R, Cootes TF, Adams JE (2010) Detection of vertebral fractures in DXA VFA images using statistical models of appearance and a semi-automatic segmentation. Osteoporos Int 21(12):2037–2046

Royal College of Physicians (1999) Oateoporosis: guidelines for prevention and treatment. Royal College of Physicians, London, pp 63–70

Salle BL, Braillon P, Glorieux FH, Brunet J, Cavero E, Meunier PJ (1992) Lumbar bone mineral content measured by dual energy X-ray absorptiometry in newborns and infants. Acta Paediatr 81: 953–958

Schoeller DA, Tylavsky FA, Baer DJ, Chumlea WC, Earthman CP, Fuerst T, Harris TB, Heymsfield SB, Horlick M, Lohman TG, Lukaski HC, Shepherd J, Siervogel RM, Borrud LG (2005) QDR 4500A dual-energy X-ray absorptiometer underestimates fat mass in comparison with criterion methods in adults. Am J Clin Nutr 81(5):1018–1025

Schousboe JT, Wilson KE, Kiel DP (2006) Detection of abdominal aortic calcification with lateral spine imaging using DXA. J Clin Densitom 9(3):302–308

Schousboe JT, Wilson KE, Hangartner TN (2007) Detection of aortic calcification during vertebral fracture assessment (VFA) compared to digital radiography. PLoS ONE 2(8):e715

Schousboe JT, Vokes T, Broy SB, Ferrar L, McKiernan F, Roux C, Binkley N (2008a) Vertebral fracture assessment: the 2007 ISCD official positions. J Clin Densitom 11(1):92–108

Schousboe JT, Taylor BC, Kiel DP, Ensrud KE, Wilson KE, McCloskey EV (2008b) Abdominal aortic calcification detected on lateral spine images from a bone densitometer predicts incident myocardial infarction or stroke in older women. J Bone Miner Res 23(3):409–416

Shepherd JA, Fan B, Lu Y, Lewiecki EM, Miller P, Genant HKW (2006) Comparison of BMD precision for Prodigy and Delphi spine and femur scans. Osteoporos Int 17(9):1303–1308

Shepherd JA, Wang L, Fan B, Gilsanz V, Kalkwarf HJ, Lappe J, Lu Y, Hangartner T, Zemel BS, Fredrick M, Oberfield S, Winer KK (2011) Optimal monitoring time interval between DXA measures in children. J Bone Miner Res 26(11):2745–2752

Silverberg SJ, Lewiecki EM, Mosekilde L, Peacock M, Rubin MR (2009) Presentation of asymptomatic primary hyperparathyroidism: proceedings of the third international workshop. J Clin Endocrinol Metab 94(2):351–365

Siris ES, Chen YT, Abbott TA, Barrett-Connor E, Miller PD, Wehren LE, Berger ML (2004) Bone mineral density thresholds for pharmacological intervention to prevent fractures. Arch Intern Med 164(10):1108–1112

Siris ES, Genant HK, Laster AJ, Chen P, Misurski DA, Krege JH (2007) Enhanced prediction of fracture risk combining vertebral fracture status and BMD. Osteoporos Int 18(6):761–770

Smyth PP, Taylor CJ, Adams JE (1999) Vertebral shape: automatic measurement with active shape models. Radiology 211:571–578

Stone KL, Seeley DG, Lui LY, Cauley JA, Ensrud K, Browner WS, Nevitt MC, Cummings SR (2003) BMD at multiple sites and risk of fracture of multiple types: long-term results from the study of osteoporotic fractures. J Bone Miner Res 18(11):1947–1954

Soininvaara T, Kroger H, Jurvelin JS, Miettinen H, Suomalainen O, Alhava E (2000) Measurement of bone density around total knee arthroplasty using fan-beam dual energy X-ray absorptiometry. Calcif Tissue Int 67:267–272

Tothill P, Pye DW (1992) Errors due to non-uniform distribution of fat in dual x-ray absorptiometry of the lumbar spine. Br J Radiol 65(777):807–813

Tothill P, Hannan WJ (2000) Comparison between Hologic QDR 1000 W, QDR 4500A, and lunar expert dual-energy X-ray absorptiometry scanners for measuring total bone and soft tissues. Ann N Y Acad Sci 904:63–71

Tuck SP, Rawlings DJ, Scane AC, Pande I, Summers GD, Woolf AD, Francis RM (2011) Femoral neck shaft angle in men with fragility fractures. J Osteoporos 2011:903726. (Epub 2011 Oct 13)

van Kuijk C (2010) Pediatric bone densitometry. Radiol Clin North Am 48(3):623–627

van Rijn RR, van der Sluis IM, Link TM, Grampp S, Guglielmi G, Imhof H, Glüer C, Adams JE, van Kuijk C (2003) Bone densitometry in children: a critical appraisal. Eur Radiolr 13(4): 700–710

Vokes T, Bachman D, Baim S, Binkley N, Broy S, Ferrar L, Lewiecki EM, Richmond B, Schousboe J (2006) International society for clinical densitometry vertebral fracture assessment: the 2005 ISCD official positions. J Clin Densitom 9(1):37–46

Ward KA, Ashby RL, Roberts SA, Adams JE, Zulf Mughal M (2007) UK reference data for the Hologic QDR Discovery dual-energy x-ray absorptiometry scanner in healthy children and young adults aged 6–17 years. Arch Dis Child 92(1):53–59

Wilkinson JM, Peel NF, Elson RA, Stockley I, Eastell R (2001) Measuring bone mineral density of the pelvis and proximal femur after total hip arthroplasty. J Bone Joint Surg Br 83:283–288

Wilson CR, Fogelman I, Blake GM, Rodin A (1991) The effect of positioning on dual-energy X-ray absorptiometry of the proximal femur. Bone Miner 13:69–76

Wishart J, Horowitz M, Need A, Nordin BE (1990) Relationship between forearm and vertebral mineral density in postmenopausal women with primary hyperparathyroidism. Arch Intern Med 150:1329–1331

World Health Organisation Study Group (1994) Assessment of fracture risk and its application to screening for postmenopausal osteoporosis. World Health Organisation, Geneva, Switzerland. (WHO Technical Report Series 843)

World Health Organization Collaborating Centre for Metabolic Bone Diseases. FRAX® WHO Fracture Risk Assessment Tool Web Version 3.2 (Internet). Sheffield, UK: University of Sheffield; 2010 Dec 8; cited 2012 November 26. http://www.shef.ac.uk/FRAX

Wren TA, Shepherd JA, Kalkwarf HJ, Zemel BS, Lappe JM, Oberfield S, Dorey FJ, Winer KK, Gilsanz V (2012) Racial disparity in fracture risk between white and nonwhite children in the United States. J Pediatr 161(6):1035–1040

Young JT, Carter K, Marion MS, Greendale GA (2000) A simple method of computing hip axis length using fan-beam densitometry and anthropomorphic measurements. J Clin Densitom 3:325–331

Zemel BS, Stallings VA, Leonard MB, Paulhamus DR, Kecskemethy HH, Harcke HT, Henderson RC (2009) Revised pediatric reference data for the lateral distal femur measured by Hologic Discovery/Delphi dual-energy X-ray absorptiometry. J Clin Densitom 12(2):207–218

Zemel BS, Kalkwarf HJ, Gilsanz V, Lappe JM, Oberfield S, Shepherd JA, Frederick MM, Huang X, Lu M, Mahboubi S, Hangartner T, Winer KK (2011) Revised reference curves for bone mineral content and areal bone mineral density according to age and sex for black and non-black children: results of the bone mineral density in childhood study. J Clin Endocrinol Metab 96(10):3160–3169

Axial and Peripheral QCT

Thomas M. Link

Contents

Abstract

While Dual X-ray absorptiometry (DXA) is considered as the standard technique to measure bone mineral density (BMD), quantitative computed tomography (QCT) measures true volumetric and not areal BMD and has a number of advantages over DXA, which makes QCT an attractive alternative technique for certain indications.

1 Introduction

While Dual X-ray absorptiometry (DXA) is considered as the standard technique to measure bone mineral density (BMD), quantitative computed tomography (QCT) measures true volumetric and not areal BMD and has a number of advantages over DXA, which makes QCT an attractive alternative technique for certain indications. Interestingly, QCT was introduced and studied prior to DXA at the end of the 1970s (Genant and Boyd 1977; Genant et al. 1983). A large number of studies were performed subsequently establishing QCT as one of the first techniques for quantitative musculoskeletal imaging (Cann and Genant 1980; Genant et al. 1982, 1983; Cann et al. 1985; Sandor et al. 1985; Firooznia et al. 1986; Kalender et al. 1987; Kalender and Süss 1987). Normative data were made available and imaging techniques were optimized with new calibration devices and better image analysis algorithms. Also in addition to single slice techniques, volumetric techniques were developed which have superior precision and thus improve monitoring of therapy.

However, with the development of DXA, QCT lost ground and the number of studies validating and establishing DXA as a standard technique has superseded these performed with QCT. QCT studies have shown the technique's ability to differentiate subjects with and without osteoporotic fractures and to monitor therapy; however, studies proving that QCT can indeed also predict osteoporotic fractures are limited and have been found to be a major

T. M. Link (✉)
Department of Radiology and Biomedical Imaging,
University of California San Francisco,
400 Parnassus Ave, A367, 0628 San Francisco,
94143 CA, USA
e-mail: Thomas.Link@ucsf.edu

G. Guglielmi (ed.), *Osteoporosis and Bone Densitometry Measurements*, Medical Radiology. Diagnostic Imaging,
DOI: 10.1007/174_2012_729, © Springer-Verlag Berlin Heidelberg 2013

limitation in evaluating the technique. Also access to CT scanners always appeared limited, while DXA scanners are now widely available in the US and Europe. An additional issue with QCT is the lack of well-established normative data allowing to define individuals as osteopenic or osteoporotic based on their BMD. The WHO criteria using T-scores of lower than −2.5 as osteoporotic are only used for DXA and not QCT nor for any other technique to assess osteoporosis.

QCT techniques are used to measure BMD at the lumbar spine and proximal femur defined as axial QCT, while peripheral QCT measures BMD at the distal radius and tibia. In the subsequent chapters, we will discuss strengths and weaknesses of both techniques and also identify specific clinical indications for QCT as compared to DXA. It should be noted that QCT is currently not the standard technique to measure BMD, but it is useful as a problem solving technique for a number of clinical indications. Also at institutions where DXA is not available, QCT will provide pertinent information on bone strength and monitoring therapy.

2   Axial QCT

QCT uniquely allows the separate estimation of trabecular and cortical BMD and provides a true volumetric density in mg/cm^3, rather than the "areal density" (mg/cm^2) of DXA. Since trabecular bone has a higher metabolic turnover, it is more sensitive to changes in BMD. A big advantage of QCT is that it is not as susceptible to degenerative changes of the spine as DXA. Osteophytes and facet joint degeneration as well as soft tissue calcifications (in particular of aortic calcification) do not falsely increase BMD in QCT. As in DXA, however, fractured or deformed vertebrae must not be used for BMD assessment since these vertebrae usually have an increased BMD.

QCT may be performed at any CT-system; however, a calibration phantom is required and dedicated software improves the precision of the examination. The patient is examined supine, lying on the phantom usually with a water or gel-filled cushion in between to avoid artifacts due to air gaps. Calibration phantoms are required to transform the attenuation measured in HU (Hounsfield units) into BMD (mg hydroxyapatite/ml). The patient and the phantom are examined at the same time, which is defined as simultaneous calibration. The Cann-Genant phantom with five cylindrical channels filled with K_2HPO_4 solutions (of known concentrations) was the first phantom in clinical use (Cann and Genant 1980; Genant et al. 1983). However, due to the limited long-term stability of these solutions solid-state phantoms with densities expressed in mg calcium hydroxyapatite/ml were developed, which do not change with time and are more resistant to damage. Two of the

most frequently used phantoms include (1) the solid-state "Cann-Genant" phantom (Arnold 1989) (Figs. 1a and 2) the phantom developed by Kalender et al. (1987; Kalender and Süss 1987) (Fig. 1b). The latter phantom has a small cross section and is constituted of only two density phases: a 200 mg/ml calcium hydroxyapatite phase and a water equivalent phase.

Thorough *quality control* is critical to acquire meaningful BMD QCT data and should be performed according to the Guidelines of the International Society of Clinical Densitometry as published by Engelke et al. (2008). This includes the following: (1) In vivo precision of new QCT techniques must be established. However, due to radiation considerations, it is not recommended to reconfirm in vivo precision for each clinical facility. Instead, precision of acquisition should be established with phantom data; analysis precision should be established by reanalysis of patient data. (2) The scanner stability should be controlled longitudinally by scanning a quality assurance (QA) phantom at least once a week whenever patients are to be scanned. (3) The scan protocol must be kept constant for all visits of an individual patient.

Currently, 2-D resp. single slice and 3-D resp. volumetric measurements are used for QCT. While the 2-D measurement is only used for the lumbar spine 3-D measurements may also be performed at the proximal femur.

2.1   Single Slice QCT

Single Slice QCT has been established for BMD measurements at the lumbar spine; using the standard technique single sections of the first to third lumbar vertebrae are scanned. Typically, slice thicknesses are in the order of 8–10 mm, the mid-vertebral portion is examined and a dedicated gantry tilt is used (Fig. 2a). Single mid-vertebral slice positions of L1-3 parallel to the vertebral endplates are selected in the lateral digital radiograph resp. scout view (Fig. 2b). An automated software, selecting the mid-vertebral planes may be useful to reduce the precision error (Kalender et al. 1988).

Low energy protocols in the order of 80 kVp (or 120 kVp) and 120 mAs (or 150–200 mAs) result in effective doses of <200 microSv (Engelke et al. 2008). Felsenberg et al. described a low energy, low dose protocol with 80 kVp, and 146 mAs resulting in effective doses down to 50–60 μSv, including the digital radiograph (Felsenberg and Gowin 1999). Bone marrow fat increases with age and may falsely decrease BMD. Thus, the actual BMD may be underestimated by 15–20 %. Due to age-matched data bases, however, the clinical relevance of this fat error is small (Glüer and Genant 1989). A dual energy QCT technique was described to reduce the fat error. However, since this technique has an increased radiation exposure and a decreased precision, its

Fig. 1 BMD calibration phantoms. **a** Shows the solid-state Mindways (*short arrow*) and Image Analysis (*long arrow*), phantoms which are based on the original "Cann-Genant" phantom. **b** Depicts the two element phantom developed by Kalender et al. (1987; Kalender and Süss 1987) (*arrow*)

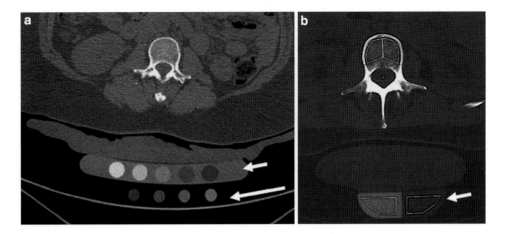

Fig. 2 Lateral digital radiogram (scout view) (**a**) shows mid-vertebral positions of the sections in L1-3, which are used to measure single slice QCT BMD. In (**b**) a mid-vertebral image of L2 demonstrates a "Pacman" or peeled region of interest (ROI) used to measure trabecular and "cortical" BMD (**b**). The cortical BMD measurement is an approximate measurement as the cortex of the vertebral body is below the spatial resolution of the axial CT image and subjected to partial volume effects

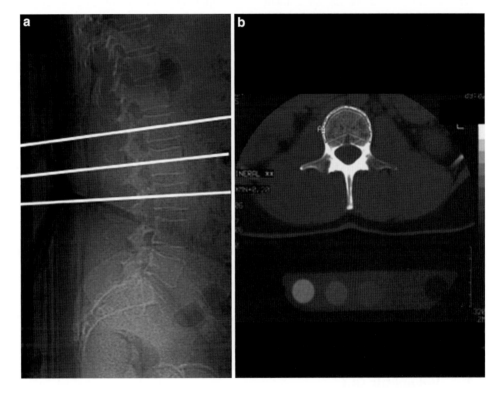

use was limited to research purposes (Genant and Boyd 1977; Felsenberg and Gowin 1999).

A number of different region of interest (ROI) shapes and techniques have been used to determine the BMD in the axial sections of the vertebral bodies. Manually, placed elliptical ROIs and automated image evaluation with elliptical and peeled or "Pacman" ROIs (Fig. 3) have been described (Kalender et al. 1987; Steiger et al. 1990). The ROI developed by Kalender et al. uses an automatic contour tracking of the cortical shell to determine a ROI analyzing trabecular and cortical (as visualized by CT) BMD separately (Kalender et al. 1987). The use of an automated ROI improves the precision of BMD measurements (Sandor et al. 1985; Kalender et al. 1987). Steiger et al. have shown

that elliptical and peeled ROIs yield similar results and have a very high correlation ($r = 0.99$) (Steiger et al. 1990).

Measurements should not be performed in fractured or deformed vertebral bodies and great care should be taken to avoid performing QCT after intravenous contrast application (e.g., after a standard contrast-enhanced CT). Also it is critical to analyze all images including the scout images for abnormalities in the bone and soft tissue windows. Vertebral fractures (scout images) and soft tissue abnormalities such as renal tumors or abnormally enlarged lymph nodes must not be missed as they may have an impact on patient management or may have legal consequences.

BMD-data obtained by QCT are compared to an age-, sex-, and race-matched database (Block et al. 1989; Kalender et al.

Fig. 3 ROIs used for BMD measurements include manually (**a**) or automatically placed (**b**) regions, which may be either oval shaped (**a**) or peeled ("Pacman" shaped ROI) (**b**)

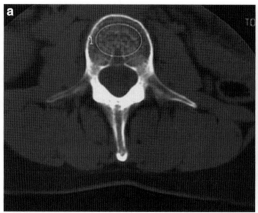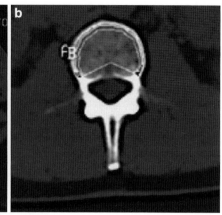

1989). T-scores used for the assessment of osteoporosis according to the WHO definition have been established for DXA but not for QCT, though they may be given by the software of the manufacturers. If these T-scores are used to diagnose osteoporosis, a substantially higher number of individuals compared to DXA will be diagnosed as osteoporotic, since BMD measured with QCT shows a faster decrease with age than DXA. In order to facilitate the interpretation of QCT results, the American College of Radiology has in 2008 published guidelines for the performance of QCT; based on these guidelines BMD values from 120 to 80 mg/ml are defined as osteopenic and BMD values below 80 mg/ml as osteoporotic, which would correspond to a T-score of approximately −3.0.

A substantial disadvantage of 2-D QCT is its lower precision compared to that of DXA (1.5–4 vs. 1 %), which results in a larger least significant change required to detect significant changes in BMD (6–11 vs. 3 %). However, since the metabolic activity of trabecular bone is higher, a lower precision is adequate for single slice QCT to monitor longitudinal changes that are in the same range as those found with DXA.

2.2 Volumetric QCT

With spiral and multislice CT acquisition of larger bone volumes, such as entire vertebrae and the proximal femur, is feasible within a few seconds (<10 s). These data sets can be used to obtain 3-D-images, which provide geometrical and volumetric density information (Fig. 4). As an alternative to volumetric QCT (vQCT) the term three dimensional (3-D) QCT may be used. Contiguous sections with a slice thickness of 1–3 mm and no CT scanner angulation are typically obtained. The lumbar spine protocols typically only include L1 and L2, as the exposure dose is relatively high. Typically, kVp is in the order of 80–120 and mAs between 100 and 200. Using these parameters, the exposure dose has been estimated to be as high as 1.5 mSv for the spine, and 2.5–3 mSv

for the hip (Engelke et al. 2008). The primary advantage of volumetric QCT of the spine is an improved precision for trabecular BMD measurements, which is in the order of 1–2.5 % (Engelke et al. 2008). Different analysis techniques have been applied to quantify BMD in the volumetric ROIs; in addition to the standard midvertebral trabecular volume of interest (VOI) that in size and location is similar to the volume analyzed in single slice mode, various additional VOI can be measured by 3-D QCT. However, to date there is no agreement on the locations, sizes, or shapes of VOIs (Engelke et al. 2008). Currently, two manufacturers offer volumetric QCT software with calibration phantoms (QCT Pro, Mindways Software, Inc., Austin, TX and Image Analysis Inc., Columbia, KY).

Because of the complex anatomy of the proximal femur, single slice QCT is not feasible but volumetric approaches have been found to have good reproducibility. The scan region typically starts 1–2 cm above the femoral head and extends a few centimeters below the lesser trochanter. Typically, kVp is in the order of 120 and mAs between 100 and 330 (Engelke et al. 2008). Algorithms to process volumetric CT images of the proximal femur and to measure BMD in the femoral neck, the total femur, and the trochanteric regions are available and include two commercial and a few advanced university-based research tools (Lang et al. 1997). Proximal femur 3-D QCT has a high precision of 0.6–1.1 % for trabecular bone and may also be used to determine geometric measures such as the cross-sectional area of the femur neck and the hip axis length. These measurements may be useful in optimizing fracture prediction of the proximal femur.

While WHO criteria are not applicable to volumetric QCT measurements of the lumbar spine, it should be noted that the American College of Radiology guidelines for the performance of QCT for single slice QCT are also applicable to volumetric QCT: BMD values of 120–80 mg/ml are defined as osteopenic and below 80 mg/ml as osteoporotic. One of the manufacturers also provides BMD ranges to quantify

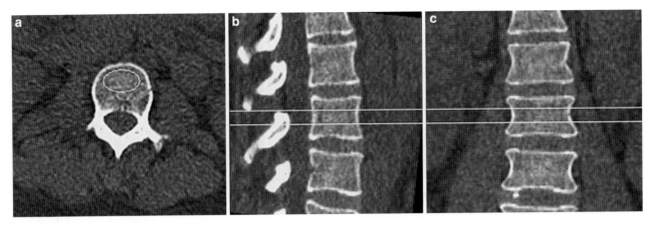

Fig. 4 Volumetric or 3-D QCT of the lumbar spine demonstrating an axial CT image of L2 (**a**) as well as sagittally (**b**) and coronally (**c**) reconstructed images indicating the volume of interest used for the volumetric BMD measurement

Fig. 5 Volumetric QCT of the hip: axial CT image of bilateral hip joints on a Mindways calibration phantom (**a**) and DXA like, 2-D, reconstructed CT image with femoral neck (*small arrow*), trochanteric (*long arrow*), and intertrochanteric ROIs (**b**)

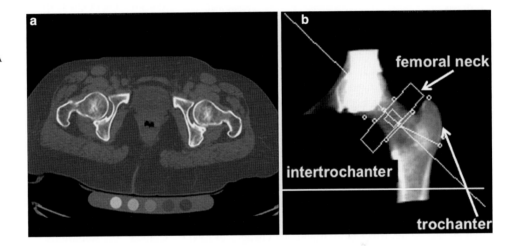

increase in fracture risk: a BMD of 110–80 mg/cc is described to indicate a mild increase in fracture risk, BMD values of 50–80 mg/cc indicate a moderate increase in fracture risk and a BMD lower than 50 mg/cc indicates a severe increase in fracture risk.

For the proximal femur, 3-D datasets may be used to derive a projectional 2-D image of the proximal femur and in this image standard DXA-equivalent ROIs may be placed (Fig. 5). This so-called QCT-derived DXA equivalent aBMD (QCT(DXA) aBMD) can be calculated using CTXA Hip software (Mindways Software Inc., Austin, TX, USA). In the ROIs, BMD values are determined in g/cm². Since the correlations between these calculated BMD values of the proximal femur and those obtained by DXA are extremely high, the WHO classification may be applied to those BMD values in post-menopausal women (Khoo et al. 2009). Thus, a T-score ≤2.5 derived from those datasets indicates osteoporotic BMD.

2.3 Advantages and Disadvantages of Axial QCT versus DXA

In addition to the true volumetric measurements, QCT has several important advantages over DXA. As DXA is a projectional technique, structures overlying the vertebral body and proximal femur will impact and limit the measurements. Thus, aortic and femoral artery calcifications will artificially increase BMD measurements, as will degenerative disc disease, diffuse idiopathic skeletal hyperostosis (DISH), and facet arthropathy. In addition surgical clips, contrast within the bowel and status post spine surgery (in particular laminectomies) will alter BMD measurements. All of this will have less impact on QCT measurements. A recent study comparing DXA and QCT in older men with DISH demonstrated that QCT was better suited to differentiate men with and without vertebral fractures (Diederichs et al. 2011); DISH is a condition which is frequently found in

Fig. 6 Volumetric QCT of the spine and hip showing nonenhanced abdominal and pelvic source images. In the para-aortic region (**a**) and the right inguinal region (**b**) there are multiple large lymph nodes (*arrows*), which were an incidental finding. Further clinical work-up led to the diagnosis of Non-Hodgkin's Lymphoma

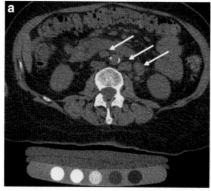
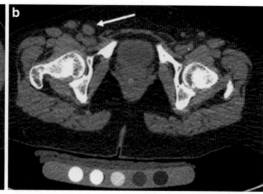

Table 1 ACR guidelines for the performance of QCT, result interpretation

Density in mg Hydroxyapatite/ml	Definition
>120 mg/ml	Normal
120–80 mg/ml	Osteopenic
<80 mg/ml	Osteoporotic

older individuals and a higher number of vertebral fragility fractures were shown in these individuals.

In addition, QCT provides purely trabecular bone measurements which are more sensitive to monitoring changes with disease and therapy. In a randomized, double-blind clinical study of parathyroid hormone and alendronate to test the hypothesis that the concurrent administration of the two agents would increase bone density more than the use of either one alone, Black et al. found that changes in BMD demonstrated with QCT in patients treated with PTH and alendronate were 2–3 times higher than those found with DXA (Black et al. 2003).

Cross-sectional studies have shown that QCT BMD of the spine allows better discrimination of individuals with and without fragility fractures (Yu et al. 1995; Bergot et al. 2001). Bergot et al. found significantly higher ($p < 0.05$) receiver operator characteristics analysis (ROC) values for QCT compared to DXA not only for vertebral fractures (0.85 vs. 0.79), but also for peripheral fractures (0.72 vs. 0.67) in 508 European women.

In addition, QCT is better suited for examining obese patients as DXA has limitations in measuring BMD in patients with a BMD over 25–30 kg/m^2; in obese patients superimposed soft tissue will elevate measured BMD due to attenuation of the X-ray beams and beam hardening artifact as shown in previous studies (Tothill et al. 1997; Weigert and Cann 1999; Binkley et al. 2003).

However, a number of pertinent disadvantages of QCT also have to be considered. Most of all, the higher radiation dose (0.06–3 mSv) is of concern in particular in

younger individuals (e.g., peri-menopausal women). Also, there are a limited number of longitudinal scientific studies assessing how QCT predicts fragility fractures and most of the pharmacological therapy studies have been performed using DXA. Another major problem with QCT is that T-scores should not be used to define osteoporosis and osteopenia. A T-score threshold of -2.5 for QCT would identify a much higher percentage of osteoporotic subjects, and has therefore never been established for clinical use. Currently, volumetric QCT techniques are state-of-the-art (Lang et al. 1999; Bousson et al. 2006; Farhat et al. 2006a, b) and in clinical routine absolute measurements of volumetric BMD to characterize fracture risk have been used (110–80 mg/cm^3 = mild increase in fracture risk, 80–50 mg/cm^3 = moderate increase in fracture risk and below 50 mg/cm^3 = severe increase in fracture risk). Also, more importantly, according to the "American College of Radiology (ACR) Guidelines for QCT" a density range of 120–80 mg/cm^3 is defined as osteopenic BMD and BMD values below 80 mg/cm^3 as osteoporotic BMD (ACR Practice Guideline for the Performance of QCT Bone Densitometry; 2008) (Table 1).

Currently, DXA of the spine and proximal femur is the preferred imaging text for making therapeutic decisions, but if not available QCT may also be used (Engelke et al. 2008). According to expert opinion from Japan, the US, the United Kingdom, and Germany for Siemens QCT scanners, a treatment threshold for spinal trabecular BMD of 80 mg/cm^3 without additional risk factors may be used (Engelke et al. 2008).

Concerning image interpretation, it should be noted that volumetric QCT takes substantially longer to report compared to DXA as the limited CT of the pelvis and abdomen may show a number of abnormalities of the internal organs, the spine, bony pelvis, and muscles, which should not be missed. Analysis of nonenhanced CT images is challenging, yet failure to report abnormalities such as kidney tumors and enlarged lymph nodes may have legal consequences (Fig. 6).

Table 2 Clinical Indications for volumetric QCT

Clinical indication for QCT	Rationale
1. Very small or large patients	Volumetric measurement, not impacted by patient size such as DXA (projectional measurement)
2. Advanced degenerative spine disease (degenerative disc disease, facet arthropathy, and DISH)	Only trabecular part of vertebral body is measured and osteophytes have limited impact on measurement
3. Obese subjects (BMI > 30)	DXA incompletely removes soft tissue
4. If high sensitivity to monitor metabolic bone change is required	Trabecular is metabolically more active

2.4 Clinical Indications for Axial QCT

The most important clinical indications for QCT are outlined in Table 2. Recommendations for the use of QCT instead of DXA are (1) very small or large individuals (DXA may suggest abnormally low BMD in small individuals), (2) older individuals with expected advanced degenerative disease of the lumbar spine or morphological abnormalities (in particular men and individuals with DISH), (3) if high sensitivity to monitor metabolic bone change is required such as in patients treated with parathyroid hormone or corticosteroids. Also, QCT should be considered and (4) in obese subjects, as dual energy in DXA only incompletely removes error due to fat.

2.5 Advanced QCT Technologies and Applications

Standard BMD measurements have limitations in assessing fracture risk; in the 2000 NIH consensus conference, the expert panel agreed to not only include BMD as a test to diagnose fracture risk, but also include measures of bone quality (NIH Consensus Development Panel on Osteoporosis Prevention 2001). Bone quality includes bone architecture, micro- and macrostructure and researchers have subsequently developed technologies to characterize bone quality. In addition to high-resolution peripheral QCT (HR-pQCT), multidetector CT (MD-CT) was investigated to image bone structure as it can be used in clinical practice and has superior spatial resolution compared to previous spiral CT scanners. For imaging of trabecular bone structure; however, spatial resolution is still limited given a minimum slice thickness in the order of 0.6 mm with minimum in plane spatial resolution of approximately $0.25–0.3$ mm^2 (Link et al. 2003). Using this spatial resolution, imaging of individual trabeculae (measuring approximately 0.05–0.2 mm in diameter) is subject to significant partial volume effects; however, it has been shown that trabecular bone parameters obtained from this technique correlate with those determined in contact radiographs from histological bone sections and μCT (Issever et al. 2002; Link et al. 2003).

An advantage of MD-CT compared to HR-pQCT is access to central regions of the skeleton such as the spine and proximal femur, sites at risk for fragility fractures, where monitoring of therapy may be most efficient. However, in order to achieve adequate spatial resolution and image quality, the required radiation exposure is substantial, which offsets the technique's applicability in clinical routine and scientific studies (Graeff et al. 2007; Damilakis et al. 2010). High-resolution MD-CT requires considerably higher radiation doses compared with standard techniques for measuring BMD. Compared with the 0.001–0.05 mSv effective dose associated with DXA in adult patients and 0.06–0.3 mSv delivered through 2-D QCT of the lumbar spine, protocols used to examine vertebral microstructure with high-resolution MD-CT provide an effective dose of approximately 3 mSv (Ito et al. 2005; Graeff et al. 2007).

Clinical studies have demonstrated that MD-CT derived structure measures at the proximal femur and lumbar spine improve differentiation of osteoporotic patients with proximal femur fractures and normal controls (Rodriguez-Soto et al. 2010) (Fig. 5) as well as individuals with and without osteoporotic spine fractures (Ito et al. 2005). In addition, the technique was shown to be well suited for monitoring teriparatide-associated changes of vertebral microstructure (Graeff et al. 2007). Recently, Keaveny et al. used finite element analysis to study vertebral body strength and therapy-related changes in MD-CT datasets of the spine and proximal femur (Keaveny et al. 2008; Mawatari et al. 2008; Keaveny 2010); the results of this work suggested improved monitoring of treatment effects compared to DXA and greater sensitivity in fracture risk assessment.

A number of studies have suggested to use clinical contrast and noncontrast-enhanced abdominal and pelvic CT to measure BMD, which would greatly enhance the availability of BMD information in larger patient populations with no extra radiation or cost. In a feasibility study, Link et al. analyzed BMD in standard single slice QCT studies and compared these measurements with those obtained in clinical spiral CT studies. They found highly significant correlations between BMD measurements using both techniques and concluded that by using a conversion factor, BMD measurements can be determined with routine abdominal spiral CT scans (Link et al. 2004). Subsequently,

BMD measurements obtained from volumetric QCT of the spine and hip were correlated with those derived from non-dedicated contrast-enhanced standard MD-CT datasets to derive a conversion factor for volumetric QCT (Bauer et al. 2007). Based on linear regression, a correlation coefficient of $r = 0.98$ was calculated for lumbar BMD with the equation BMD(QCT) $= 0.96 \times$ BMD(MD-CT) -20.9 mg/mL and a coefficient of $r = 0.99$ was calculated for the proximal femur with the equation BMD(QCT) $= 0.99 \times$ BMD(MD-CT) -12 mg/cm2 ($p < 0.01$). Both standard volumetric QCT and contrast-enhanced MD-CT datasets could be used to differentiate post-menopausal women with and without fragility fractures; no significant differences were found between both techniques' performance in differentiating fracture and nonfracture cohorts. The investigators concluded that with the conversion factors, reliable volumetric BMD measurements can be calculated for the hip and the spine from routine abdominal and pelvic MD-CT datasets (Bauer et al. 2007). Similar results were also found by other studies (Lenchik et al. 2004; Papadakis et al. 2009; Baum et al. 2011, 2012), which confirms the potential of standard MD-CT abdominal and pelvic studies to provide clinically pertinent BMD information if performed with the patient located on a calibration phantom.

3 Peripheral QCT

Dedicated peripheral QCT (pQCT) scanners have been developed to assess the BMD of the distal radius and tibia (Butz et al. 1994). These scanners have a low radiation dose, a high precision with a short examination time, but have the same limitations as peripheral DXA in the monitoring of patients with osteoporosis. While this technique is potentially suited to predict fracture risk, studies have shown the limitations of this technique in predicting spine fractures and proximal hip fractures compared to other bone densitometry techniques (Grampp et al. 1997; Augat et al. 1998a, b).

Standard pQCT scanners work in step and scan mode, operating either with single slice or multislice acquisition. The forearm measurement locations are defined with respect to the length of the radius and measured from the radio-carpal joint surface to the olecranon. Typically, scan locations with single slice CT scanners are distal sites (4% of radius length) containing mainly trabecular bone and a shaft location (15%–65% of radius length) consisting predominantly of cortical bone, while multislice scanners use a distal site between 4 and 10 % of the length of the radius and also a shaft location (Engelke et al. 2008). The most frequently used peripheral scanners for the distal radius are the Stratec Scanners (Stratec Medizintechnik, Pforzheim, Germany).

Previous cross-sectional studies have demonstrated that pQCT can differentiate patients with hip fragility fractures and normal controls (Augat et al. 1998a, b), while findings were more controversial for spine fragility fractures (Formica et al. 1998; Clowes et al. 2005). While absolute BMD threshold values are available for axial QCT to differentiate patients with normal, osteopenic, and osteoporotic BMD, those threshold values are not available for pQCT. Given these limitations, using pQCT to initiate osteoporosis treatment is problematic; however, once initiated, pQCT can be used to monitor treatment (Engelke et al. 2008). Please note that as in axial QCT, measurements between different scanners should not be compared.

3.1 HR-pQCT

One of the most promising developments to assess bone architecture over the last 10 years has been the introduction of high-resolution peripheral QCT (HR-pQCT) (Boutroy et al. 2005; Burghardt et al. 2008; Burrows et al. 2009; Burghardt et al. 2010a; Krug et al. 2010) (Fig. 7). The dedicated extremity imaging system designed for imaging of trabecular and cortical bone architecture is currently available from a single manufacturer (Xtreme CT, Scanco Medical AG, Brüttisellen, Switzerland) and was developed based on experimental MicroCT technology. This device has the advantage of significantly higher signal to noise ratio (SNR) and spatial resolution compared to MD-CT, MRI, and other pQCT devices (nominal isotropic voxel dimension of 82 μm) (Krug et al. 2010). By comparison, MD-CT has a maximum in plane spatial resolution of 250–300 and MRI of 150–200 μm with slice thicknesses of 0.5–0.7 and 0.3–0.5 mm, respectively. Furthermore, the effective radiation dose is substantially lower compared to whole-body MD-CT, and primarily does not involve critical, radiosensitive organs (effective dose <3 microSv). The scan time for HR-pQCT is approximately 3 min for each scan of the tibia and femur.

There are several disadvantages to this technology; most notably, that it is limited to peripheral skeletal sites, and therefore can provide no direct insight into bone quality in the lumbar spine or proximal femur—common sites for osteoporotic fragility fractures (Krug et al. 2010). Only a limited region of the distal radius and tibia may be scanned in one pass (9.02 mm in length with 110 slices). In addition, the scanner tube has a limited life span and motion artifacts sometimes limit morphological analysis of the bone architecture.

The advantages of the system are that it allows acquisition of BMD, trabecular, and cortical bone architecture at the same time. A semi-automatic standard protocol provided by the manufacturer is used for image analysis; the segmentation

Fig. 7 HR-pQCT images of the distal radius (**a**) and the distal tibia (**b**). Images impressively demonstrate trabecular bone architecture, which is well interconnected in (**a**) and shows central loss of trabeculae in (**b**)

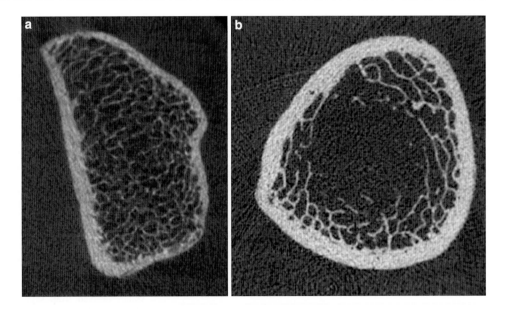

Fig. 8 HR-pQCT images of the distal tibia in a healthy control (**a**) and a patient with Diabetes and a fragility fracture in (**b**), note impressive increase in cortical porosity in the fracture patient (*arrows*)

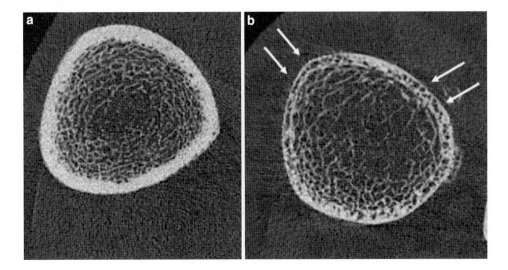

process is initiated by the operator and automatically adjusted using an edge detection process to precisely identify the periosteal boundary. The cortical bone compartment is segmented using a 3-D Gaussian smoothing filter followed by a simple fixed threshold. The trabecular compartment is identified by digital subtraction of the cortical bone from the region enclosed by the periosteal contours. Based on this semi-automated contouring and segmentation process, the trabecular, and cortical compartments are segmented automatically for subsequent densitometric, morphometric, and biomechanical analyses (Link 2012).

A 5 cylinder hydroxyapatite calibration phantom is used to generate volumetric BMD separately for cortical and trabecular bone compartments, similarly to central QCT. Morphometric indices analogous to classical histomorphometry as well as connectivity, structure model index (a measure of the rod or plate-like appearance of the structure), and

anisotropy can be calculated from the binary images of the trabecular bone (Link 2012). In addition, finite element analysis (FEA) can be applied to these datasets and apparent biomechanical properties (e.g., stiffness, elastic modulus) can be computed by decomposing the trabecular bone structure into small cubic elements (i.e., the voxels) with assumed mechanical properties (Macneil and Boyd 2008a; Burghardt et al. 2010b; Liu et al. 2010). Reproducibility of HR-pQCT densitometric measures is high (coefficient of variation <1 %), while biomechanical and morphometric measures typically have a coefficient of variation of 4–5 % (Boutroy et al. 2005; MacNeil and Boyd 2008b; Burghardt et al. 2010b).

A number of clinical studies have been performed which have shown promising results in differentiating post-menopausal females and older men with and without fragility fractures (Boutroy et al. 2005; Szulc et al. 2010) as well as in monitoring therapeutic interventions (Burghardt et al. 2010c; Li et al. 2010). It was also found that trabecular and cortical subregional analysis may provide additional information in characterizing gender and age-related bone changes (Sode et al. 2010).

Recently, structural analysis of cortical bone has been introduced to the study of HR-pQCT datasets and cortical porosity measurements have been developed (Burghardt et al. 2010d). A recent study suggested that cortical porosity measurements may be useful to assess increased fracture risk in patients with diabetes (Burghardt et al. 2010d) (Fig. 8). Patients with type II diabetes are at higher risk for fragility fractures, yet DXA BMD in diabetes patients is increased, and is therefore not well suited to diagnose fracture risk (Schwartz and Sellmeyer 2004).

4 Conclusion and Future Developments

In summary, while DXA is the standard technique to measure BMD, QCT has some important advantages over DXA which are useful for a number of clinical applications including (1) BMD in small, large, or obese patients, (2) when rapid information on treatment effects is required and (3) when degenerative disease, arterial calcifications, or artifacts limit evaluation of DXA scans. QCT also has a number of disadvantages including the higher radiation dose, limited applicability of WHO criteria, and overall less experience with fracture prediction, treatment initiation, and response with QCT compared to DXA.

Given the deficits of QCT in relation to DXA, future research needs to focus on prospective studies clearly providing evidence that QCT also predicts fragility fractures of the spine, proximal femur, and appendicular skeleton and better treatment thresholds need to be defined; those for spine QCT are currently based on expert opinion and for pQCT no good recommendations exist. While central QCT of the spine is relatively well-established QCT of the hip and pQCT of the distal radius and tibia are still substantially less developed. HR-pQCT is currently a promising research tool, but not suited for larger scale clinical applications.

Research currently targets improved evaluation of bone strength using structure analysis techniques and finite element modeling has a central role in this arena; in addition, there is an increasing body of knowledge on cortical bone structure and its significance in predicting bone strength, which may change our algorithms in how to interpret the risk of fragility fractures in individual patients.

References

Arnold B (1989) Solid phantom for QCT bone mineral analysis. Proceedings of the 7th international workshop on bone densitometry, Palm, Springs, California, 17–21 Sept 1989

Augat P, Fan B, Lane N et al (1998a) Assessment of bone mineral at appendicular sites in females with fractures of the proximal femur. Bone 22:395–402

Augat P, Fuerst T, Genant H (1998b) Quantitative bone mineral assessment at the forearm: a review. Osteoporos Int 8:299–310

Bauer JS, Henning TD, Mueller D et al (2007) Volumetric quantitative CT of the spine and hip derived from contrast-enhanced MDCT: conversion factors. AJR Am J Roentgenol 188(5):1294–1301

Baum T, Muller D, Dobritz M et al (2011) BMD measurements of the spine derived from sagittal reformations of contrast-enhanced MDCT without dedicated software. Eur J Radiol 80(2):e140–145

Baum T, Muller D, Dobritz M et al (2012) Converted lumbar BMD values derived from sagittal reformations of contrast-enhanced MDCT predict incidental osteoporotic vertebral fractures. Calcif Tissue Int 90(6):481–487

Bergot C, Laval-Jeantet A, Hutchinson K et al (2001) A comparison of spinal quantitative computed tomography with dual energy X-ray absorptiometry in European women with vertebral and nonvertebral fractures. Calcif Tissue Int 68:74–82

Binkley N, Krueger D, Vallarta-Ast N (2003) An overlying fat panniculus affects femur bone mass measurement. J Clin Densitom 6(3):199–204

Black DM, Greenspan SL, Ensrud KE et al (2003) The effects of parathyroid hormone and alendronate alone or in combination in postmenopausal osteoporosis. N Engl J Med 349(13):1207–1215

Block J, Smith R, Glüer CC et al (1989) Models of spinal trabecular bone loss as determined by quantitative computed tomography. J Bone Miner Res 4:249–257

Bousson V, Le Bras A, Roqueplan F et al (2006) Volumetric quantitative computed tomography of the proximal femur: relationships linking geometric and densitometric variables to bone strength. Role for compact bone. Osteoporos Int 17(6):855–864

Boutroy S, Bouxsein ML, Munoz F et al (2005) In vivo assessment of trabecular bone microarchitecture by high-resolution peripheral quantitative computed tomography. J Clin Endocrinol Metab 90(12):6508–6515

Burghardt AJ, Buie HR, Laib A et al (2010a) Reproducibility of direct quantitative measures of cortical bone microarchitecture of the distal radius and tibia by HR-pQCT. Bone 47(3):519–528

Burghardt AJ, Dais KA, Masharani U et al (2008) In vivo quantification of intra-cortical porosity in human cortical bone using hr-pQCT in patients with type II diabetes. J Bone Miner Res 23:S450

Burghardt AJ, Issever AS, Schwartz AV et al (2010b) High-resolution peripheral quantitative computed tomographic imaging of cortical and trabecular bone microarchitecture in patients with type 2 diabetes mellitus. J Clin Endocrinol Metab 95(11):5045–5055

Burghardt AJ, Kazakia GJ, Ramachandran S et al (2010c) Age- and gender-related differences in the geometric properties and biomechanical significance of intracortical porosity in the distal radius and tibia. J Bone Miner Res 25(5):983–993

Burghardt AJ, Kazakia GJ, Sode M et al (2010d) A longitudinal HR-pQCT study of alendronate treatment in post-menopausal women with low bone density: Relations between density, cortical and trabecular micro-architecture, biomechanics, and bone turnover. J Bone Miner Res 25:2282–2295

Burrows M, Liu D, McKay H (2009) High-resolution peripheral QCT imaging of bone micro-structure in adolescents. Osteoporos Int 21(3):515–520

Butz S, Wüster C, Scheidt-Nave C et al. (1994) Forearm BMD as measured by peripheral quantitative computed tomography (pQCT) in a German reference population. Osteoporos Int (4):179–184

Cann C, Genant H (1980) Precise measurement of vertebral mineral content using computed tomography. J Comput Assist Tomogr 4:493–500

Cann C, Genant H, Kolb F et al (1985) Quantitative computed tomography for the prediction of vertebral body fracture risk. Bone 6:1–7

Clowes JA, Eastell R, Peel NF (2005) The discriminative ability of peripheral and axial bone measurements to identify proximal femoral, vertebral, distal forearm and proximal humeral fractures: a case control study. Osteoporos Int 16(12):1794–1802

Damilakis J, Adams JE, Guglielmi G et al (2010) Radiation exposure in X-ray-based imaging techniques used in osteoporosis. Eur Radiol 20(11):2707–2714

Diederichs G, Engelken F, Marshall LM et al (2011) Diffuse idiopathic skeletal hyperostosis (DISH): relation to vertebral fractures and bone density. Osteoporos Int 22(6):1789–1797

Engelke K, Adams JE, Armbrecht G et al (2008) Clinical use of quantitative computed tomography and peripheral quantitative computed tomography in the management of osteoporosis in adults: the 2007 ISCD official positions. J Clin Densitom 11(1):123–162

Farhat GN, Cauley JA, Matthews KA et al (2006a) Volumetric BMD and vascular calcification in middle-aged women: the study of women's health across the nation. J Bone Miner Res 21(12):1839–1846

Farhat GN, Strotmeyer ES, Newman AB et al (2006b) Volumetric and areal bone mineral density measures are associated with cardio-vascular disease in older men and women: the health, aging, and body composition study. Calcif Tissue Int 79(2):102–111

Felsenberg D, Gowin W (1999) Knochendichtemessung mit Zwei-Spektren-Methoden. Radiologe 39:186–193

Firooznia H, Rafii M, Golimbu C et al (1986) Trabecular mineral content of the spine in women with hip fracture: CT measurement. Musculoskel Rad 159:737–740

Formica CA, Nieves JW, Cosman F et al (1998) Comparative assessment of bone mineral measurements using dual X-ray absorptiometry and peripheral quantitative computed tomography. Osteoporos Int 8(5):460–467

Genant H, Cann C, Ettinger B et al (1982) Quantitative computed tomography of vertebral spongiosa: a sensitive method for detecting early bone loss after oophorectomy. Ann Int Med 97:699–704

Genant HK, Boyd DP (1977) Quantitative bone mineral analysis using dual energy computed tomography. Invest Radiol 12:545–551

Genant HK, Cann CE, Pozzi-Mucelli RS et al (1983) Vertebral mineral determination by quantitative computed tomography: clinical feasibility and normative data. J Comput Assist Tomogr 7:554

Glüer C, Genant H (1989) Impact of marrow fat in accuracy of quantitative CT. J Comput Assist Tomogr 13:1023–1035

Graeff C, Timm W, Nickelsen TN et al (2007) Monitoring teriparatide-associated changes in vertebral microstructure by high-resolution CT in vivo: results from the EUROFORS study. J Bone Miner Res 22(9):1426–1433

Grampp S, Genant H, Mathur A et al (1997) Comparisons of noninvasive bone mineral measurements in assessing age-related loss, fracture discrimination, and diagnostic classification. J Bone Miner Res 12:697–711

Issever AS, Vieth V, Lotter A et al (2002) Local differences in the trabecular bone structure of the proximal femur depicted with high-spatial-resolution MR imaging and multisection CT. Acad Radiol 9(12):1395–1406

Ito M, Ikeda K, Nishiguchi M et al (2005) Multi-detector row CT imaging of vertebral microstructure for evaluation of fracture risk. J Bone Miner Res 20(10):1828–1836

Kalender W, Brestowsky H, Felsenberg D (1988) Bone mineral measurements: automated determination of the mitvertebral CT section. Radiology 168:219–221

Kalender W, Felsenberg D, Louis O et al (1989) Reference values for trabecular and cortical vertebral bone density in single and dual-energy quantitative computed tomography. Europ J Radiol 9:75–80

Kalender WA, Klotz E, Süss C (1987) Vertebral bone mineral analysis: an integrated approach. Radiology 164:419–423

Kalender WA, Süss C (1987) A new calibration phantom for quantitative computed tomography. Med Phys 9:816–819

Keaveny TM (2010) Biomechanical computed tomography-noninvasive bone strength analysis using clinical computed tomography scans. Ann N Y Acad Sci 1192:57–65

Keaveny TM, Hoffmann PF, Singh M et al (2008) Femoral bone strength and its relation to cortical and trabecular changes after treatment with PTH, alendronate, and their combination as assessed by finite element analysis of quantitative CT scans. J Bone Miner Res 23(12):1974–1982

Khoo BC, Brown K, Cann C et al (2009) Comparison of QCT-derived and DXA-derived areal bone mineral density and T scores. Osteoporos Int 20(9):1539–1545

Krug R, Burghardt AJ, Majumdar S et al (2010) High-resolution imaging techniques for the assessment of osteoporosis. Radiol Clin North Am 48(3):601–621

Lang T, Keyak J, Heitz M et al (1997) Volumetric quantitative computed tomography of the proximal femur: precision and relation to bone strength. Bone 21:101–108

Lang T, Li J, Harris S et al (1999) Assessment of vertebral bone mineral density using volumetric quantitative CT. J Comput Assist Tomogr 23:130–137

Lenchik L, Shi R, Register TC et al (2004) Measurement of trabecular bone mineral density in the thoracic spine using cardiac gated quantitative computed tomography. J Comput Assist Tomogr 28(1):134–139

Li EK, Zhu TY, Hung VY et al (2010) Ibandronate increases cortical bone density in patients with systemic lupus erythematosus on long-term glucocorticoid. Arthritis Res Ther 12(5):R198

Link T, Vieth V, Stehling C et al (2003) High resolution MRI versus Multislice spiral CT—which technique depicts the trabecular bone structure best? Eur Radiol 13:663–671

Link TM (2012) Osteoporosis imaging: state of the art and advanced imaging. Radiology 263(1):3–17

Link TM, Koppers BB, Licht T et al (2004) In vitro and in vivo spiral CT to determine bone mineral density: initial experience in patients at risk for osteoporosis. Radiology 231(3):805–811

Liu XS, Zhang XH, Sekhon KK et al (2010) High-resolution peripheral quantitative computed tomography can assess micro-structural and mechanical properties of human distal tibial bone. J Bone Miner Res 25(4):746–756

Macneil JA, Boyd SK (2008a) Bone strength at the distal radius can be estimated from high-resolution peripheral quantitative computed tomography and the finite element method. Bone 42(6):1203–1213

MacNeil JA, Boyd SK (2008b) Improved reproducibility of high-resolution peripheral quantitative computed tomography for measurement of bone quality. Med Eng Phys 30(6):792–799

Mawatari T, Miura H, Hamai S et al (2008) Vertebral strength changes in rheumatoid arthritis patients treated with alendronate, as assessed by finite element analysis of clinical computed tomography scans: a prospective randomized clinical trial. Arthritis Rheum 58(11):3340–3349

NIH Consensus Development Panel on Osteoporosis Prevention, D., and Therapy (2001) Osteoporosis prevention, diagnosis, and therapy. JAMA 285:785–795

Papadakis AE, Karantanas AH, Papadokostakis G et al (2009) Can abdominal multi-detector CT diagnose spinal osteoporosis? Eur Radiol 19(1):172–176

Rodriguez-Soto AE, Fritscher KD, Schuler B et al (2010) Texture analysis, bone mineral density, and cortical thickness of the proximal femur: fracture risk prediction. J Comput Assist Tomogr 34(6):949–957

Sandor T, Kalender WA, Hanlon WB et al (1985) Spinal bone mineral determination using automated contour detection: application to single and dual—energy CT. SPIE Med Imaging Instrum 555:188–194

Schwartz AV, Sellmeyer DE (2004) Women, type 2 diabetes, and fracture risk. Curr Diab Rep 4(5):364–369

Sode M, Burghardt AJ, Kazakia GJ et al (2010) Regional variations of gender-specific and age-related differences in trabecular bone structure of the distal radius and tibia. Bone 46(6):1652–1660

Steiger P, Block J, Steiger S (1990) Spinal bone mineral density measured with quantitative CT: effect of region of interest, vertebral level and techniques. Radiology 175:537–543

Szulc P, Boutroy S, Vilayphiou N et al. (2010) Cross-sectional analysis of the association between fragility fractures and bone microarchitecture in older men—the STRAMBO study. J Bone Miner Res. epub ahead of print

Tothill P, Hannan WJ, Cowen S et al (1997) Anomalies in the measurement of changes in total-body bone mineral by dual-energy X-ray absorptiometry during weight change. J Bone Miner Res 12(11):1908–1921

Weigert J, Cann C (1999) DXA in obese patients: are normal values really normal. J Women's Imaging 1:11–17

Yu W, Gluer C, Grampp S et al (1995) Spinal bone mineral assessment in postmenopausal women: a comparison between dual X-ray absorptiometry and quantitative computed tomography. Osteoporos Int 5:433–439

Quantitative Ultrasound and Fracture Risk Assessment

Giuseppe Guglielmi and Michelangelo Nasuto

Contents

G. Guglielmi (✉) · M. Nasuto
Department of Radiology, University of Foggia,
Viale Luigi Pinto 1, 71100 Foggia, Italy
e-mail: g.guglielmi@unifg.it

G. Guglielmi
Department of Radiology, Scientific Institute
"Casa Sollievo della Sofferenza" Hospital,
Viale Cappuccini 1, 71013 San Giovanni Rotondo, Foggia, Italy

Abstract

Quantitative ultrasound (QUS) is a non-invasive technique for the investigation of bone tissue used in several pathologies and clinical conditions, especially for the identification of bone changes connected with menopause, osteoporosis and bone fragility. The versatility of the method, its low cost and lack of ionising radiation have led to a worldwide diffusion with an increasing interest among clinicians. In the last years several studies have been conducted to investigate the potential of QUS in various pathologies of bone metabolism, in secondary osteoporosis, paediatrics, neonatology, genetics and other fields. The results have confirmed the ability of the technique in the prediction of fracture risk; studies in paediatrics led to the establishment of reference curves for some QUS devices and other promising results have been reported in several conditions involving metabolic bone disorders.

1   Introduction

The first attempts to quantitatively evaluate bone tissue with ultrasound date back to 20 years ago, although the potential of ultrasonography (US) in investigating bone has been recognized and proposed as a method for monitoring fractures healing since the early 1950s (Siegel et al. 1958). The immaturity of technology and the poor knowledge of physical interactions between US and bone led to set aside this technique until Langton et al. in 1984 demonstrated that bone ultrasound at the heel was useful in the assessment of osteoporosis in women (Langton et al. 1984).

The aim to deepen the knowledge in this technique resulted in several in vitro and clinical studies with different quantitative ultrasound (QUS) approaches that measured

G. Guglielmi (ed.), *Osteoporosis and Bone Densitometry Measurements*, Medical Radiology. Diagnostic Imaging,
DOI: 10.1007/174_2012_751, © Springer-Verlag Berlin Heidelberg 2013

parameters related to the velocity and attenuation of US waves as they passed through bone in order to estimate the probability of future fractures.

Clinical results confirmed that QUS are capable to detect osteoporosis and can be used to measure a variety of parameters related not only with bone density, but even to bone quality.

In fact, QUS devices have found a clinical use in fields different from osteoporosis, predicting bone fragility in a wider context of pathologies related to mineral metabolism in female, male, and pediatric populations.

Today this inexpensive, transportable, and ionizing radiation free technique represents an effective method to evaluate bone tissue in all the cases where avoiding ionizing radiation is mandatory (pregnant women) or preferable (newborns, infants) and all the patients needing continuous assessment of bone status (e.g., growth evaluation, results of treatment).

The aim of this chapter is to describe the physical principles of bone ultrasound and the related technological developments, to review the literature through the most recent and important in vivo and in vitro study and to analyze the clinical experience in the assessment of fracture risk, underlying limitations, and potentials of the technique.

2 Ultrasound and Bone: Interactions and Physical Principles

2.1 Ultrasound Waves

Unlike medical ultrasonography, QUS methods are in general not used for the reconstruction of an image from the inner human body but to obtain parameters by which to assess tissue properties. (Laugier et al. 1994).

The term ultrasound describes the propagation of a mechanical wave at frequencies above the range of human hearing (conventionally 20 kHz).

During the propagation in fluids and solids, the mechanical vibration provokes tiny disturbances of the medium particles from their resting position. Due to the interaction between the particles, the vibration induces a displacement transmitted step by step to other parts of the medium. This propagation depends on the intrinsic elastic properties of the medium as well as on its mass density. In perfect fluids (gases or liquids) only sound waves that make the particles oscillating in the longitudinal axis or the direction of wave can propagate: these are called *compression* or *longitudinal waves*.

However, longitudinal elastic waves can also propagate in solids. Unlike in fluids, a shearing strain can be transmitted to adjacent layers due to the strong binding between particles. Since the motion of the particles is perpendicular to the direction of propagation, these are called *transverse* or *shear waves*.

Even if both compression and shear waves can propagate in biological soft tissues (viscoelastic solids), at ultrasonic frequencies shear waves are usually highly attenuated and consequently neglected. However, in hard tissues like bone, both compression and shear waves have to be considered.

2.2 Frequency–Period–Wavelength

Physical parameters that describe the propagation of the wave in time and space are frequency f or period T and wavelength λ. Medical ultrasound devices usually employ frequencies in the range of 2–15 MHz. On the contrary, due to the frequency dependence of ultrasound attenuation and to high attenuation values in bone, frequency range in quantitative bone ultrasound lies between 200 kHz and 1.5 MHz.

2.3 Sound Pressure–Acoustic Impedance–Intensity

Other properties of ultrasound waves are: the *sound pressure*, which describes pressure changes due to the compressions and rarefactions produced by a compression wave; the *acoustic impedance*, which explains the strict relationship between sound pressure and acoustic particle velocity (specific vibrations of particles about their resting positions caused by the propagation of the wave); the *intensity*, which describes the energy carried by the ultrasound wave.

2.4 Speed of Sound

Sound waves are propagated with a definite velocity (higher in solids and lower in gases) which is the result of interactions between a given type of wave (longitudinal or transverse) and elastic characteristics that determine the stiffness of the medium. Due to this relationship, the measurement of *speed of sound* has a great practical importance in determining elastic properties of materials. Lang was the first to use ultrasound in measuring elastic properties of bone (Lang 1970). The speed of ultrasound in bone can be higher in compact bone (similar to the velocity in solids) and gradually lower in cancellous bone (similar to the velocity in soft tissue) and in high porous bone (Evans et al. 1990).

2.5 Tissue Interactions

Some of the fundamental aspects of ultrasound techniques comprehend tissue interactions with the ultrasound wave. *Reflection* and *refraction* occur at the boundary between two media with different characteristic acoustic impedances or different speeds of sound. Specular reflections constitute the basis of pulse-echo ultrasonic imaging (echography) and contribute to image formation displaying the boundaries of organs.

Scattering is the result from the interaction between a primary ultrasonic wave and the boundaries of particles (inhomogeneities) with physical properties (density or elasticity) different from those of the surrounding medium. As a result, the oscillatory movement of the scatterer is different from that of the surrounding medium and leads to the emission of a secondary wave denoted scattered wave. Due to the alternance of bone marrow (soft-tissue like medium) and trabeculae (solid medium), the cancellous bone can be considered a highly–inhomogeneous scattering medium (Katz et al. 1987).

Attenuation is characterized by a decrease of intensity of ultrasound wave with traveling distance due to absorption phenomena (which turn the ultrasonic wave directly into heat) and scattering (Njeh et al. 1999a, b).

Since bone mass has good absorption capabilities, the attenuation of ultrasound waves in bone will increase with frequency.

Further important factors that contribute to the total wave intensity attenuation are diffraction, reflection, and refraction.

3 Quantitative Bone Ultrasound Parameters

The QUS method involves generating ultrasound impulses that are transmitted (transversally or longitudinally) through the bone of study. The ultrasound wave is produced in the form of a sinusoid impulse by distinct piezoelectric probes (emitting and receiving) and is detected once it has passed through the skeletal segment placed between them.

The most important parameters, commonly adopted by QUS devices manufacturers, include speed of sound (SoS) and broadband ultrasound attenuation (BUA).

3.1 Speed of Sound

Speed of Sound (SoS unit: m/s) is the result of the influence on ultrasound propagation through bone in terms of velocity of transmission (arrival time of the signal at the receiving transducer) and amplitude. This parameter is also affected by the velocities of propagation in the overlying soft tissue and the coupling medium (Chappard et al. 2000).

3.2 Broadband Ultrasound Attenuation

As mentioned before, the attenuation of ultrasound waves in cancellous bone increases with frequency, at first in a linear way. The slope of the attenuation curve related to the frequency is represented by the BUA (BUA unit: dB/MHz). As an increased bone mass causes greater attenuation of higher frequencies, BUA is higher in healthy bone and typically lower in osteoporotic bone (Fig. 1a, b).

3.3 Amplitude Dependent-Speed of Sound, Stiffness Index and Quantitative Ultrasound Index

Both SoS and BUA are influenced by the coupling medium (temperature of water, type of gel) and by the properties of soft tissue layers like temperature and/or edema (Barkmann and Glüer 1999; Johansen and Stone 1997).

As a consequence, more complex parameters like Amplitude Dependent-Speed of Sound (AD-SoS), Stiffness Index (SI), and Quantitative Ultrasound Index (QUI) have been developed to obtain higher precision and less pronounced sensitivity to external influencing factors (Gluer 1997).

These new parameters have proved to be useful not only in the identification of subjects with low bone mineral density and at high risk for fracture (Hans et al. 1996; Guglielmi et al. 2003), but also, and above all, in the investigation of the significant alterations in bone elasticity and structure in metabolic pathologies affecting the skeleton. This new approach to the interaction between ultrasound and bone tissue has led to the availability of complementary data to those provided by densitometry techniques (Roben et al. 2001; Zitmann et al. 2002; Passeri et al. 2003).

4 QUS Measurement Sites and Approaches

The most common skeletal sites currently studied by QUS techniques are the calcaneus, the distal metaphysis of the phalanx, the radius, and the tibia.

4.1 Calcaneus

In 1984 Langton, in his first pioneering model (Langton et al. 1984), suggested transverse transmission in cancellous bone basing on the principle that the site of measurement

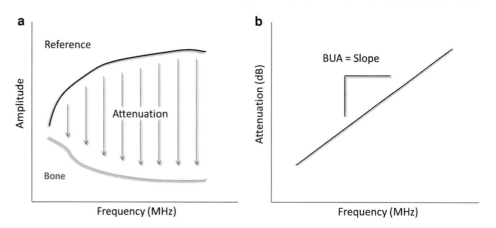

and the transducers had to be immersed in a temperature controlled water bath to ensure proper coupling of the acoustic wave into the skin.

The most preferred site become the calcaneus, which is made up almost entirely of trabecular bone and has the advantage of featuring two flat, parallel surfaces that reduce repositioning errors and are very useful for optimizing the geometry of transmission of the ultrasound band through it.

Therefore a variety of devices measuring ultrasound transmission through the human calcaneus have been developed with several differences regarding to the coupling of the ultrasound wave into the body and the selection of the region to be measured.

Recent Achilles (GE Healthcare, Madison, USA) models, which use water encapsulated in compliant membranes that conform closely to the patient's foot through a temperature-controlled medium, have left the UBIS 5000 (Diagnostic Medical Systems, Pérois, France) and the DTU-One (Osteometer MediTech, Hawthorne, USA) as the main water-bath systems actually on the market.

In fact the greater part of manufacturers adopted the gel as a coupling medium in order to avoid water reservoirs. A proper coupling into the skin has been reached with the use of transducers which are pressed against the skin, usually with the help of rubber pads (CUBA Clinical, McCue—Sahara, Hologic, Bedford, USA).

Several in vitro studies demonstrated that within the same measurement site (i.e. the calcaneus) there is a pronounced variation in BUA and SOS depending upon the localization of the region of interest (Damilakis et al. 2000).

The importance to avoid measurement errors due to variable positioning caused by different foot sizes led to the introduction of several techniques capable to obtain an image of the calcaneus.

An adjustable region of interest (ROI) shown on the display lets the operator confirm the approximate location of where the ultrasound beam will enter the heel during measurement, ensuring optimal positioning and increasing confidence in measurement.

Although numerous devices for QUS measurement of calcaneus are available on the market, few of these have attained an acceptable level of scientific validation in the prediction of fracture risk.

4.2 Phalanx

The metaphysis of the phalanx is consisting of trabecular (at about 40 %) and cortical component, the main determinant of biomechanical bone strength (Fig. 2).

Transverse transmission of cortical bone has been chosen at that level for its high bone turnover and for the sensitivity to changes regarding the skeleton: growth and aging (natural causes), metabolic diseases (hyperparathyroidism…) or drugs (glucocorticoids) (Montagnani et al. 2002) (Fig. 3).

The DBM Sonic Bone Profiler (Igea, Carpi, Italy), unique device that uses this method, measures proximal finger phalanges from II–V by a hand-held caliper with two transducers positioned on opposite sites of the metaphysis and acting as transmitter and receiver respectively.

4.3 Tibia, Radius and Other Sites

Axial transmission of ultrasound through tibia and radius is actually available in only one device (Omnisense, Beam-Med-Sunlight Ultrasound Technologies, Rehovot, Israel). Unlike all the other products, the one side approach offers the potential to measure a variety of bones (metacarpus, humerus, and others), even if tibia and radius remain the most validated skeletal sites demonstrating a good sensitivity to endosteal reabsorption phenomena (Barkmann et al. 2000a). Since propagation occurs mainly along the external surface of the bone, this technique provides indications mostly on the intrinsic material properties of cortical bone (Raum et al. 2005) (Fig. 4).

Other skeletal sites like femur and spine have been suggested for evaluation of bone tissue for the assessment of

Fig. 2 Picture of human phalanx showing the trabecular and cortical component

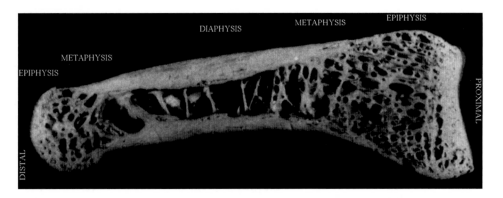

axial BMD at the most common and important sites of fragility fractures.

5   Quality Assurance

The quantitative study of bone tissue requires an adequate reproducibility in terms of reproducibility of measurements performed by different operators with the same medical device and the reproducibility of the measurement performed with different devices of the same model.

First of all a comprehensive training program for the staff is necessary because the apparent fast and easy method of assessing bone status can give the false impression that measurement is always adequately performed. On the contrary, the absence of an immediate feedback on the quality of examination (as it is for DXA) requires a careful adherence to protocol by the operator.

Second, to limit all possible sources of errors, it is fundamental to strictly follow the quality assurance procedures developed for QUS devices.

A constant check of the calibration of the apparatus is mandatory to ensure correct emission of the ultrasound signal by the transducers (i.e., a check of correct functioning of the probes) and the determination of the speed of propagation of the impulse emitted. All devices on the market usually require routine testing for probes and calibration with specific phantoms (usually composed of plastic material or of plexiglass) and own procedures capable of recognize and signal any kind of malfunction problems (Thijssen et al. 2007).

Since QUS devices are portable, environmental conditions become extremely important particularly for calcaneus devices that use water as the coupling medium between transducers. The dependence of the measurement on variations in the temperature of the water is more evident with the use of phantom and has been well-observed by several authors (Chappard et al. 1999; Barkmann et al. 1996; Paggiosi et al. 2005; Krieg et al. 2002; Ikeda and Iki 2004; Mentzel et al. 2009).

Various longitudinal studies attempted to establish quality control for the calcaneus devices proposing a combination of external phantom and internal indicators based on the water measurements (Barkmann and Gluer 1998). Langton (Langton 1997) proposed an external electronic phantom in order to reach a better stability and to reduce the influence of external factors while Laugier et al. (1996) suggested the use of internal digital phantoms; this system has been adopted by the UBIS 5000 (Diagnostic Medical Systems, Pérois, France) showing encouraging results (Hans et al. 2005) but the overall complexity of these quality assurance procedures still results poorly suitable for clinical practice (Hans et al. 2002; Chen et al. 2012).

The issue of cross calibration between different QUS devices assumes determining importance not only in case of equipment change in a single clinic, but most of all in multicenter clinical studies where data are to be collected in different places with several devices, even from the same manufacturer. In the osteoporosis and ultrasound (OPUS) European multicenter clinical study Gluer and colleagues (2004) proposed a single specific phantom for all the devices and a monitor subject who underwent periodic tests at all the centers involved in the study with the aim to check the agreement and calculate the error of reproducibility among the devices.

Although several progresses have been achieved in this field, at the moment there are not yet adequate procedures for standardizing QUS devices, even in those that perform measurements on the same skeletal site.

An important point of discussion is related to the population-based geographic variations in bone density in Europe. Although the OPUS study, the Network in Europe on Male Osteoporosis (NEMO) study (Kaptoge et al. 2008) and the European Vertebral Osteoporosis (EVOS) study (Lunt et al. 1997) have shown between-center differences in hip bone mineral density in European women, an appropriate knowledge on the international geographical heterogeneity of QUS measurement variables has not been reached yet (Paggiosi et al. 2011).

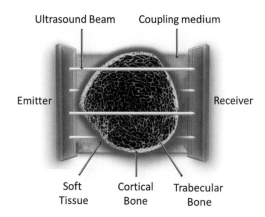

Fig. 3 Transversal ultrasound transmission

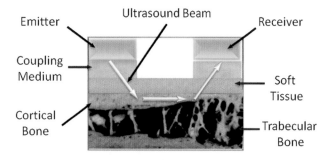

Fig. 4 Axial ultrasound transmission

Recently, Pye et al. (2010) described significant between–center differences in BUA, SOS, and QUI in the European Male Aging Study (EMAS) with no consistent geographical trends in results between North-western, Southern or Eastern Europe. However data have been acquired with a single manufacturer type of device (Sahara, Hologic, USA). In order to avoid these limitations, Paggiosi and colleagues (2012) have recently examined the data acquired with a different range of QUS devices during the OPUS study. The aim was to demonstrate a significant geographical variation in QUS measurement variables, to compare them with hip BMD and to analyze the influence of anthropometric characteristics on the heterogeneity of QUS parameters. The results suggested that QUS measurement variables vary between European countries in a different way to those for hip BMD. These variations may be explained by the influence of anthropometric characteristics, the heterogeneity of QUS devices and other factors that still remain difficult to assess and quantify.

Although a validated cross-calibration procedure still remains elusive, a statistical approach to achieve a standardization of data can be adopted to reduce any between–center differences in QUS measurement variables. However, a widely application of this method still needs further validation.

6   Experience In Vitro and In Vivo

6.1   Ultrasonic Propagation Models

A detailed understanding of ultrasound parameters and their relations with bone characteristics is a key to the development of bone QUS.

Historical models of ultrasonic propagation revealed the importance of both the viscous effects of bone marrow and the anisotropy of the porous microstructure.

Considering the elastic modulus of the cancellous framework as a major determinant of ultrasound speed, Biot developed a wide applicable theory that predicts wave propagation in a two phase heterogeneous media (fluid saturated porous solid). First Taking into account the motion of the fluid and the solid independently and second the viscoelastic coupling between them, two longitudinal waves, fast wave and slow wave are observed. The fast wave moves within the mineralized materials and the slower one moves through the inter trabecular medullar structure (McKelvie and Palmer 1991).

However in practice it has been notified that, due to superimposition phenomena, it is difficult to identify these waves in the received signal and the extraction of information can be difficult to achieve. To obtain a proper separation of the waves Grimes et al. used a space alternating generalized expectation maximization (SAGE) algorithm and got parameters such as arrival time, center frequency, bandwidth, amplitude, phase and velocity of each wave (Grimes et al. 2012).

In these years other important limitations of classical wave propagation theories have been notified (Leclaire et al. 1997). These considerations have induced the development of several studies employing wave equations as alternative formulation of Biot's theory (Gautier et al. 2011; Hughes et al. 2007) or other numerical modeling methods (Ha et al. 2007; Nelson et al. 2011; Lawrence et al. 2010).

Although the results seem to be promising, no single model is actually capable to explain the acoustic behavior of bone; future developments should consider additional attenuation mechanisms as scattering, local flow in microcracks and surface roughness of the trabeculae in a fully comprehensive theory (Haire et al. 1999).

6.2   Cancellous Bone

Although the influence on speed of sound of both mineral content and porosity still remains to be deeply elucidated, several in vivo clinical trials and in vitro laboratory measurements have confirmed a good correlation between SoS and density (r^2 0.78–0.91) (de Terlizzi et al. 2000). On the other hand BUA seems to have a stronger correlation with trabecular porosity and can be a useful indicator of bone structural changes (Gluer et al. 2004; Tavakoli and Evans 1991, 1992).

It has been observed that SoS are strongly dependent on the orientation of the measurement in the same skeletal site (Strelitzki et al. 1997). This element suggested that, even though is greatly influenced by the mineral density, SoS reflects other properties as the degree of alignment of the trabecular structure and the elastic modulus of bone (Yamamoto et al. 2012; Hans et al. 1999; Wear et al. 2012; Grondin et al. 2012). Nicholson and Bouxsein (2000) studied human calcaneus bones to evaluate QUS variables before and after the compression of the specimens without finding differences between elastic modulus and measurements. However it has been observed that SoS reflects bone density independently of the bone elastic constants and that the slope of the BUA versus frequency reflects bone elastic constants independently of bone density (Grimm and Williams 1997). Other analysis of different models of trabecular bone demonstrated a better correlation of the SoS with bone volume rather than other structural or elastic components, whereas the BUA appeared to be more influenced by scattering and viscoelastic mechanisms (Sasso et al. 2008).

Other studies showed that SoS and BUA seem not to be capable to provide different and/or complementary characteristics of the bone tissue from those obtained with densitometry techniques.

6.3 Cortical Bone

The bone architecture of the phalanx can be described with a micromechanical model of cortical bone made of two-phase composite material consisting of an anisotropic mineralized matrix pervaded by cylindrical pores. This model influences the characteristics of the ultrasound wave that have propagated through it: the SoS, the shape (number of peaks) and the amplitude of the ultrasound signal (fast wave amplitude) (Cadossi and Canè 1996).

Wuster and colleagues (2005), in a study performed on human phalanges of cadavers analyzed by bone ultrasound, dual-energy X-ray absorptiometry (DXA), and micro quantitative computed tomography, showed a close correlation of SoS and fast wave amplitude with the mineralized spaces of the trabecular and cortical structure. The frequency content of the signal, calculated by Fourier analysis, has been correlated with the inter trabecular spaces occupied by the marrow and the organic matrix.

In a clinical study on human phalanges, Barkmann and colleagues demonstrated that the duration (microseconds) of the fast ultrasound signal and the ADSoS are able to reveal endosteal bone absorption and are correlated with the cortical area and strength (Barkmann et al. 2000b).

Grondin and colleagues (2012) investigated the relative contributions of porosity and mineralized matrix properties to the bulk compressional wave velocity (BCV) along the long bone axis and confirmed the hypothesis that the intracortical porosity strongly influences the mesoscopic elasticity (Granke et al. 2011).

Recent studies on excised human radii suggested a sophisticated multimodal approach with several propagating models in order to collect different elements on bone strength and to achieve a more complete status of cortical bone (Muller et al. 2008).

Other authors (Sievänen et al. 2001; Tatarinov et al. 2005; Njeh et al. 1999b) have found an independent contribution to SoS of cortical thickness and cortical BMD at different sites as radius (Bosisio et al. 2007; Muller et al. 2005; Bossy et al. 2004) and tibia (Prevrhal et al. 2001; Tatarinov et al. 2011; Määttä et al. 2009).

6.4 Future Approaches

In the past years a growing attention to new QUS methods of investigation at femur and spinal level have been developed as a response to the lack of direct measurements in the most common sites of fragility fractures (Barkmann et al. 2007; Dencks et al. 2007; Serra-Hsu et al. 2011; Nicholson and Alkalay 2007). Studies in vitro in samples of human femur have shown a high correlation between QUS measurement and bone mineral density (BMD) with a good level of accuracy (Grondin et al. 2010; Bossy et al. 2007; Zebaze et al. 2010).

Machado et al. proposed the evaluation of fracture healing measuring the time of flight (TOF) of ultrasound wave by axial transmission at cortical bovine femur sample. The results have shown that SoS was affected by local changes in mineralization and therefore is sensitive to callus changes during the regeneration process (Machado et al. 2011).

Nauleau and colleagues focused their attention to the characterization of thickness and elastic properties of femur applying an algorithm to measure the wavenumbers of several circumferential guided modes in a cylindrical cortical bone-mimicking phantom. The results open interesting perspectives for the ultrasonic characterization of one of the most important site of osteoporosis fracture: the femoral neck (Nauleau et al. 2012).

7 Clinical Experience: Fracture Risk and Further Applications

7.1 Primary Osteoporosis and Fracture Risk

At the beginning the clinical interest in quantitative bone ultrasound centered mainly on the problem of diagnosing osteoporosis. In fact several studies evaluated the performance of ultrasound devices and their ability to discriminate subjects with osteoporotic fractures, especially in the elderly female population and it has been widely demonstrated how the correlation between ultrasound and densitometry values is statistically significant. However, the lack of ultrasound measurement at axial BMD (rachis or femur) and the QUS capability to provide some information about bone quality without ionizing radiation have shifted the attention to the assessment of fracture risk.

In recent years, numerous prospective prospective studies of great importance have been performed to assess fracture risk by QUS at the calcaneus (Bauer et al. 1997; Hans et al. 1996; Krieg et al. 2006) showing a significant association between heel QUS and fracture prediction. One of the latest, the EPIC-Norfolk prospective population study, has been conducted on a British male and female population of 14,824 subjects in an age range of 42–82 years, with a mean follow-up of 1.9 (0.7) years and definitely proved the efficacy of QUS at the calcaneus in predicting fracture risk (Khaw et al. 2004).

A European cross-sectional multicentre study (phalangeal osteoporosis study PhOS) performed on over 10,000 women provided important confirmation and clinical validation of the QUS method at the phalanx. It demonstrated the high precision (coefficient of variation CV below 1 % in both the short- and long -term) of QUS performed at phalanx and the ability to detect osteoporotic subjects with vertebral or hip fractures (Wuster et al. 2000).

Guglielmi and colleagues compared QUS at the phalanges with X-ray methods (DXA and QCT) and morphometric analysis of hand radiographs. Adopting receiver operating characteristic (ROC) analysis, no differences between the two techniques have been found (Guglielmi et al. 2003). Similar studies conducted by other authors, have also shown similar results (Boonen et al. 2005).

In the Basel Osteoporosis Study (BOS) for detecting vertebral fractures, Hartl and colleagues have shown that QUS at the calcaneus and phalanx has comparable performances with the results obtained with axial DXA (Hartl et al. 2002).

Krieg and colleagues performed a retrospective and cross-sectional study conducted on an elderly (70–80 years of age) Swiss population assessing the ability of calcaneal and phalangeal QUS in discriminating subjects with hip fracture. Although both methods showed encouraging results, QUS at calcaneus proved more effective in the elderly population (Krieg et al. 2003). To this regard, a small but interesting Italian study has highlighted that QUS at phalanx is more sensitive in discriminating subjects with vertebral fracture immediately post-menopause (Camozzi et al. 2007).

As mentioned before, the OPUS study has shown that QUS at the phalanx and calcaneus is effective in identifying subjects with vertebral fractures in a large European population.

Kanis et al. have identified the criteria for risk assessment based on QUS at the phalanx and age and published tables for calculating fracture risk at 10 years (Kanis et al. 2005).

Recently, a large cross-sectional population-based survey called European Male Ageing Study (EMAS) tried to demonstrate the influence of sex hormones on markers of bone turnover and to explore the association between these markers and bone health in middle-aged and elderly European men (Boonen et al. 2011). The results have shown a suggestive evidence of association between a single nucleotide polymorphism with SoS and BUA measured at the calcaneus.

The International Society for Clinical Densitometry (ISCD) has recently published the new position of the society regarding QUS outlining a high level of evidence of heel QUS in osteoporotic fracture prediction. However, as reported by Hans and Krieg in a review article, although several QUS models are available on the market, especially for measurement at the calcaneus, only a small minority of these have a scientific validity confirmed by clinical studies published in literature. Furthermore, the level of evidence in the assessment of osteoporotic fracture risk can be quite different for each device and has been validated in some, but not all populations (Table 1).

Considering these aspects, QUS cannot be claimed to replace densitometry, but rather combines with it; specific algorithms combining instrumental (DXA or QUS) and clinical risk factors should be used to identify women to be treated to avoid future fracture and pathologic ultrasound values must be considered an independent factor of fracture risk.

Several European scientific societies have included QUS in their national guidelines for the assessment of fracure risk for post-menopausal osteoporosis in women who are in the perspective of treatment (National Osteoporosis Society 2002; Schattauer GmbH 2006). In Italy, "note 79" regarding the prescription of anti-osteoporosis drugs has included QUS in the model for estimating fracture risk at 10 years, using the combination of clinical risk factors and T-score values (Agenzia Italiana Del Farmaco 2007).

7.2 Secondary Osteoporosis

The studies of QUS applied in causes of secondary osteoporosis have proved to be useful in characterization of metabolic bone pathologies such as: osteoporosis induced by glucocorticoids (Gonnelli et al. 2010), hyperparathyroidism (Gonnelli et al. 2000), osteomalacia (Luisetto et al. 2000), thalassemia (Filosa and de Terlizzi 2002), osteogenesis imperfecta (Kutilek and Bayer 2010), rheumatoid arthritis

Table 1 Evidences in fracture risk assessment for available QUS devices

Manufacturer	Model	Site of measurement	Ability to assess hip fracture risk	Ability to assess spine fracture risk
GE-medical	Achilles	Calcaneus	Proven in most populations	Proven in most populations
DMS	UBIS 3000/5000	Calcaneus	Some evidence	Some evidence
Hologic	Sahara	Calcaneus	Proven in Caucasian	Proven in Caucasian
McCue-Norland	Cuba clinical	Calcaneus	Proven in Caucasian	Some evidence
IGEA	DBM sonic BP	Phalanx	Proven in Caucasian	Proven in Caucasian
BeamMed	Omnisense	Radius, Tibia	Some evidence	Some evidence
Meditech	DTU-One	Calcaneus	No evidence	Some evidence
Aloka	AOS-100	Calcaneus	Some evidence	No evidence
Elk Co	CM-100/200	Calcaneus		No evidence

(Cryer et al. 2007), psoriatic arthritis (Frediani et al. 2003), epilepsy (Pluskiewicz and Nowakowska 1997), and cystic fibrosis (Rossini et al. 2007; Lopez-Rodriguez et al. 2012).

The technique has also been used in nephrology for some years; several studies have applied it in populations of uremic subjects on chronic dialysis and demonstrated that QUS parameters (phalanx, tibia, calcaneus) can be used in combination with biochemical markers of bone turnover in the follow-up of uremic patients who present pathologies or alterations affecting bone. Different characteristics of parameters found in menopause, osteoporosis and azotaemic osteodystrophy could be ascribed to each bone tissue property, enabling a clear differentiation of bone tissue changes occurring in each pathology (Pluskiewicz et al. 2002; Guglielmi et al. 2006; Peretz et al. 2000).

QUS studies have yielded very promising results in patient affected by Paget disease, HIV-infected patients (Cournil et al. 2012), survivors of malignant bone tumors or acute lymphoblastic leukemia (Azcona et al. 2003), women with breast cancer (Langmann et al. 2012), Down's syndrome, Martin Bell syndrome, acromegalic patients (Padova et al. 2011), Marfan Mass phenotype, and genetic disorders (Halaba et al. 2006).

7.3 Treatment Monitoring

The QUS parameters [Bone Transmission Time (BTT); pure Speed of Sound (pSoS)] have shown characteristics of accuracy, stability in time, and independence of the presence of soft tissue, enabling an effective follow-up during osteotrophic treatments.

Mauloni and colleagues evaluated the accuracy of the method and the variations expected in time in a longitudinal study of subjects on hormone replacement therapy and calculated that an interval of 18 months between one measurement and the next is required (Mauloni et al. 2000).

Similar studies by ultrasound at the calcaneus about the effects of calcitonin therapy or hormone replacement

therapy after 2 years have shown good results (Giorgino et al. 1996; Gonnelli et al. 1996).

It is also possible to monitor treatment with alendronate (Ingle et al. 2005), raloxifene (Agostinelli and de Terlizzi 2007), and teriparatide (Gonnelli et al. 2006) by bone ultrasound at the calcaneus and at the phalanx.

However, due to the lack of large population studies describing the efficacy of QUS in monitoring the effects of treatments, according to the ISCD official positions (Krieg et al. 2008), QUS cannot be recommended for the monitoring of treatment response in patients with osteoporosis.

However, as the effect of different treatments can affect trabecular and cortical bone differently, this aspect can be monitored by different QUS devices. As an example, QUS at the calcaneus seems to be not effective in monitoring teriparatide treatment because its effects have been shown to affect particularly the cortical bone.

7.4 Children

In the pediatric field the possibilities of the technique for studying skeletal maturation without ionizing radiation have been considered appealing. Since bone status can be assessed comparing QUS variables of an individual with the population, reference growth charts at the level of phalanx, radius, tibia, and calcaneus have been produced for European and American children ranging from 3 to 18 years of age (Halaba and Pluskiewicz 1997; Gimeno-Ballester et al. 2001). As initial requirement to test the usefulness of QUS in this field, main anthropometric findings including pubertal stages and body mass index (BMI expressed as centiles) have been recently collected as reference database for phalangeal QUS (Barkmann et al. 2002; Baroncelli et al. 2006).

According to these anthropometric parameters, the Z-score for QUS can be calculated for the clinical use of reference curves: a Z-score below −2.0 could refer to a condition of "low bone mineral status".

The effectiveness of the QUS technique in the study of pediatric diseases regarding the skeleton has been assessed by several researchers (Baroncelli et al. 2003; Sundberg et al. 1998). QUS can be used to estimate bone mineral status and fragility similarly to DXA. Furthermore QUS parameters, as descripted before, give additional information on bone quality because influenced not only by bone density, as occurs for DXA, but also by bone structure and composition (Williams et al. 2012).

T scores significantly below the normal values have been found performing QUS to populations of children and adolescents affected by type 1 diabetes (Chobot et al. 2012), congenital heart defects (Laura Gabriela et al. 2012), severe untreated bronchial asthma (Mainz et al. 2009), disturbances of growth and other disorders of bone and mineral metabolism (Hartman et al. 2004).

Although large databases according to the main anthropometric findings from early childhood to young-adulthood are needed for a correct interpretation of the results in clinical setting, QUS methods in children should be considered similar to DXA in the diagnosis of a reduced bone mineral status and can be a useful radiation-free screening method for osteopenia. However, the Paediatric Positions of the International Society for Clinical Densitometry do not recognize at all QUS techniques applied to children and only refer to X-ray-based methods.

7.5 Neonates

In neonatology, the increasing survival rate of very low birth weight (VLBW) preterm infants (Meadow et al. 2004) led to the necessity to explore non-invasive and affordable methods for assessing bone health in these patients. The measurement is currently performed at humerus and tibia; several studies (Rubinacci et al. 2003; Ritschl et al. 2005) in preterm newborns and infants have shown significant relationships with gestational age, axiometric parameters, and postnatal age: in fact QUS parameters were significantly lower in preterm infants compared to term infants ($r = 0.4$–0.84, $p < 0.05$) (McDevitt and Ahmed 2007). Similar results have been found by Rosso et al. in perinatally HIV-Infected children (Rosso et al. 2005).

8 Conclusions

Clinical experience has shown that quantitative bone ultrasound provides a valid support for the study of a large variety of pathologies involving the bone tissue.

QUS techniques are useful tool particularly where the determination of bone fragility and fracture risk cannot be completely reached with the evaluation of bone mass alone.

The versatility of the method makes it applicable not only to the adult population but to also to children, newborns, and preterm infants.

Although based on similar physical principles, QUS techniques still have a high variability in terms of skeletal site of measurement, precision, accuracy, parameters, and normative data. In addition, not all ultrasound devices have reached a significant and sufficient level of clinical validation.

When technology improvements will solve most of the issues related to QUS technique, a deeper assessment of bone quality will be granted in the clinical practice.

References

Agenzia Italiana del Farmaco (2007) Note AIFA 2006–2007 per l'uso appropriato dei farmaci. Supplemento ordinario alla "Gazzetta Ufficiale" n. 7 del 10 gennaio 20-Serie generale, Nota 79

Agostinelli D, de Terlizzi F (2007) QUS in monitoring raloxifene and estrogen-progestogens: a 4-year longitudinal study. Ultrasound Med Biol 33(8):1184–1190

Azcona C, Burghard E, Ruza E et al (2003) Reduced bone mineralization in adolescent survivors of malignant bone tumors: comparison of quantitative ultrasound and dual-energy X-ray absorptiometry. J Pediatr Hematol Oncol 25(4):297–302

Barkmann R, Heller M, Gluer CC (1996) The influence of soft tissue and waterbath temperature on quantitative ultrasound transmission parameters: an in vivo study. Osteoporos Int 6:181

Barkmann R, Gluer CC (1998) Factors influencing QUS parameters of the calcaneum: suggestions for an improved measurment procedure. J Clin Densitom 1:93–94

Barkmann R, Glüer CC (1999) Error sources in quantitative ultrasound measurement. In: Njeh CF, Hans D (eds) Quantitative ultrasound: assessment of osteoporosis and bone status. Martin Dunitz, London, pp 101–108

Barkmann R, Kantorovich E, Singal C et al (2000a) A new method for quantitative ultrasound measurements at multiple skeletal sites. J Clin Densitom 3:1–7

Barkmann R, Lüsse S, Stampa B et al (2000b) Assessment of the geometry of human finger phalanges using quantitative ultrasound in vivo. Osteoporos Int 11:745–755

Barkmann R, Rohrschenider W, Vierling M et al (2002) German pediatric reference data for quantitative transverse transmission ultrasound of finger phalanges. Osteoporos Int 13:55–61

Barkmann R, Laugier P, Moser U et al (2007) A method for the estimation of femoral bone mineral density from variables of ultrasound transmission through the human femur. Bone 40(1):37–44

Baroncelli GI, Federico G, Bertelloni S et al (2003) Assessment of bone quality by quantitative ultrasound of proximal phalanges of the hand and fracture rate in children and adolescents with bone and mineral disorders. Pediatr Res 54:125–136

Baroncelli GI, Federico G, Vignolo M et al (2006) The phalangeal quantitative ultrasound group. Cross-sectional reference data for phalangeal quantitative ultrasound from early childhood to young-adulthood according to gender, age, skeletal growth, and pubertal development. Bone 39:159–173

Bauer DC, Gluer CC, Cauley JA et al (1997) Broadband ultrasound attenuation predict fractures strongly and independently of densitometry in older women: a prospective study. Arch Intern Med 157:629–634

Boonen S, Nijs J, Borghs H, Peeters H, Vanderschueren D, Luyten FP (2005) Identifying postmenopausal women with osteoporosis by calcaneal ultrasound, metacarpal digital X-ray radiogrammetry and phalangeal radiographic absorptiometry: a comparative study. Osteoporos Int 16:93–100

Boonen S, Pye SR, O'Neill TW et al (2011) Influence of bone remodelling rate on quantitative ultrasound parameters at the calcaneus and DXA BMDa of the hip and spine in middle-aged and elderly European men: the European Male Ageing Study (EMAS). Eur J Endocrinol 165(6):977–986

Bosisio MR, Talmant M, Skalli W, Laugier P, Mitton D (2007) Apparent Young's modulus of human radius using inverse finite-element method. J Biomech 40(9):2022–2028

Bossy E, Talmant M, Peyrin F, Akrout L, Cloetens P, Laugier P (2004) An in vitro study of the ultrasonic axial transmission technique at the radius: 1-MHz velocity measurements are sensitive to both mineralization and intracortical porosity. J Bone Miner Res 19(9):1548–1556

Bossy E, Laugier P, Peyrin F, Padilla F (2007) Attenuation in trabecular bone: a comparison between numerical simulation and experimental results in human femur. J Acoust Soc Am 122:2469–2475

Cadossi R, Cané V (1996) Pathways of transmission of ultrasound energy through the distal metaphysis of the second phalanx of pigs: an in vitro study. Osteoporos Int 6:196–206

Camozzi V, De Terlizzi F, Zangari M et al (2007) Quantitative bone ultrasound at phalanges and calcaneus in osteoporotic postmenopausal women: influence of age and measurement site. Ultrasound Med Biol 33(7):1039–1045

Chappard C, Berger G, Roux C, Laugier P (1999) Ultrasound measurement on the calcaneus: influence of immersion time and rotation of the foot. Osteoporos Int 9:318–326

Chappard C, Camus E, Lefebvre F et al (2000) Evaluation of error bounds on calcaneal speed of sound caused by surrounding soft tissue. J Clin Densitom 3:121–131

Chen YY, Xu YB, Zhan LK, Ma ZC, Sun YN (2012) Reducing temperature influence on dry quantitative ultrasound bone assessment with constant temperature control. Ultrasonics 52(2):276–280

Chobot AP, Haffke A, Polanska J et al (2012) Quantitative ultrasound bone measurements in pre-pubertal children with type 1 diabetes. Ultrasound Med Biol 38(7):1109–1115

Cournil A, Eymard-Duvernay S, Diouf A et al (2012) Reduced quantitative ultrasound bone mineral density in HIV-infected patients on antiretroviral therapy in Senegal. PLoS ONE 7(2):e31726

Cryer JR, Otter SJ, Bowen CJ (2007) Use of quantitative ultrasound scans of the calcaneus to diagnose osteoporosis in patients with rheumatoid arthritis. J Am Podiatr Med Assoc 97(2):108–114

Damilakis J, Perisinakis K, Gourtsoyiannis N (2000) Imaging ultrasonometry of the calcaneus: dependence on calcaneal area. Calcif Tissue Int 67:24–28

De Terlizzi F, Battista S, Cavani F et al (2000) Influence of bone tissue density and elasticity on ultrasound propagation: an in vitro study. J Bone Miner Res 15:2458–2466

Dencks S, Barkmann R, Padilla F et al (2007) Wavelet based signal processing of in vitro ultrasonic measurements at the proximal femur. Ultrasound Med Biol 33(6):970–980

Evans JA, Tavakoli MB (1990) Ultrasonic attenuation and velocity in bone. Phys Med Biol 35:1387–1396

Filosa A, de Terlizzi F (2002) Quantitative ultrasound (QUS): a new approach to evacuate bone status in thalassemic patients. Ital J Pediatr 28:310–318

Frediani B, Falsetti P, Baldi F et al (2003) Effects of 4-year treatment with once-weekly clodronate on prevention of corticosteroid-induced bone loss and fractures in patients with arthritis: evaluation with dual-energy X-ray absorptiometry and quantitative ultrasound. Bone 33(4):575–581

Gautier G, Kelders L, Groby JP, Dazel O, De Ryck L, Leclaire P (2011) Propagation of acoustic waves in a one-dimensional macroscopically inhomogeneous poroelastic material. J Acoust Soc Am 130(3):1390–1398

Gimeno-Ballester J, Azcona San Julian C, Sierrasesumaga Ariznabarreta L (2001) Bone mineral density determination by osteosonography in healthy children and adolescents: normal values. An Esp Pediatr 54(6):540–546

Giorgino R, Lorusso D, Paparella P (1996) Ultrasound bone densitometry and 2-year hormonal replacement therapy efficacy in the prevention of early postmenopausal bone loss. Osteoporos Int 6(Suppl 1):S341

Gluer CC (1997) The international quantitative ultrasound consensus group. Quantitative ultrasound techniques for the assessment of osteoporosis: expert agreement on current status. J Bone Miner Res 12:1280–1288

Gluer CC, Eastell R, Reid DM et al (2004) Association of five quantitative ultrasound devices and bone densitometry with osteoporotic vertebral fractures in a population-based sample: the OPUS study. J Bone Miner Res 19(5):782–793

Gonnelli S, Cepollaro C, Pondrelli C (1996) Ultrasound parameters in osteoporotic patients treated with salmon calcitonin: a longitudinal study. Osteoporos Int 6:303–307

Gonnelli S, Montagnani A, Cepollaro C et al (2000) Quantitative ultrasound and bone mineral density in patients with primary hyperparathyroidism before and after surgical treatment. Osteoporos Int 11:255–260

Gonnelli S, Martini G, Caffarelli C et al (2006) Teriparatide's effects on quantitative ultrasound parameters and bone density in women with established osteoporosis. Osteoporos Int 17(10):1524–1531

Gonnelli S, Caffarelli C, Maggi S et al (2010) Effect of inhaled glucocorticoids and beta (2) agonists on vertebral fracture risk in COPD patients: the EOLO study. Calcif Tissue Int 87(2):137–143

Granke M, Grimal Q, Sa A, Nauleau P, Peyrin F, Laugier P (2011) Change in porosity is the major determinant of the variation of cortical bone elasticity at the millimeter scale in aged women. Bone 49(5):1020–1026

Grimes M, Bouhadjera A, Haddad S, Benkedidah T (2012) In vitro estimation of fast and slow wave parameters of thin trabecular bone using space-alternating generalized expectation-maximization algorithm. Ultrasonics 52(5):614–621

Grimm MJ, Williams JL (1997) Assessment of bone quantity and quality by ultrasound attenuation and velocity in the heel. Clin Biomech 12:281–285

Grondin J, Grimal Q, Engelke K, Laugier P (2010) Potential of first arriving signal to assess cortical bone geometry at the hip with QUS: a model based study. Ultrasound Med Biol 36:656–666

Grondin J, Grimal Q, Yamamoto K et al (2012) Relative contributions of porosity and mineralized matrix properties to the bulk axial ultrasonic wave velocity in human cortical bone. Ultrasonics 52:467–471

Guglielmi G, Njeh CF, de Terlizzi F et al (2003) Phalangeal quantitative ultrasound, phalangeal morphometric variables and vertebral fracture discrimination. Calcif Tissue Int 72:469–477

Guglielmi G, de Terlizzi F, Aucella F et al (2006) Quantitative ultrasound technique at the phalanges in discriminating between uremic and osteoporotic patients. Eur J Radiol 60(1):108–114

Ha G, Padilla F, Peyrin F, Laugier P (2007) Variation of ultrasonic parameters with microstructure and material properties of trabecular bone: a 3D model simulation. J Bone Miner Res 22(5):665–674

Haire TJ, Langton CM (1999) Biot theory: a review of its application to ultrasound propagation through cancellous bone. Bone 24(4):291–295

Halaba Z, Pluskiewicz W (1997) The assessment of development of bone mass in children by quantitative ultrasound through the proximal phalanxes of the hand. Ultrasound Med Biol 23:1331–1335

Halaba Z, Pyrkosz A, Adamczyk P et al (2006) Longitudinal changes in ultrasound measurements: a parallel study in subjects with genetic disorders and healthy controls. Ultrasound Med Biol 32:409–413

Hans D, Dargent-Molina P, Schott AM et al (1996) Ultrasonographic heel measurements to predict hip fracture in elderly women: the EPIDOS prospective study. Lancet 348:511–514

Hans D, Wu C, Njeh CF et al (1999) Ultrasound velocity of trabecular cubes reflects mainly bone density and elasticity. Calcif Tissue Int 64:18–23

Hans D, Wacker W, Genton L et al (2002) Longitudinal quality control methodology for the quantitative ultrasound Achilles in clinical trial settings. Osteoporos Int 13(10):788–795

Hans D, Alekxandrova I, Njeh C et al (2005) Appropriateness of internal digital phantoms for monitoring the stability of the UBIS 5000 quantitative ultrasound device in clinical trials. Osteoporos Int 16(4):435–445

Hartl F, Tyndall A, Kraenzlin M et al (2002) Discriminatory ability of quantitative ultrasound parameters and bone mineral density in a population-based sample of postmenopausal women with vertebral fractures: result of the Basel Osteoporosis Study. J Bone Miner Res 17:321–330

Hartman C, Shamir R, Eshach-Adiv O, Iosilevsky G, Brik R (2004) Assessment of osteoporosis by quantitative ultrasound versus dual energy X-ray absorptiometry in children with chronic rheumatic diseases. J Rheumatol 31:981–985

Hughes ER, Leighton TG, White PR, Petley GW (2007) Investigation of an anisotropic tortuosity in a biot model of ultrasonic propagation in cancellous bone. J Acoust Soc Am 121(1):568–574

Ikeda Y, Iki M (2004) Precision control and seasonal variations in quantitative ultrasound measurement of the calcaneus. J Bone Miner Metab 22(6):588–593

Ingle BM, Machado ABC, Pereda CA et al (2005) Monitoring alendronate and oestradiol therapy with quantitative ultrasound and bone mineral density. J Clin Densitom 8:278–286

Johansen A, Stone MD (1997) The effect of ankle oedema on bone ultrasound assessment at the heel. Osteoporos Int 7:44–47

Kanis JA, Johnell O, Oden A et al (2005) Ten-year probabilities of clinical vertebral fractures according to phalangeal quantitative ultrasonography. Osteoporos Int 16:1065–1070

Kaptoge S, da Silva JA, Brixen K et al (2008) Geographical variation in DXA bone mineral density in young European men and women. Results from the Network in Europe on Male Osteoporosis (NEMO) study. Bone 43:332–339

Katz J, Meunier A (1987) The elastic anisotropy of bone. J Biomech 20:1063–1070

Khaw KT, Reeve J, Luben R et al (2004) Prediction of total and hip fracture risk in men and women by quantitative ultrasound of the calcaneus: EPIC-Norfolk prospective population study. Lancet 363:197–202

Krieg MA, Cornuz J, Hartl F et al (2002) Quality controls for two heel bone ultrasounds used in the swiss evaluation of the methods of measurement of Osteoporotic fracture risk study. J Clin Densitom 5(4):335–341

Krieg MA, Cornuz J, Ruffieux C et al (2003) Comparison of three bone ultrasounds for the discrimination of subjects with and without osteoporotic fractures among 7,562 elderly women. J Bone Miner Res 18:1261–1266

Krieg MA, Cornuz J, Ruffieux C et al (2006) Prediction of hip fracture risk by quantitative ultrasound in more than 7,000 Swiss women > or = 70 years of age: comparison of three technologically different bone ultrasound devices in the SEMOF study. J Bone Miner Res 21:1457–1463

Krieg MA, Hans D, Gonnelli S et al (2008) Quantitative ultrasound in the management of osteoporosis: the 2007 ISCD official positions. J Clin Densitom 11:163–187

Kutilek S, Bayer M (2010) Quantitative ultrasonometry of the calcaneus in children with osteogenesis imperfecta. J Paediatr Child Health 46(10):592–594

Lang SB (1970) Ultrasonic method for measuring elastic coefficients of bone and results on fresh bovine bones. IEEE Trans Biomed Eng 17:101–105

Langmann GA, Vujevich KT, Medich D (2012) Heel ultrasound can assess maintenance of bone mass in women with breast cancer. J Clin Densitom 15(3):290–294

Langton CM, Palmer SB, Porter RW (1984) The measurement of broadband ultrasonic attenuation in cancellous bone. Eng Med 13:89–91

Langton CM (1997) Development of an electronic phantom for calibration, cross-correlation, and quality assurance of BUA measurement in the calcaneus. Osteoporos Int 7:309

Laugier P, Giat P, Berger G (1994) Broadband ultrasonic attenuation imaging: a new imaging technique of the os calcis. Calcif Tiss Int 54:83–86

Laugier P, Fournier B, Berger G (1996) Ultrasound parametric imaging of the calcaneus: in vivo results with a new device. Calcif Tissue Int 58:326–331

Laura Gabriela CB, Nalleli VM, Dalia Patricia AT et al (2012) Bone quality and nutritional status in children with congenital heart defects. J Clin Densitom 15(2):205–210

Lawrence HL, Yu JG, Yuping L, Chan Z (2010) Probing long bones with ultrasonic body waves. Appl Phys Lett 96:14102–14103

Leclaire P, Kelders L, Lauriks W, Glorieux C, Thoen J (1997) Ultrasonic wave propagation in porous media: determination of acoustic parameters and high frequency limit of the classical models. Stud Health Technol Inform 40:139–155

Lopez-Rodriguez MJ, Lavado-Garcia JM, Canal-Macias ML et al (2012) Quantitative ultrasound in Spanish children and young adults with cystic fibrosis. Biol Res Nurs 32(16):5553–5561

Luisetto G, Camozzi V, De Terlizzi F (2000) Use of quantitative ultrasonography in differentiating osteomalacia from osteoporosis: preliminary study. J Ultrasound Med 19(4):251–256

Lunt M, Felsenberg D, Adams J et al (1997) Population-based geographic variations in DXA bone density in Europe: the EVOS study. Osteoporos Int 7:175–189

Machado CB, Pereira WC, Granke M et al (2011) Experimental and simulation results on the effect of cortical bone mineralization in ultrasound axial transmission measurements: a model for fracture healing ultrasound monitoring. Bone 48(5):1202–1209

Määttä M, Moilanen P, Nicholson P, Cheng S, Timonen J, Jämsä T (2009) Correlation of tibial low-frequency ultrasound velocity with femoral radiographic measurements and BMD in elderly women. Ultrasound Med Biol 35(6):903–911

Mauloni M, Rovati LC, Cadossi R et al (2000) Monitoring bone effect of transdermal hormone replacement therapy by ultrasound investigation at the phalanx. A four year follow up study. Menopause 7:402–412

Mainz JG, Kaiser WA, Beck JF, Mentzel HJ (2009) Substantially reduced calcaneal bone ultrasound parameters in severe untreated asthma. Respiration 78(2):230–233

McDevitt H, Ahmed SF (2007) Quantitative ultrasound assessment of bone health in the neonate. Neonatology 91:2–11

McKelvie ML, Palmer SB (1991) The interaction of ultrasound with cancellous bone. Phys Med Biol 36:1331–1340

Meadow W, Lee G, Lin K, Lantos J (2004) Changes in mortality for extremely low birth weight infants in the 1990s: implications for treatment decisions and resource use. Pediatrics 113:1223–1229

Mentzel HJ, Reusch R, Kaiser WA (2009) Seasonal dependence of the parameters of quantitative ultrasonic measurements on the peripheral skeleton. Rofo 181(8):760–766

Montagnani A, Gonnelli S, Cepollaro C et al (2002) Graphic trace analysis of ultrasound at the phalanges may differentiate between subjects with primary hyperparathyroidism and with osteoporosis: a pilot study. Osteoporos Int 13:222–227

Muller M, Moilanen P, Bossy E et al (2005) Comparison of three ultrasonic axial transmission methods for bone assessment. Ultrasound Med Biol 31(5):633–642

Muller M, Mitton D, Moilanen P et al (2008) Prediction of bone mechanical properties using QUS and pQCT: study of the human distal radius. Med Eng Phys 30(6):761–767

National Osteoporosis Society (2002) The use of quantitative ultrasound in the management of osteoporosis. Position statement of 31st January 2002

Nauleau P, Cochard E, Minonzio JG et al (2012) Characterization of circumferential guided waves in a cylindrical cortical bone-mimicking phantom. J Acoust Soc Am 131(4):289–294

Nelson AM, Hoffman JJ, Anderson CC et al (2011) Determining attenuation properties of interfering fast and slow ultrasonic waves in cancellous bone. J Acoust Soc Am 130(4):2233–2240

Nicholson PH, Bouxsein ML (2000) Quantitative ultrasound does not refl ect mechanically induced damage in human cancellous bone. J Bone Miner Res 15:2467–2472

Nicholson PH, Alkalay R (2007) Quantitative ultrasound predicts bone mineral density and failure load in human lumbar vertebrae. Clin Biomech 22(6):623–629

Njeh CF, Hans D, Fuerst T et al (1999a) Quantitative ultrasound: assessment of osteoporosis and bone status. Martin Dunitz, London

Njeh CF, Hans D, Wu C et al (1999b) An in vitro investigation of the dependence on sample thickness of the speed of sound along the specimen. Med Eng Phys 21:651–659

Padova G, Borzì G, Incorvaia L et al (2011) Prevalence of osteoporosis and vertebral fractures in acromegalic patients. Clin Cases Miner Bone Metab 8(3):37–43

Paggiosi MA, Blumsohn A, Barkmann R et al (2005) Effect of temperature on the longitudinal variability of quantitative ultrasound variables. J Clin Densitom 8(4):436–444

Paggiosi MA, Glüer CC, Roux C et al (2011) International variation in proximal femur bone mineral density. Osteoporos Int 22:721–729

Paggiosi MA, Barkmann R, Glüer CC et al. (2012) A European multicenter comparison of quantitative ultrasound measurement variables: The OPUS study. Osteoporos Int [Epub a head of print]

Passeri G, Pini G, Troiano L et al (2003) Low vitamin D status, high bone turnover, and bone fractures in centenarians. J Clin Endocrinol Metab 88(11):5109–5115

Peretz A, Penaloza A, Mesquita M et al (2000) Quantitative ultrasound and dual X-ray absorptiometry measurements of the calcaneus in patients on maintenance hemodialysis. Bone 27:287–292

Pluskiewicz W, Nowakowska J (1997) Bone status after long-term anticonvulsant therapy in epileptic patients: evaluation using quantitative ultrasound of calcaneus and phalanges. Ultrasound Med Biol 23(4):553–558

Pluskiewicz W, Adamczyk P, Drozdzowska B et al (2002) Skeletal status in children, adolescents and young adults with end-stage renal failure treated with hemo- or peritoneal dialysis. Osteoporos Int 13:353–357

Prevrhal S, Fuerst T, Fan B et al (2001) Quantitative ultrasound of the tibia depends on both cortical density and thickness. Osteoporos Int 12:28–34

Pye SR, Devakumar V, Boonen S et al (2010) Influence of lifestyle factors on quantitative heel ultrasound measurements in middle-aged and elderly men. Calcif Tissue Int 86:211–219

Raum K, Leguerney I, Chandelier F et al (2005) Bone microstructure and elastic tissue properties are reflected in QUS axial transmission measurements. Ultrasound Med Biol 31:1225–1235

Ritschl E, Wehmeijer K, De Terlizzi F et al (2005) Assessment of skeletal development in preterm and term infants by quantitative ultrasound. Pediatr Res 58:341–346

Roben P, Barkmann R, Ullrich S et al (2001) Assessment of phalangeal bone loss and erosions in patients with rheumatoid arthritis by quantitative ultrasound. Ann Rheum Dis 60:670–677

Rossini M, Viapiana O, Del Marco A et al (2007) Quantitative ultrasound in adults with cystic fibrosis: correlation with bone mineral density and risk of vertebral fractures. Calcif Tissue Int 80(1):44–49

Rosso R, Vignolo M, Parodi A et al (2005) Bone quality in perinatally HIV-infected children: role of age, sex, growth, HIV infection, and antiretroviral therapy. AIDS Res Hum Retroviruses 21(11):927–932

Rubinacci A, Moro GE, Noehm G et al (2003) Quantitative ultrasound for the assessment of osteopenia in preterm infants. Eur J Endocrinol 149:307–315

Sasso M, Ha G, Yamato Y et al (2008) Dependence of ultrasonic attenuation on bone mass and microstructure in bovine cortical bone. J Biomech 41(2):347–355

Serra-Hsu F, Cheng J, Lynch T, Qin YX (2011) Evaluation of a pulsed phase-locked loop system for noninvasive tracking of bone deformation under loading with finite element and strain analysis. Physiol Meas 32(8):1301–1313

Schattauer GmbH (2006) Evidence-based DVO guidelines osteoporosis in Germany; prophylaxis, diagnosis and therapy in postmenopausal women and men over 60 years. Verlag fur medizin und naturwissenschaften Stuttgart

Siegel IM, Anast GT, Fields T (1958) The determination of fracture healing by measurement of sound velocity across the fracture site. Surg Gynecol Obstet 107:327–332

Sievänen H, Cheng S, Ollikainen S et al (2001) Ultrasound velocity and cortical bone characteristics in vivo. Osteoporos Int 12:399–405

Strelitzki R, Evans JA, Clarke AJ (1997) The influence of porosity and pore size on the ultrasonic properties of bone investigated using a phantom material. Osteoporos Int 7:370–375

Sundberg M, Gardsell P, Johnell O et al (1998) Comparison of quantitative ultrasound measurements in calcaneus with DXA and SXA at other skeletal sites:a population-based study on 280 children aged 11–16 years. Osteoporos Int 8:410–427

Tavakoli MB, Evans JA (1991) Dependence of the velocity and attenuation of ultrasound in bone on the mineral content. Phys Med Biol 36(11):1529–1537

Tavakoli MB, Evans JA (1992) The effect of bone structure on ultrasonic attenuation and velocity. Ultrasonics 30(6):389–395

Tatarinov A, Sarvazyan N, Sarvazyan A (2005) Use of multiple acoustic wave modes for assessment of long bones: model study. Ultrasonics 43(8):672–680

Tatarinov A, Sarvazyan A, Beller G, Felsenberg D (2011) Comparative examination of human proximal tibiae in vitro by ultrasonic guided waves and pQCT. Ultrasound Med Biol 37(11):1791–1801

Thijssen JM, Weijers G, de Korte CL (2007) Objective performance testing and quality assurance of medical ultrasound equipment. Ultrasound Med Biol 33(3):460–471

Wear KA, Nagaraja S, Dreher ML, Gibson SL (2012) Relationships of quantitative ultrasound parameters with cancellous bone microstructure in human calcaneus in vitro. J Acoust Soc Am 131(2):1605–1612

Williams JE, Wilson CM, Biassoni L, Suri R, Fewtrell MS (2012) Dual energy X-ray absorptiometry and quantitative ultrasound are not interchangeable in diagnosing abnormal bones. Arch Dis Child [Epub a head of print]

Wuster C, Albanese C, de Aloysio D et al (2000) Phalangeal osteosonogrammetry study (PhOS): age related changes, diagnostic sensitivity and discrimination power. J Bone Miner Res 15(8):1603–1614

Wuster C, de Terlizzi F, Becker S et al (2005) Usefulness of quantitative ultrasound in evaluating structural and mechanical properties of bone: comparison of ultrasound, dual-energy X-ray absorptiometry, microcomputed tomography, and mechanical testing of human phalanges in vitro. Technol Health Care 13:1–14

Yamamoto K, Nakatsuji T, Yaoi Y et al (2012) Relationships between the anisotropy of longitudinal wave velocity and hydroxyapatite crystallite orientation in bovine cortical bone. Ultrasonics 52:377–386

Zebaze RM, Ghasem-Zadeh A, Bohte A et al (2010) Intracortical remodelling and porosity in the distal radius and post-mortem femurs of women: a cross-sectional study. Lancet 375:1729–1736

Zitzmann M, Brune M, Vieth V et al (2002) Monitoring bone density in hypogonadal men by quantitative phalangeal ultrasound. Bone 31:422–429

High-Resolution Imaging

Janina M. Patsch and Jan S. Bauer

Contents

Abstract

In the last two decades, high-resolution imaging of the skeleton has emerged as a growing field of research. Techniques such as high-resolution peripheral quantitative computed tomography (HR-pQCT) and high-resolution magnetic resonance imaging (HR-MRI) provide noninvasive access to bone microarchitecture, an important determinant of bone quality. High-resolution images can be processed by a multitude of techniques such as compartment-specific morphometric analyses including the quantification of cortical porosity, finite element analyses (FEA), decomposition techniques, and texture analysis.

1 Introduction

In the past, bone mineral density (BMD) has been established as the main surrogate marker for bone strength. In clinical routine, fracture risk is typically assessed by BMD-based techniques such as DXA and quantitative computed tomography (QCT). However, bone strength does not only result from BMD, it also depends on bone quality. Bone quality refers to a wide range of skeletal tissue properties such as trabecular and cortical bone microarchitecture, bone turnover, bone matrix status (e.g., collagen properties, mineralization), and the accumulation of microdamage (Anonymous 2001). In the past, most of these features were only quantifiable by tissue analyses of bone biopsies. Nowadays, noninvasive imaging techniques are available to study bone microarchitecture in vivo. This chapter will focus on some of the most common high-resolution imaging techniques used by bone researchers and is aimed at providing a basic overview of this growing field of research.

J. M. Patsch (✉)
Department of Radiology and Biomedical Imaging, University of California, San Francisco, 185 Berry Street, Suite 350, San Francisco, CA 94107, USA
e-mail: janina.patsch@meduniwien.ac.at;
janina.patsch@ucsf.edu

J. S. Bauer
Department of Radiology,
Technische Universität München,
Ismaninger Str. 22, 81675 Munich, Germany

G. Guglielmi (ed.), *Osteoporosis and Bone Densitometry Measurements*, Medical Radiology. Diagnostic Imaging,
DOI: 10.1007/174_2012_755, © Springer-Verlag Berlin Heidelberg 2013

2   Computed Tomography

2.1   Multidetector Computed Tomography

Multidetector computed tomography (MDCT) can achieve a spatial resolution of $\sim 250 \times 250 \times 500$ µm at the appendicular skeleton and ~ 500 µm isotropic at the spine and the proximal femur. Although this resolution is not sufficient to reveal true details of trabecular bone structure, MDCT can capture certain microstructural image features. These features, depicted by MDCT, were highly correlated with morphometric measures as quantified by a high-resolution gold standard technique (i.e., microcomputed tomography; μ-CT) (Bauer et al. 2007). Coherently, Ito et al. demonstrated that MDCT was able to depict certain aspects of trabecular microarchitecture at the thoracic spine (T12). They found that MDCT-derived indirect microstructural analysis was able to discriminate patients with and without prevalent vertebral fractures which was not possible according to DXA (Ito et al. 2005; Graeff et al. 2007). Graeff et al. also showed in the EUROFORS study that high-resolution MDCT could capture PTH-induced improvements in spinal bone microarchitecture beyond changes in BMD. However, a considerable radiation dose of about 3 mSv was applied in both studies.

2.2   Flat-Panel C-arm-Based Computed Tomography

Recently, fluoroscopic devices with a flat-panel detector have been developed, that are capable of cross-sectional 3D imaging like conventional CT devices. In contrast to MDCT, these systems use a large flat-panel detector with a high number of pixels and thus can achieve higher resolutions than MDCT of up to 150 µm isotropic both at the appendicular and central skeleton (Walsh et al. 2010; Mulder et al. 2012). Using μ-CT as a standard of reference, Mulder et al. recently showed that the true bone structure can be revealed at clinically relevant bone sites as the upper spine and proximal femur (Mulder et al. 2012). In contrast, for the lower spine, where trabeculae are thin and there is much noise related to soft tissue, image quality was insufficient to analyze trabecular microarchitecture by flat-panel CT. In a clinical setting, flat-panel CT has successfully been applied at the distal radius (Walsh et al. 2010).

2.3   High Resolution-Peripheral Quantitative Computed Tomography

As opposed to quantitative bone imaging with MDCT or fluoroscopic devices, high resolution-peripheral quantitative computed tomography (HR-pQCT) imaging requires a dedicated scanner specifically built for the noninvasive imaging of bone microstructure of the distal extremities. Standard imaging regions of HR-pQCT are located proximal to the radiocarpal joint at the ultradistal radius and proximal to the ankle joint at the ultradistal tibia. To obtain a 3D stack of images with an isotropic voxel size of 82 µm (110 slices, 9 mm scan length), HR-pQCT exposes the patient to a radiation dose of <4 µSv. Compared to a clinical abdominal CT scan, the radiation dose of HR-pQCT is about 500–1000-fold smaller (Damilakis et al. 2010). Motion artifacts were shown to have major impact on most parameters obtained from HR-pQCT imaging, thus visual motion grading according has been introduced as a central step in quality control prior to quantitative image analyses (Pialat et al. 2012).

HR-pQCT has been shown to discriminate patients with and without prevalent fragility fractures based on bone microstructure but irrespective of their BMD. Specifically, Boutroy et al. found significantly lower trabecular density (−12.3 %), lower trabecular number (−8.5 %), and higher standard deviations in trabecular separation (+25.6 %) in osteopenic women with fractures when compared to non-fractured subjects with identical BMD (Boutroy et al. 2005). Several other HR-pQCT studies also found poor peripheral bone microarchitecture to be a characteristic skeletal feature of male and female fracture patients (Vico et al. 2008; Stein et al. 2010, 2011; Vilayphiou et al. 2011). Moreover, HR-pQCT parameters appear to deteriorate along with increasing severity of spine fractures (Sornay-Rendu et al. 2009).

Especially at the ultradistal radius, there is good agreement between volumetric density and microstructure by HR-pQCT and areal BMD (aBMD) by DXA. Correlations are also significant, but slightly weaker for tibial HR-pQCT parameters and aBMD by hip DXA (Sornay-Rendu et al. 2007). In general, peripheral measurements by HR-pQCT were shown to correlate well with aBMD, volumetric BMD (vBMD), and biomechanical properties of the central skeleton (Vico et al. 2008; Liu et al. 2010a, b).

Cross-sectional HR-pQCT studies have provided insight into disease-, age- and gender-specific aspects of peripheral bone microstructure (Khosla et al. 2006; Burghardt et al. 2010c, d; Macdonald et al. 2011a, b) (Fig. 1). Compartment-specifc analyses of bone density and microarchitecture by HR-pQCT seem to be of particular relevance in understanding osteologic paradoxes with discrepancies between fracture prevalence and densitometric risk prediction such as low fracture rates in Asians or high fracture risk in diabetic bone disease. Asian men and women were shown to have smaller bones, thus aBMD as measured by DXA tends to underestimate their real bone density. Clinically, Asians sustain fewer fractures. Using HR-pQCT,

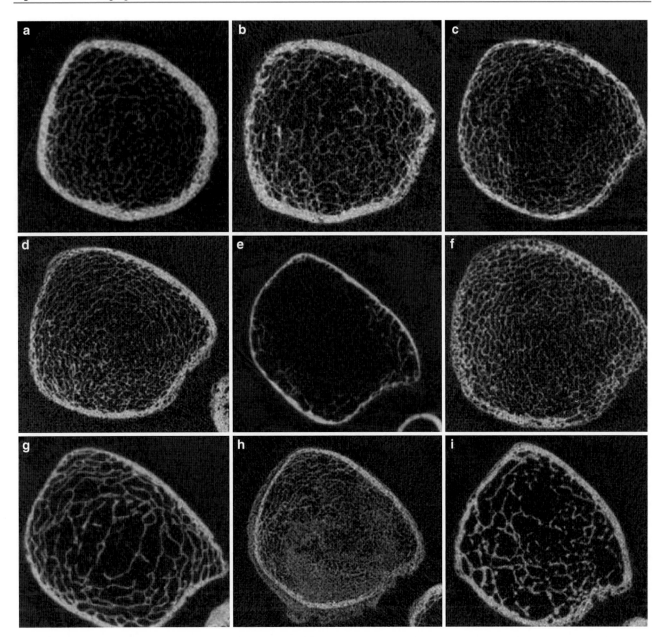

Fig. 1 HR-pQCT. Normal morphology and pathologic examples of the ultradistal tibia. **a** Normal tibial bone microstructure in a middle-aged woman; **b + c** postmenopausal osteoporosis; **d** premenopausal osteoporosis; **e** young patient with post-traumatic paralysis of lower limbs; **f** postmenopausal women with type-2 diabetes mellitus and fractures; **g** renal osteodystrophy; **h** healing insufficiency fracture; **i** osteogenesis imperfecta (Sillence type 1)

Wang et al. found that in spite of relatively low total bone area, premenopausal Asian women displayed significantly thicker cortices and a richer trabecular microarchitecture than Caucasians (Wang et al. 2009). μ-FE analyses also yielded higher estimates of bone stiffness/strength (Liu et al. 2011). Patients with type-2 diabetes mellitus tend to have relatively high BMD. Nevertheless, they exhibit a disproportionally high fracture risk. HR-pQCT has been particularly helpful in identifying cortical porosity as a key

pathomorphology overtly found in diabetics with prevalent fragility fractures (Patsch 2012). Moreover, HR-pQCT has been used to address gender-specific research questions (Macdonald et al. 2011b). In accordance with previous biopsy studies, Khosla et al. confirmed by noninvasive imaging that trabecular bone volume and trabecular thickness were significantly higher in young men than in young women (Khosla et al. 2006). They further observed that that the rate of age-related decline in trabecular bone volume

Fig. 2 3D visualization of μCT scans of a healthy (*left*) and an osteoporotic (*right*) vertebral specimen. The dimensionality of every single trabecula is color coded, as determined by the scaling index method: rods are *blue* and *green*, plates are red and *yellow*

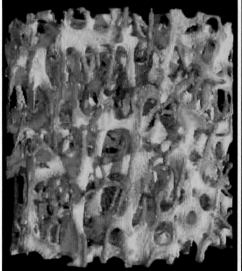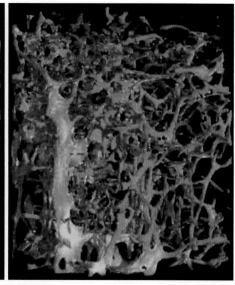

seemed independent of gender, but also reaffirmed that in aging but otherwise healthy men trabecular thinning seemed to predominate over actual loss of trabeculae.

Somewhat surprisingly, the interpretation of longitudinal HR-pQCT studies has been challenging (Burghardt et al. 2010c, d; Li et al. 2010; Seeman 2010; Seeman et al. 2010; Macdonald et al. 2011a; Rizzoli et al. 2012). Only a few studies have used data acquired at multiple imaging centers (Seeman et al. 2010). As with DXA, the utility of HR-pQCT to address important questions related to the epidemiology of osteoporosis, the antifracture efficacy of certain drugs, and the development of normative databases for clinical assessment of skeletal health requires scalability of imaging parameters to standardized multicenter data pools. In particular, cross-calibration procedures are needed to account for sources of intrinsic data variability between scanners and time points. To address these issues, Burghardt et al. proposed the use of structure- and composition-realistic anthropomorphic phantoms constructed from static cadaveric bone tissue (Burghardt et al. 2012). Based on phantom measurements at nine different imaging centers, they reported inters-canner variability comparable in magnitude to short term in vivo reproducibility reported elsewhere (MacNeil and Boyd 2007; Kazakia et al. 2008). Resembling reproducibility results from single scanner studies, densitometric measures were also highly reproducible in this multiscanner study [root mean square coefficient of variation (RMSCV) approximately 1 %]. Likewise, geometric and microstructural measures were less precise (4–6 % RMSCV). Sources of error were found to be variable and scanner specific, including differences in resolution and signal-to-noise ratios, geometric, and density calibration, or related to post-processing factors. Among other caveats in longitudinal HR-pQCT studies, the assumption of a fixed

bone matrix mineralization has to be considered. Many drugs with proven antifracture efficacy significantly affect tissue mineralization which could per se lead to small, false positive increases in vBMD, and the derived structural parameters such as relative trabecular bone volume (BV/TV), trabecular thickness, or trabecular separation (Boivin et al. 2000; Roschger et al. 2010).

2.3.1 μ-CT

Micro-computed tomography (μ-CT) is a high-resolution imaging technique for small objects such as bone biopsies (Muller 2002). It does not allow in vivo imaging of human bone tissue but has been widely used as a validation tool for techniques such as HR-pQCT (Cohen et al. 2010; Liu et al. 2010c) or HR-MRI (Bauer et al. 2009; Bae et al. 2012). The spatial resolution of μ-CT reaches up to a few micron, therefore imaging of trabecular structures is well feasible (trabecular diameter = approx. 100–200 μm). μ-CT does not only allow for 3D (global) morphometry of bone samples but also provides access to structural properties of individual trabeculae [e.g. Stauber and Muller 2006; Scaling Index Method (SIM)] (Fig. 2). Morphometric indices are determined by using a direct 3D approach (Hildebrand et al. 1999) and typically include (BV/TV), trabecular thickness (TbTh), trabecular separation (TbSp), trabecular number (TbN), connectivity density (Conn.D), and the structure model index (SMI). μ-CT and other high-resolution techniques that provide even higher spatial resolution (e.g. synchrotron imaging) have become essential tools that support various scientific disciplines such as osteology, tissue engineering (Peyrin 2011), anthropology (Benazzi et al. 2011), geophysics, and material testing. For more details on μ-CT and its state of the art use, the reader is referred elsewhere (Muller 2002; Bouxsein et al. 2010)

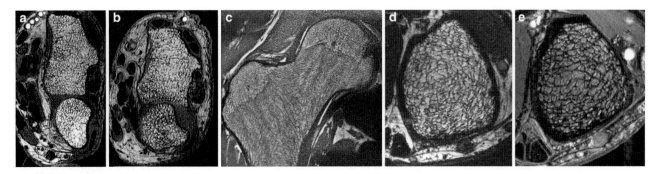

Fig. 3 HR-MRI of trabecular structure, visualized at 3T (**a–d**) and 7T (**e**), at the distal radius (**a, b**), the proximal femur (**c**), and the distal tibia (**d, e**). Differences between postmenopausal women without (**a**) and with (**b**) vertebral fractures are obvious

3   Magnetic Resonance Imaging

Like in CT, technical innovations have pushed the limits in high-resolution magnetic resonance imaging (HR-MRI). With phased array coils, parallel imaging, stronger gradients, and magnets as well as improved pulse sequences and postprocessing software, clinical scanners provide an in vivo spatial resolution close to the diameter of single trabeculae (Techawiboonwong et al. 2005; Krug et al. 2006; Phan et al. 2006; Wehrli 2007). Ultra short TE imaging opens the possibility to directly visualize cortical bone. Additionally, even functional parameters like bone marrow perfusion can be assessed by MRI. However, difficulties in standardization, fluctuations in image quality have impeded broader use and often lead to HR-pQCT being the preferred imaging modality for the noninvasive assessment of bone microarchitecture (Bauer and Link 2009; Ito 2011).

3.1   High Resolution-Magnetic Resonance Imaging of Trabecular Bone

Compared to CT, mechanisms of image generation differ completely in high resolution-magnetic resonance imaging (HR-MRI). It lacks ionizing radiation, an advantage both for clinical screening and scientific studies. On the other hand, one must be aware that trabeculae appear as signal voids within the high-intensity fatty bone marrow—not the mineralized tissue itself is visualized by conventional MRI, but only an artifact due to the very short T2 relaxation time and off-resonance effects at the bone—bone marrow interfaces. The appearance of these signal voids is determined by many imaging parameters: gradient echo sequences, longer TE, and higher field strengths increase susceptibility artifacts, and consequently the overestimation of the trabecular thickness and bone volume fraction (Majumdar et al. 1995; Bauer et al. 2009). Thus, a similar acquisition technique is essential to compare trabecular

bone measurements across different patients and studies (Fig. 3).

HR-MRI has mostly been performed in the peripheral skeleton, as these sites are easily accessible with small coils, contain a high amount of trabeculae and the bone marrow consists of fat, resulting in high bone–bone marrow contrast. However, using SNR efficient sequences, high magnetic field strength (3 Tesla), and phased array coils, HR-MRI has been shown to be feasible at the proximal femur, a skeletal site frequently affected by osteoporotic fractures (Krug et al. 2005). However, spatial resolution was limited, and persistent hematopoietic bone marrow obscured the visualization of single trabeculae in some patients at the femoral neck. Comparing trabecular bone architecture at the distal radius and tibia, Wehrli et al. could demonstrate treatment effects and age-related changes only at the lower extremity, suggesting that the distal tibia might be the best site to measure bone microarchitecture by HR-MRI techniques currently available (Wehrli et al. 2008) (Fig. 3).

Many ex vivo studies demonstrated a high correlation between biomechanical strength and MR-derived measures of trabecular structure at different skeletal sites (Majumdar et al. 1996; Hwang et al. 1997; Pothuaud et al. 2002; Ammann and Rizzoli 2003; Link et al. 2004). In most studies, the combination of density measurements with parameters of the trabecular architecture yielded best results and significantly improved correlations of BMD alone. In vivo, many cross-sectional and longitudinal HR-MRI studies have been conducted (Majumdar et al. 1999; Cortet et al. 2000; Wehrli et al. 2001; Laib et al. 2002; Link et al. 2002; Rietbergen et al. 2002; Boutry et al. 2003; Benito et al. 2005; Chesnut et al. 2005; Ladinsky et al. 2008). Postmenopausal women with and without osteoporotic insufficiency fractures were better separated using MR-derived structure measures compared to BMD alone (Link et al. 1998; Majumdar et al. 1999; Cortet et al. 2000; Wehrli et al. 2001). Similar results were obtained for HR-MRI in hypogonadal men, patients with renal osteodystrophy, and patients with cardiac and renal transplants (Link et al. 2000,

2002; Link 2002; Benito et al. 2003; Wehrli et al. 2004). Treatment effects and age-related changes were quantified in longitudinal studies and demonstrated the feasibility of HR-MRI to reproducibly quantify changes of trabecular architecture noninvasively and without ionizing radiation (Rietbergen et al. 2002; Benito et al. 2003; Chesnut et al. 2005; Wehrli et al. 2008; Folkesson et al. 2011).

3.2 Magnetic Resonance Imaging of Cortical Bone

While vertebral fracture risk is determined predominantly by trabecular bone architecture, cortical bone geometry, thickness, and porosity are important predictors for hip fractures. Cortical bone can be assessed, visualized, and quantified in several ways by MRI. Several studies focused predominantly on geometric parameters (Woodhead et al. 2001; Sievanen et al. 2007). They showed that MRI provides a feasible tool for the assessment of cortical bone at the femur and may be of clinical utility in assessing hip fragility, as the thin cortical bone at the narrowest location of the femoral neck could be delineated precisely and accurately with a standard clinical 1.5 T MRI device (Gomberg et al. 2005; Sievanen et al. 2007). In other studies, osteoporotic patients with vertebral or femoral fractures could be distinguished based on proximal femur geometry and femoral geometry improved the prediction of bone strength in biomechanical studies (Beck et al. 1990; Alonso et al. 2000; Gnudi et al. 2004; Louis et al. 2010). A more sophisticated approach to characterize cortical bone is the visualization and quantification by ultrashort echo time pulse sequences (UTE) (Du et al. 2011; Krug et al. 2011; Rad et al. 2011; Bae et al. 2012; Biswas et al. 2012). Due to the short T1 and T2* relaxation times of bone tissue, such special sequences are needed to retrieve any signal from bone tissue (Reichert et al. 2005). Despite the challenging pulse sequence design, studies showed that a quantification of bone water content is possible and correlates with cortical porosity and biomechanical properties (Bae et al. 2012; Biswas et al. 2012). Also treatment effects could be detected (Anumula et al. 2010). However, the significance of these findings is not completely understood and future research will have to study cortical porosity using both MR and HR-pQCT, what may be interesting in particular in diabetic patients (Burghardt et al. 2010b; Patsch 2012) or patients with renal osteodystrophy.

3.3 Functional Magnetic Resonance Imaging

The viability of bone relies on bone cells, mineralized tissue properties, and bone marrow function. Several diseases, as diabetes mellitus, immobility, and glucocorticoid therapy are associated with high bone marrow fat fraction and increased fracture risk (Rosen and Bouxsein 2006). Thus, MR spectroscopy and dynamic contrast-enhanced MR perfusion imaging have been used to investigate bone marrow composition and function (Schellinger et al. 2004; Griffith et al. 2005, 2006, 2008; Shen et al. 2007). MR perfusion showed a decrease in vertebral marrow maximum enhancement and enhancement slope in patients with low BMD. An increase in marrow fat content measured with spectroscopy was also associated with lower BMD.

4 Basic Principles of Quantifying Bone Structure in High-Resolution Bone Imaging

4.1 Image Preprocessing

To calculate quantitative parameters of trabecular or cortical bone, the processing of images usually consists of several steps, like normalization or binarization, resolution enhancement, registration, and segmentation. To ensure a high degree of reproducibility, human interaction has to be limited to a minimum and each step needs to be standardized (Newitt et al. 2002; Valentinitsch et al. 2012). Different morphometric analysis techniques have been applied with the most common approaches yielding a reproducibility of 2–4 % for MRI and <4.5 % for HR-pQCT parameters (Ouyang et al. 1997; Newitt et al. 2002b; Gomberg et al. 2004; MacNeil and Boyd 2007; Burghardt et al. 2010a; Baum et al. 2012). In case of HR-pQCT, prior to the application of a fixed segmentation threshold, a smoothing and edge enhancement procedure is performed on grayscale images. Afterwards, the periosteal contours are drawn in a semiautomatic manner. In case of MRI, registration can be included in the image acquisition already. Resolution enhancement usually is performed before images are binarized with a dual reference thresholding technique that uses the signal intensity of the cortex as a reference (Majumdar et al. 1995). Segmentation of the trabecular bone compartment is mostly done either manually or semiautomatically (Mueller et al. 2006; Phan et al. 2006; Wehrli 2007). A more recent approach used in HR-pQCT is fully automated (Valentinitsch et al. 2012).

4.2 Morphometric Parameters

In high-resolution bone imaging, standard morphometric parameters are named in analogy to those used in microscopy-based, static histomorphometry (Parfitt et al. 1987). In HR-pQCT, parameters of bone microstructure are mostly

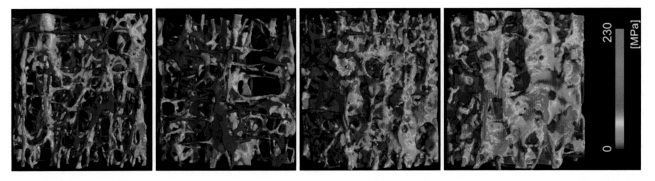

Fig. 4 Color-coded local van-Mises stress in four different vertebral bone samples scanned by μ-CT as determined by FEA

derived from compartment-specific bone density. Specifically, BV/TV is derived from trabecular vBMD assuming a fixed mineralization of 1,200 mg HA/cm^3 for compact bone. Tb.N and network heterogeneity are directly measured by 3D distance transformations (Hildebrand and Ruegsegger 1997). Tb.Th (in μm) and Tb.Sp (in μm) are derived from Tb.N and/or trabecular density using stereological standard relations assuming a plate-model geometry (Laib et al. 1998).

4.3 Advanced Parameters

HR-pQCT also provides morphologic measures of cortical bone including cortical porosity (Burghardt et al. 2010a; Nishiyama et al. 2010). Although cortical porosity is increasingly recognized as a pathomorphologic surrogate of poor bone quality (Holzer et al. 2009; Burghardt et al. 2010c, d; Zebaze et al. 2010), it remains to be stressed that noninvasive imaging techniques only capture relatively large pores (>82 μm) (Nishiyama et al. 2010).

Parameters describing trabecular shape and anisotropy can also be estimated in vivo. They include measures of the surface curvature or the differentiation of plates and rods by decomposition technique-based analyses (Boutry et al. 2003; Pothuaud et al. 2004; Liu et al. 2010a, b; Pialat et al. 2012). The anisotropy and preferred orientation of the trabeculae were first quantified by the mean intercept length method (MIL) in histological sections (Whitehouse 1974). In ex vivo applications, 3D techniques such as the scaling vector method or gabor filtering have been proposed to quantify trabecular orientations (Monetti et al. 2005).

While most of these measures require a binarization of the grayscale image data, several methods have been proposed to account for the partial volume effects due to the limited spatial resolution in MDCT and MRI and use the full grayscale data. Autocorrelation functions and fuzzy logic methods were used to determine parameters of scale and connectivity, while the SIM was used to determine the dimensionality of the single trabeculae as a parameter of

shape (Mueller et al. 2006; Räth et al 2008; Monetti et al. 2011; Sidorenko et al. 2011). These parameters demonstrated benefits regarding the prediction of biomechanical strength in particular for osteoporotic bone (Räth et al 2008).

MDCT, HR-pQCT, and HR-MRI data can also be subjected to FE modeling. FE modeling is a well-established biomechanical computation method that yields loading scenario-specific, image-based estimates of bone strength (e.g., ultimate force required to fracture upon a certain type of fall) (Newitt et al. 2002a; Chevalier et al. 2010; Genant et al. 2010; Rajapakse et al. 2012) (Fig. 4). HR-pQCT-based μ-FE analyses have been shown to discriminate men and postmenopausal women with and without fragility fractures independent of BMD (Boutroy et al. 2008; Vilayphiou et al. 2010, 2011). MDCT-based FEA better estimated proximal femoral strength as compared to DXA and explained differences between men and women (Keyak et al. 2011). Also treatment effects were characterized by FE analysis (van Rietbergen et al. 2002; Jayakar et al. 2012; Keaveny et al. 2012). In experimental studies, very high correlations ($R^2 > 0.93$) were observed between biomechanical experiments and FE analysis by combining bone density and measures of trabecular anisotropy (Trabelsi et al. 2011). By separately modeling cortical and trabecular bone, such high correlations were also observed in resolution regimes available by in vivo MDCT imaging (Eswaran et al. 2009; Pahr and Zysset 2009) .

5 Conclusion

In conclusion, flat-panel CT, HR-pQCT, and HR-MRI provide novel, noninvasive, and accurate options for the quantification of bone microarchitecture. Although current research focusing on potential clinical applications seems promising, both techniques are still limited to research use. The results of high-resolution imaging studies should be interpreted with respect to technical caveats of these techniques.

6   Key Points

- High-resolution imaging techniques allow the noninvasive quantification of bone microarchitecture in research settings.
- HR-pQCT involves very low radiation doses but dedicated scanners are needed.
- HR-MRI is a technically challenging method which is somewhat hard to standardize, but allows the quantification of trabecular microarchitecture noninvasively without ionizing radiation.
- Advanced structural and biomechanical metrics of trabecular and cortical bone structure are promising research parameters for the quantification of drug effects and patient-specific fracture risk.
- Prospective studies, tight quality control, and standardized approaches are required for HR imaging to transition from a promising research method into a clinical tool.

References

Alonso CG, Curiel MD et al (2000) Femoral bone mineral density, neck-shaft angle and mean femoral neck width as predictors of hip fracture in men and women. Multicenter Project for Research in Osteoporosis. Osteoporos Int J Established Result Cooper Eur Found Osteoporos Natl Osteoporos Found USA 11(8):714–720

Ammann P, Rizzoli R (2003) Bone strength and its determinants. Osteoporos Int J Established Result Cooper Eur Found Osteoporos Natl Osteoporos Found USA 14(Suppl 3):13–18

Anonymous (2001) Osteoporosis prevention, diagnosis, and therapy. JAMA 285(6):785–795

Anumula S, Wehrli SL et al (2010) Ultra-short echo-time MRI detects changes in bone mineralization and water content in OVX rat bone in response to alendronate treatment. Bone 46(5):1391–1399

Bae WC, Chen PC et al (2012) Quantitative ultrashort echo time (UTE) MRI of human cortical bone: correlation with porosity and biomechanical properties. J Bone Miner Res Off J Am Soc Bone Miner Res 27(4):848–857

Bauer JS, Link TM (2009) Advances in osteoporosis imaging. Eur J Radiol 71(3):440–449

Bauer JS, Link TM et al (2007) Analysis of trabecular bone structure with multidetector spiral computed tomography in a simulated soft-tissue environment. Calcif Tissue Int 80(6):366–373

Bauer JS, Monetti R et al (2009) Advances of 3T MR imaging in visualizing trabecular bone structure of the calcaneus are partially SNR-independent: analysis using simulated noise in relation to micro-CT, 1.5T MRI, and biomechanical strength. J Magn Reson Imaging 29(1):132–140

Baum T, Dütsch Y et al (2012) Reproducibility of trabecular bone structure measurements of the distal radius at 1.5 and 3.0 T magnetic resonance imaging. J Comput Assist Tomogr 36(5):623–626

Beck TJ, Ruff CB et al (1990) Predicting femoral neck strength from bone mineral data. A structural approach. Invest Radiol 25(1):6–18

Benazzi S, Douka K et al (2011) Early dispersal of modern humans in Europe and implications for Neanderthal behaviour. Nature 479(7374):525–528

Benito M, Gomberg B et al (2003) Deterioration of trabecular architecture in hypogonadal men. J Clin Endocrinol Metab 88(4):1497–1502

Benito M, Vasilic B et al (2005) Effect of testosterone replacement on trabecular architecture in hypogonadal men. J Bone Miner Res Off J Am Soc Bone Miner Res 20(10):1785–1791

Biswas R, Bae W et al (2012) Ultrashort echo time (UTE) imaging with bi-component analysis: bound and free water evaluation of bovine cortical bone subject to sequential drying. Bone 50(3):749–755

Boivin GY, Chavassieux PM et al (2000) Alendronate increases bone strength by increasing the mean degree of mineralization of bone tissue in osteoporotic women. Bone 27(5):687–694

Boutroy S, Bouxsein ML et al (2005) In vivo assessment of trabecular bone micro architecture by high-resolution peripheral quantitative computed tomography. J Clin Endocrinolo Metab 90(12):6508–6515

Boutroy S, Van Rietbergen B et al (2008) Finite element analysis based on in vivo HR-pQCT images of the distal radius is associated with wrist fracture in postmenopausal women. J Bone Miner Res Off J Am Soc Bone Miner Res 23(3):392–399

Boutry N, Cortet B et al (2003) Trabecular bone structure of the calcaneus: preliminary in vivo MR imaging assessment in men with osteoporosis. Radiology 227(3):708–717

Bouxsein ML, Boyd SK et al (2010) Guidelines for assessment of bone microstructure in rodents using micro-computed tomography. J Bone Miner Res Off J Am Soc Bone Miner Res 25(7):1468–1486

Burghardt AJ, Buie HR et al (2010a) Reproducibility of direct quantitative measures of cortical bone microarchitecture of the distal radius and tibia by HR-pQCT. Bone 47(3):519–528

Burghardt AJ, Pialat JB, Kazakia GJ, Boutroy S, Engelke K, Patsch JM, Valentinitsch A, Liu D, Szabo E, Bogado CE, Zanchetta MB, McKay HA, Shane E, Boyd SK, Bouxsein ML, Chapurlat R, Khosla S, Majumdar S. (2012) Multi-center precision of cortical and trabecular bone quality measures assessed by HR-PQCT. J Bone Miner Res. doi:10.1002/jbmr.1795. [Epub ahead of print]

Burghardt AJ, Issever AS et al (2010b) High-resolution peripheral quantitative computed tomographic imaging of cortical and trabecular bone microarchitecture in patients with type 2 diabetes mellitus. J Clin Endocrinol Metab 95(11):5045–5055

Burghardt AJ, Kazakia GJ et al (2010c) Age- and gender-related differences in the geometric properties and biomechanical significance of intracortical porosity in the distal radius and tibia. J Bone Miner Res 25(5):983–993

Burghardt AJ, Kazakia GJ et al (2010d) A longitudinal HR-pQCT study of alendronate treatment in postmenopausal women with low bone density: relations among density, cortical and trabecular microarchitecture, biomechanics, and bone turnover. J Bone Miner Res 25(12):2282–2295

Chesnut CH 3rd, Majumdar S et al (2005) Effects of salmon calcitonin on trabecular microarchitecture as determined by magnetic resonance imaging: results from the QUEST study. J Bone Miner Res Off J Am Soc Bone Miner Res 20(9):1548–1561

Chevalier Y, Quek E et al (2010) Biomechanical effects of teriparatide in women with osteoporosis treated previously with alendronate and risedronate: results from quantitative computed tomography-based finite element analysis of the vertebral body. Bone 46(1):41–48

Cohen A, Dempster DW et al (2010) Assessment of trabecular and cortical architecture and mechanical competence of bone by high-resolution peripheral computed tomography: comparison with transiliac bone biopsy. Osteoporos Int J Established Result Cooper Eur Found Osteoporos Natl Osteoporos Found USA 21(2):263–273

Cortet B, Boutry N et al (2000) In vivo comparison between computed tomography and magnetic resonance image analysis of the distal radius in the assessment of osteoporosis. J Clin Densitom Off J Int Soc Clin Densitom 3(1):15–26

Damilakis J, Adams JE et al (2010) Radiation exposure in X-ray-based imaging techniques used in osteoporosis. Eur Radiol 20(11):2707–2714

Du J, Bydder M et al (2011) Short T2 contrast with three-dimensional ultrashort echo time imaging. Magn Reson Imaging 29(4):470–482

Eswaran SK, Fields AJ et al (2009) Multi-scale modeling of the human vertebral body: comparison of micro-CT based high-resolution and continuum-level models. In: Pacific symposium on biocomputing, pp 293–303

Folkesson J, Goldenstein J et al (2011) Longitudinal evaluation of the effects of alendronate on MRI bone microarchitecture in postmenopausal osteopenic women. Bone 48(3):611–621

Genant HK, Engelke K et al (2010) Denosumab improves density and strength parameters as measured by QCT of the radius in postmenopausal women with low bone mineral density. Bone 47(1):131–139

Gnudi S, Malavolta N et al (2004) Differences in proximal femur geometry distinguish vertebral from femoral neck fractures in osteoporotic women. Br J Radiol 77(915):219–223

Gomberg BR, Wehrli FW et al (2004) Reproducibility and error sources of micro-MRI-based trabecular bone structural parameters of the distal radius and tibia. Bone 35(1):266–276

Gomberg BR, Saha PK et al (2005) Method for cortical bone structural analysis from magnetic resonance images. Acad Radiol 12(10):1320–1332

Graeff C, Timm W et al (2007) Monitoring teriparatide-associated changes in vertebral microstructure by high-resolution CT in vivo: results from the EUROFORS study. J Bone Miner Res Off J Am Soc Bone Miner Res 22(9):1426–1433

Griffith JF, Yeung DK et al (2005) Vertebral bone mineral density, marrow perfusion, and fat content in healthy men and men with osteoporosis: dynamic contrast-enhanced MR imaging and MR spectroscopy. Radiology 236(3):945–951

Griffith JF, Yeung DK et al (2006) Vertebral marrow fat content and diffusion and perfusion indexes in women with varying bone density: MR evaluation. Radiology 241(3):831–838

Griffith JF, Yeung DK et al (2008) Compromised bone marrow perfusion in osteoporosis. J Bone Miner Res Off J Am Soc Bone Miner Res 23(7):1068–1075

Hildebrand T, Ruegsegger P (1997) A new method for the model-independent assessment of thickness in three-dimensional images. J Microsc (Oxford) 185:67–75

Hildebrand T, Laib A et al (1999) Direct three-dimensional morphometric analysis of human cancellous bone: Microstructural data from spine, femur, iliac crest, and calcaneus. J Bone Miner Res 14(7):1167–1174

Holzer G, von Skrbensky G et al (2009) Hip fractures and the contribution of cortical versus trabecular bone to femoral neck strength. J Bone Miner Res Off J Am Soc Bone Miner Res 24(3):468–474

Hwang SN, Wehrli FW et al (1997) Probability-based structural parameters from three-dimensional nuclear magnetic resonance images as predictors of trabecular bone strength. Med Phys 24(8):1255–1261

Ito M (2011) Recent progress in bone imaging for osteoporosis research. J Bone Miner Metab 29(2):131–140

Ito M, Ikeda K et al (2005) Multi-detector row CT imaging of vertebral microstructure for evaluation of fracture risk. J Bone Miner Res Off J Am Soc Bone Miner Res 20(10):1828–1836

Jayakar RY, Cabal A et al (2012) Evaluation of high-resolution peripheral quantitative computed tomography, finite element analysis and biomechanical testing in a pre-clinical model of osteoporosis: a study with odanacatib treatment in the ovariectomized adult rhesus monkey. Bone 50(6):1379–1388

Kazakia GJ, Hyun B et al (2008) In vivo determination of bone structure in postmenopausal women: a comparison of HR-pQCT and high-field MR imaging. J Bone Miner Res 23(4):463–474

Keaveny TM, McClung MR et al (2012) Femoral strength in osteoporotic women treated with teriparatide or alendronate. Bone 50(1):165–170

Keyak JH, Sigurdsson S et al (2011) Male-female differences in the association between incident hip fracture and proximal femoral strength: a finite element analysis study. Bone 48(6):1239–1245

Khosla S, Riggs BL et al (2006) Effects of sex and age on bone microstructure at the ultradistal radius: a population-based noninvasive in vivo assessment. J Bone Miner Res Off J Am Soc Bone Miner Res 21(1):124–131

Krug R, Banerjee S et al (2005) Feasibility of in vivo structural analysis of high-resolution magnetic resonance images of the proximal femur. Osteoporos Int J Established Result Cooper Eur Found Osteoporos Natl Osteoporos Found USA 16(11):1307–1314

Krug R, Han ET et al (2006) Fully balanced steady-state 3D-spin-echo (bSSSE) imaging at 3 Tesla. Magn Reson Med Off J Soc Magn Reson Med/Soc Magn Reso Med 56(5):1033–1040

Krug R, Larson PE et al (2011) Ultrashort echo time MRI of cortical bone at 7 tesla field strength: a feasibility study. J Magn Reson Imaging 34(3):691–695

Ladinsky GA, Vasilic B et al (2008) Trabecular structure quantified with the MRI-based virtual bone biopsy in postmenopausal women contributes to vertebral deformity burden independent of areal vertebral BMD. J Bone Miner Res Off J Am Soc Bone Miner Res 23(1):64–74

Laib A, Hauselmann HJ et al (1998) In vivo high resolution 3D-QCT of the human forearm. Technol Health Care Off J Eur Soc Eng Med 6(5–6):329–337

Laib A, Newitt DC et al (2002) New model-independent measures of trabecular bone structure applied to in vivo high-resolution MR images. Osteoporos Int J Established Result Cooper Eur Found Osteoporos Natl Osteoporos Found USA 13(2):130–136

Li EK, Zhu TY et al (2010) Ibandronate increases cortical bone density in patients with systemic lupus erythematosus on long-term glucocorticoid. Arthritis Res Ther 12(5):R198

Link TM (2002) High-resolution magnetic resonance imaging to assess trabecular bone structure in patients after transplantation: a review. Top Magn Reson Imaging 13(5):365–375

Link TM, Majumdar S et al (1998) In vivo high resolution MRI of the calcaneus: differences in trabecular structure in osteoporosis patients. J Bone Miner Res Off J Am Soc Bone Miner Res 13(7):1175–1182

Link TM, Lotter A et al (2000) Changes in calcaneal trabecular bone structure after heart transplantation: an MR imaging study. Radiology 217(3):855–862

Link TM, Saborowski et al (2002) Changes in calcaneal trabecular bone structure assessed with high-resolution MR imaging in patients with kidney transplantation. Osteoporos Int J Established Result Cooper Eur Found Osteoporos Natl Osteoporos Found USA 13(2):119–129

Link TM, Bauer J et al (2004) Trabecular bone structure of the distal radius, the calcaneus, and the spine: which site predicts fracture status of the spine best? Invest Radiol 39(8):487–497

Liu XS, Cohen A et al (2010a) Individual trabeculae segmentation (ITS)-based morphological analysis of high-resolution peripheral quantitative computed tomography images detects abnormal trabecular plate and rod microarchitecture in premenopausal women with idiopathic osteoporosis. J Bone Miner Res 25(7):1496–1505

Liu XS, Cohen A et al (2010b) Bone density, geometry, microstructure, and stiffness: Relationships between peripheral and central skeletal sites assessed by DXA, HR-pQCT, and cQCT in premenopausal women. J Bone Miner Res Off J Am Soc Bone Miner Res 25(10):2229–2238

Liu XS, Zhang XH et al (2010c) High-resolution peripheral quantitative computed tomography can assess microstructural and mechanical properties of human distal tibial bone. J Bone Miner Res Off J Am Soc Bone Miner Res 25(4):746–756

Liu XS, Walker MD et al (2011) Better skeletal microstructure confers greater mechanical advantages in Chinese-American women versus white women. Osteoporos Int J Established Result Cooper Eur Found Osteoporos Natl Osteoporos Found USA 26(8):1783–1792

Louis O, Cattrysse E et al (2010) Accuracy of peripheral quantitative computed tomography and magnetic resonance imaging in assessing cortical bone cross-sectional area: a cadaver study. J Comput Assist Tomogr 34(3):469–472

Macdonald HM, Nishiyama KK et al (2011a) Changes in trabecular and cortical bone microarchitecture at peripheral sites associated with 18 months of teriparatide therapy in postmenopausal women with osteoporosis. Osteoporos Int 22(1):357–362

Macdonald HM, Nishiyama KK et al (2011b) Age-related patterns of trabecular and cortical bone loss differ between sexes and skeletal sites: a population-based HR-pQCT study. J Bone Miner Res Off J Am Soc Bone Miner Res 26(1):50–62

MacNeil JA, Boyd SK (2007) Accuracy of high-resolution peripheral quantitative computed tomography for measurement of bone quality. Med Eng Phys 29(10):1096–1105

Majumdar S, Newitt D et al (1995) Evaluation of technical factors affecting the quantification of trabecular bone structure using magnetic resonance imaging. Bone 17(4):417–430

Majumdar S, Newitt D et al (1996) Magnetic resonance imaging of trabecular bone structure in the distal radius: relationship with X-ray tomographic microscopy and biomechanics. Osteoporos Int J Established Result Cooper Eur Found Osteoporos Natl Osteoporos Found USA 6(5):376–385

Majumdar S, Link TM et al (1999) Trabecular bone architecture in the distal radius using magnetic resonance imaging in subjects with fractures of the proximal femur. Magnetic Resonance Science Center and Osteoporosis and Arthritis Research Group. Osteoporos Int J Established Result Cooper Eur Found Osteoporos Natl Osteoporos Found USA 10(3):231–239

Monetti RA, Boehm H et al (2005) Structural analysis of human proximal femur for the prediction of biomechanical strength in vitro: the locally adapted scaling vector method. In: Fitzpatrick JM, Reinhardt JM (eds) Proceedings of the SPIE medical imaging 2005: Image processing, vol 5747, pp 231–239

Monetti R, Bauer J et al (2011) The locally adapted scaling vector method: a new tool for quantifying anisotropic structures in bone images. In: Saba L (ed) Computed tomography—special applications. InTech. http://www.intechopen.com/articles/show/title/the-locally-adapted-scaling-vector-method-a-new-tool-for-quantifying-anisotropic-structures-in-bone-

Mueller D, Link TM et al (2006) The 3D-based scaling index algorithm: a new structure measure to analyze trabecular bone architecture in high-resolution MR images in vivo. Osteoporos Int J Established Result Cooper Eur Found Osteoporos Natl Osteoporos Found USA 17(10):1483–1493

Mulder L, van Rietbergen B et al (2012) Determination of vertebral and femoral trabecular morphology and stiffness using a flat-panel C-arm-based CT approach. Bone 50(1):200–208

Muller R (2002) The Zurich experience: one decade of three-dimensional high-resolution computed tomography. Top Magn Reson Imaging 13(5):307–322

Newitt DC, Majumdar S et al (2002a) In vivo assessment of architecture and micro-finite element analysis derived indices of mechanical properties of trabecular bone in the radius. Osteoporos Int J established Result Cooper Eur Found Osteoporos Natl Osteoporos Found USA 13(1):6–17

Newitt DC, van Rietbergen B et al (2002b) Processing and analysis of in vivo high-resolution MR images of trabecular bone for longitudinal studies: reproducibility of structural measures and micro-finite element analysis derived mechanical properties. Osteoporos Int J Established Result Cooper Eur Found Osteoporos Natl Osteoporos Found USA 13(4):278–287

Nishiyama KK, Macdonald HM et al (2010) Postmenopausal women with osteopenia have higher cortical porosity and thinner cortices at the distal radius and tibia than women with normal aBMD: an in vivo HR-pQCT study. J Bone Miner Res Off J Am Soc Bone Miner Res 25(4):882–890

Ouyang X, Selby K et al (1997) High resolution magnetic resonance imaging of the calcaneus: age-related changes in trabecular structure and comparison with dual X-ray absorptiometry measurements. Calcif Tissue Int 60(2):139–147

Pahr DH, Zysset PK (2009) A comparison of enhanced continuum FE with micro FE models of human vertebral bodies. J Biomech 42(4):455–462

Parfitt AM, Drezner MK et al (1987) Bone histomorphometry: standardization of nomenclature, symbols, and units. Report of the ASBMR Histomorphometry Nomenclature Committee. J Bone Miner Res Off J Am Soc Bone Miner Res 2(6):595–610

Patsch JM (2012) Increased cortical porosity in type-2 diabetic postmenopausal women with fragility fractures. J Bone Miner Res. doi:10.1002/jbmr.1763. [Epub ahead of print]

Peyrin F (2011) Evaluation of bone scaffolds by micro-CT. Osteoporos Int J Established Result Cooper Eur Found Osteoporos Natl Osteoporos Found USA 22(6):2043–2048

Phan CM, Matsuura M et al (2006) Trabecular bone structure of the calcaneus: comparison of MR imaging at 3.0 and 1.5 T with micro-CT as the standard of reference. Radiology 239(2):488–496

Pialat JB, Burghardt AJ, Sode M, Link TM, Majumdar S (2012) Visual grading of motion induced image degradation in high resolution peripheral computed tomography: impact of image quality on measures of bone density and micro-architecture. Bone 50(1):111–118

Pialat JB, Vilayphiou N et al (2012) Local topological analysis at the distal radius by HR-pQCT: application to in vivo bone microarchitecture and fracture assessment in the OFELY study. Bone 51(3):362–368

Pothuaud L, Laib A et al (2002) Three-dimensional-line skeleton graph analysis of high-resolution magnetic resonance images: a validation study from 34-microm-resolution microcomputed tomography. J Bone Miner Res Off J Am Soc Bone Miner Res 17(10):1883–1895

Pothuaud L, Newitt DC et al (2004) In vivo application of 3D-line skeleton graph analysis (LSGA) technique with high-resolution magnetic resonance imaging of trabecular bone structure. Osteoporos Int J Established Result Cooper Eur Found Osteoporos Natl Osteoporos Found USA 15(5):411–419

Rad HS, Lam SC et al (2011) Quantifying cortical bone water in vivo by three-dimensional ultra-short echo-time MRI. NMR Biomed 24(7):855–864

Rajapakse CS, Leonard MB et al (2012) Micro-MR imaging-based computational biomechanics demonstrates reduction in cortical and trabecular bone strength after renal transplantation. Radiology 262(3):912–920

Räth C, Monetti R et al (2008) Strength through structure: visualization and local assessment of the trabecular bone structure. New J Phys 10(12): 125010 (122008)

Reichert IL, Robson MD et al (2005) Magnetic resonance imaging of cortical bone with ultrashort TE pulse sequences. Magn Reson Imaging 23(5):611–618

Rizzoli R, Chapurlat RD, Laroche JM, Krieg MA, Thomas T, Frieling I, Boutroy S, Laib A, Bock O (2012) Effects of strontium ranelate and alendronate on bone microstructure in women with osteoporosis: results of a 2-year study. Osteoporos Int 23(1):305–315

Roschger P, Manjubala I et al (2010) Bone material quality in transiliac bone biopsies of postmenopausal osteoporotic women after 3 years of strontium ranelate treatment. J Bone Miner Res Off J Am Soc Bone Miner Res 25(4):891–900

Rosen CJ, Bouxsein ML (2006) Mechanisms of disease: is osteoporosis the obesity of bone? Nat Clin Pract Rheumatol 2(1):35–43

Schellinger D, Lin CS et al (2004) Bone marrow fat and bone mineral density on proton MR spectroscopy and dual-energy X-ray absorptiometry: their ratio as a new indicator of bone weakening. Am J Roentgenol 183(6):1761–1765

Seeman E (2010) Bone morphology in response to alendronate as seen by high-resolution computed tomography: through a glass darkly. J Bone Miner Res 25(12):2277–2281

Seeman E, Delmas PD et al (2010) Microarchitectural deterioration of cortical and trabecular bone: differing effects of denosumab and alendronate. J Bone Miner Res 25(8):1886–1894

Shen W, Chen J et al (2007) MRI-measured bone marrow adipose tissue is inversely related to DXA-measured bone mineral in Caucasian women. Osteoporos Int J Established Result Cooper Eur Found Osteoporos Natl Osteoporos Found USA 18(5):641–647

Sidorenko I, Monetti R et al (2011) Assessing methods for characterising local and global structural and biomechanical properties of the trabecular bone network. Curr Med Chem 18(22):3402–3409

Sievanen H, Karstila T et al (2007) Magnetic resonance imaging of the femoral neck cortex. Acta Radiol 48(3):308–314

Sornay-Rendu E, Boutroy S et al (2007) Alterations of cortical and trabecular architecture are associated with fractures in postmenopausal women, partially independent of decreased BMD measured by DXA: the OFELY study. J Bone Miner Res 22(3):425–433

Sornay-Rendu E, Cabrera-Bravo JL et al (2009) Severity of vertebral fractures is associated with alterations of cortical architecture in postmenopausal women. J Bone Miner Res 24(4):737–743

Stauber M, Muller R (2006) Volumetric spatial decomposition of trabecular bone into rods and plates–a new method for local bone morphometry. Bone 38(4):475–484

Stein EM, Liu XS et al (2010) Abnormal microarchitecture and reduced stiffness at the radius and tibia in postmenopausal women with fractures. J Bone Miner Res Off J Am Soc Bone Miner Res 25(12):2572–2581

Stein EM, Liu XS et al (2011) Abnormal microarchitecture and stiffness in postmenopausal women with ankle fractures. J Clin Endocrinol Metab 96(7):2041–2048

Techawiboonwong A, Song HK et al (2005) Implications of pulse sequence in structural imaging of trabecular bone. J Magn Reson Imaging 22(5):647–655

Trabelsi N, Yosibash Z et al (2011) Patient-specific finite element analysis of the human femur–a double-blinded biomechanical validation. J Biomech 44(9):1666–1672

Valentinitsch A, Patsch JM et al (2012) Automated threshold-independent cortex segmentation by 3D-texture analysis of HR-pQCT scans. Bone

van Rietbergen B, Majumdar S et al (2002) High-resolution MRI and micro-FE for the evaluation of changes in bone mechanical properties during longitudinal clinical trials: application to calcaneal bone in postmenopausal women after one year of idoxifene treatment. Clin Biomech 17(2):81–88

Vico L, Zouch M et al (2008) High-resolution pQCT analysis at the distal radius and tibia discriminates patients with recent wrist and femoral neck fractures. J Bone Miner Res 23(11):1741–1750

Vilayphiou N, Boutroy S et al (2010) Finite element analysis performed on radius and tibia HR-pQCT images and fragility fractures at all sites in postmenopausal women. Bone 46(4):1030–1037

Vilayphiou N, Boutroy S et al (2011) Finite element analysis performed on radius and tibia HR-pQCT images and fragility fractures at all sites in men. J Bone Miner Res 26(5):965–973

Walsh CJ, Phan CM et al (2010) Women with anorexia nervosa: finite element and trabecular structure analysis by using flat-panel volume CT. Radiology 257(1):167–174

Wang XF, Wang Q et al (2009) Differences in macro- and microarchitecture of the appendicular skeleton in young Chinese and white women. J Bone Miner Res Off J Am Soc Bone Miner Res 24(12):1946–1952

Wehrli FW (2007) Structural and functional assessment of trabecular and cortical bone by micro magnetic resonance imaging. J Magn Reson Imaging 25(2):390–409

Wehrli FW, Gomberg BR et al (2001) Digital topological analysis of in vivo magnetic resonance microimages of trabecular bone reveals structural implications of osteoporosis. J Bone Miner Res Off J Am Soc Bone Miner Res 16(8):1520–1531

Wehrli FW, Leonard MB et al (2004) Quantitative high-resolution magnetic resonance imaging reveals structural implications of renal osteodystrophy on trabecular and cortical bone. J Magn Reson Imaging 20(1):83–89

Wehrli FW, Ladinsky GA et al (2008) In vivo magnetic resonance detects rapid remodeling changes in the topology of the trabecular bone network after menopause and the protective effect of estradiol. J Bone Miner Res Off J Am Soc Bone Miner Res 23(5):730–740

Whitehouse WJ (1974) The quantitative morphology of anisotropic trabecular bone. J Microsc 101(Part 2):153–168

Woodhead HJ, Kemp AF et al (2001) Measurement of midfemoral shaft geometry: repeatability and accuracy using magnetic resonance imaging and dual-energy X-ray absorptiometry. J Bone Miner Res Off J Am Soc Bone Miner Res 16(12):2251–2259

Zebaze RM, Ghasem-Zadeh A et al (2010) Intracortical remodelling and porosity in the distal radius and post-mortem femurs of women: a cross-sectional study. Lancet 375(9727):1729–1736

Vertebroplasty and Kyphoplasty

Lotfi Hacein-Bey, Ali Guermazi, and Alexander M. Norbash

Contents

L. Hacein-Bey (✉)
Interventional Neuroradiology and Neuroradiology,
Radiological Associates of Sacramento Medical Group, Inc,
1500 Expo Parkway, Sacramento, CA 95815, USA
e-mail: haceinbeyl@radiological.com

A. Guermazi
Quantitative Imaging Center, Musculoskeletal Imaging,
Department of Radiology, Boston University School of Medicine,
820 Harrison Avenue, Boston, MA 02118, USA

A. M. Norbash
Department of Radiology, Boston University Medical Center,
820 Harrison Avenue, Boston, MA 02118, USA

Abstract

Vertebroplasty has had a major impact on the management of vertebral compression fractures of all etiologies in the past 20 years. A number of variations of the technique initially described by Deramond have been described, including kyphoplasty, lordoplasty, and device-implanting procedures, all of which appear to provide similar pain relief rates as vertebroplasty, commonly in the 90 % range. Although the effectiveness of vertebroplasty (and other vertebral augmentation procedures) has been challenged, there is *significant* evidence for its effectiveness. Given the economic pressures involved in health care, the effectiveness of any procedure will be scrutinized. Further analyses of vertebroplasty will most likely result in establishing the appropriateness, clinical effectiveness, and cost-effectiveness of vertebral augmentation.

1 Introduction

Although vertebral augmentation procedures are relatively recent, their therapeutic impact and benefit to patients has been measurable. Hervé Deramond, a French neuroradiologist, is credited with performing the first vertebroplasty in 1984 on a young woman with a destructive hemangioma of the dens axis causing intractable cervical pain and instability (Galibert et al. 1987). In that patient, percutaneous injection of acrylic cement in the vertebra both improved craniocervical stability and provided profound lasting pain relief. In the ensuing few years, Deramond and his group successfully applied the technique to the treatment of painful, osteoporosis-induced or cancer-related vertebral fractures, which resulted in rapid worldwide adoption of vertebroplasty (Grados et al. 2000). In the mid 1990s, the procedure was introduced in the United States by Lee Jensen and the University of Virginia group (Jensen et al. 1997).

G. Guglielmi (ed.), *Osteoporosis and Bone Densitometry Measurements*, Medical Radiology. Diagnostic Imaging,
DOI: 10.1007/174_2012_702, © Springer-Verlag Berlin Heidelberg 2013

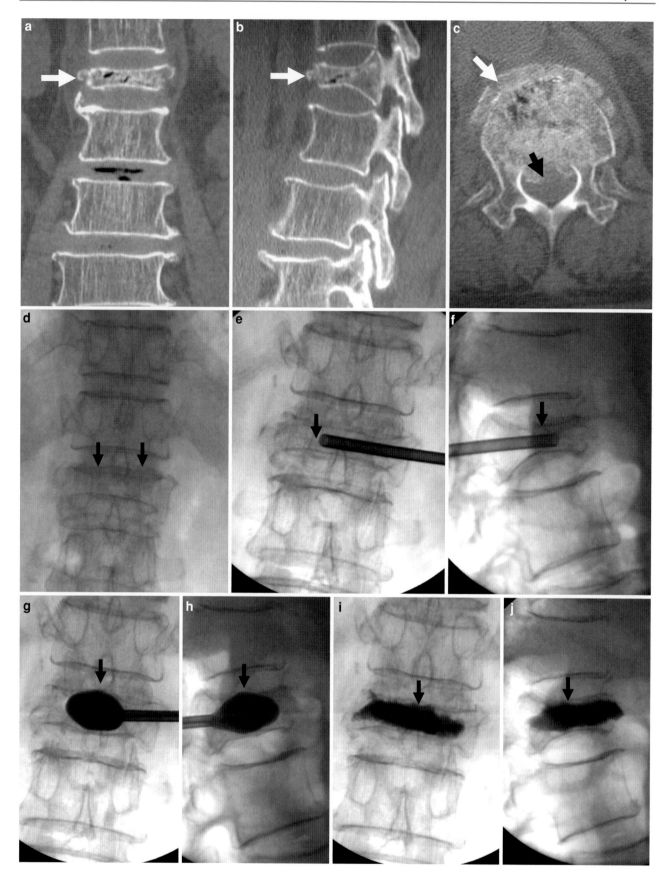

◄ **Fig. 1** 85-year-old woman with severe back pain from L1 fracture with mild retropulsion. Unilateral transpedicular kyphoplasty results in pain relief. CT of the lumbar spine, coronal (**a**) and sagittal (**b**) reconstruction images show fracture of the L1 vertebra with vacuum phenomenon and severe height loss. Axial imaging (**c**) also confirms retropulsion. X-ray (**d**) shows 70 % height loss (arrows). Kyphoplasty trocar (*arrows*) has been introduced into the vertebral body of L1 through a right transpedicular approach visible on AP (**e**) and lateral (**f**) views. AP (**g**) and lateral (**h**) views show that single balloon (*arrow*) positioned in the center of the vertebral body provides significant height recovery. AP (**i**) and lateral (**j**) views show that moderate reduction has been obtained with cement injection (*arrows*). The posterior wall is not compromised

Vertebroplasty has made a major difference for patients with vertebral compression fractures, whether from cancer or osteoporosis, and has contributed in many instances to improved quality of life while decreasing, replacing, or delaying further pain and disability.

A number of variations on the initial procedure described by Deramond have been developed. Kyphoplasty, which uses a dilatation balloon to restore some degree of height to the treated vertebra and reduce angular kyphosis, was initially marketed as an improvement over vertebroplasty for the treatment of osteoporotic fractures (Lieberman et al. 2001). A number of other variations followed, most of which involve implantation in the vertebra of metallic or plastic devices (Kiva™, Optimesh®, StatXx-FX®) (Ortiz and Mathis 2010).

Despite recent controversy as to the effectiveness of vertebroplasty in pain relief, which was generated by two articles published in the same August 2009 issue of the *New England Journal of Medicine* (Kallmes et al. 2009; Buchbinder et al. 2009), there is strong evidence to support the role of vertebroplasty and other augmentation procedures in properly selected patients.

2   Patient Selection

Vertebral compression fractures are most commonly the result of osteoporosis. In addition, vertebral fractures are the most common osteoporosis-related fracture. Osteoporosis constitutes a significant burden to society, with more than 700,000 vertebral fractures in the United States per year and an annual cost estimated at several billion dollars (Riggs and Melton 1995). Although osteoporosis affects predominantly women in the post-menopausal period, men are almost as equally affected by standards of bone mass measurement.

While there is no single method for predicting which patients will be most at risk for fractures, some observations may be helpful. Siminoski et al. (2005) have pointed out that patients who lose significant height (4 cm or more) within a short period of time are very likely to have experienced a vertebral compression fracture. When a vertebral fracture occurs, there is a significant increase in load on muscles, ligaments, and facets, which can cause muscle spasms and precipitate facet arthropathy, triggering additional pain-generating mechanisms. The center of gravity is displaced forward with angular kyphosis, causing an increased risk of falls, and therefore an increased risk for additional axial and appendicular fractures.

The goals of treatment are pain relief, fracture reduction, and vertebral reconstruction.

Vertebral body fractures that are associated with compromise of the posterior wall and retropulsion, particularly if associated with neurological deficit, are traditionally considered best treated by conventional surgical techniques. However, percutaneous vertebral augmentation procedures may be performed successfully in selected cases (Fig. 1).

Extreme compression fractures (vertebra plana) make the procedure technically difficult, although not impossible if the endplates are intact (Fig. 2). Traumatic fractures not associated with osteoporosis that cause recurrent severe pain may be considered for vertebroplasty, particularly if relatively recent and if surgery is not a reasonable consideration (Fig. 3). Kyphoplasty has also been reported in the successful treatment of a vertebral fracture associated with Guillain-Barré syndrome, promoting significant improvement in functional activity and neurological function by allowing the patient to enroll immediately in a rehabilitation program (Masala et al. 2004).

3   Vertebroplasty, Kyphoplasty, and Newer Vertebral Augmentation Procedures

Vertebroplasty, the first vertebral augmentation procedure described, involved the direct injection of bone cement within the spongious bone of the vertebral body through needles inserted through one or both pedicles. The first variation of the technique was to use a unilateral transpedicular approach to increase the safety and decrease the duration of the procedure. Technical improvements to the vertebroplasty procedure soon took place, the most notable being curved and directional needles (Cook®, DePuy Osseon®, AvaFlex®), bone filler needles (CareFusion®, Stryker®), cavity creating devices (Latitude®), and newer cements with higher viscosity containing bioceramics (Cortoss®) or calcium phosphate hydroxyapatite (Actos®).

The concept of inserting and inflating a balloon into a vertebral body was first developed in the mid-1980s by an orthopedic surgeon, Dr. Mark Reiley and an engineer, Arie Scholten. It was not until 1994 that Dr. Reiley was able to find investors interested in his "balloons in bones" idea.

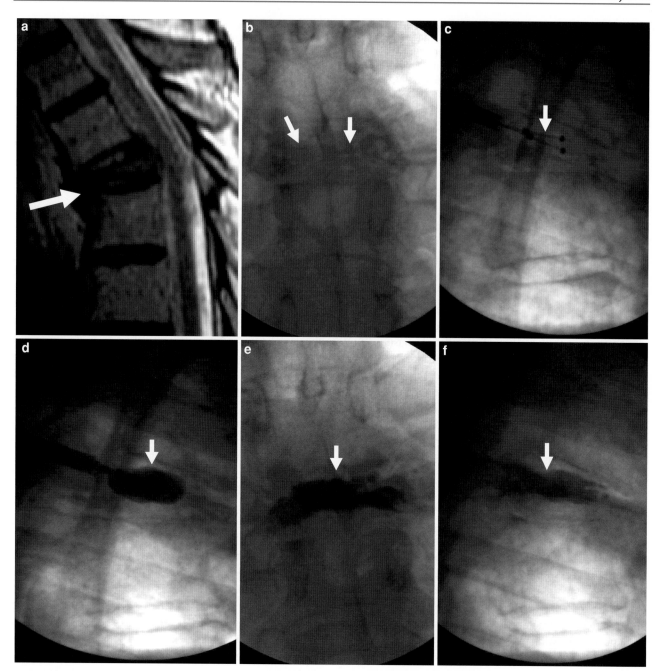

Fig. 2 Kyphoplasty for painful T5 vertebra plana fracture in a 67-year-old man with multiple myeloma. Excellent pain relief. **a** Sagittal T2 weighted MRI shows T5 fracture with severe anterior wedging and height loss (*arrow*) in a vertebra plana pattern. **b** X-ray, anteroposterior view shows severe height loss of T5 (*arrows*). **c** X-ray, lateral view shows deflated kyphoplasty balloons placed within the vertebral body of T5 (*arrow*). **d** X-ray, lateral view shows inflated kyphoplasty balloons within T5 (*arrow*). **e** X-ray, anteroposterior view shows excellent cement filling in T5 (*arrow*). **f** Lateral X-ray shows excellent reduction of T5 (*arrow*)

The newly formed Kyphon Corporation (Sunnyvale, CA) succeeded in developing a balloon capable of displacing bone. The KyphX® Inflatable Bone Tamp™ received 510(k) clearance from the United States Food and Drug Administration (FDA) in July 1998 (Fig. 4).

Lordoplasty is a variation of vertebroplasty which reportedly has similar pain relief rates (in the 90 % range), and has the theoretical advantage of reducing vertebral and segmental kyphosis by 10–15° (Orler et al. 2006). Lordoplasty uses cannulas in the fractured and adjacent vertebrae, which function as internal fixators; a lordotic moment is applied via the cannulas, allowing reduction of the lordosis while the fractured vertebra is simultaneously filled with cement.

Vertebral body remodeling devices all differ from vertebroplasty, lordoplasty, or kyphoplasty as they involve the permanent implantation within the vertebral body of a device in addition to bone cement. Whether implantable devices have greater effectiveness and safety over vertebroplasty and kyphoplasty is not known at this time.

The Kiva^{TM} device (Benvenue Medical Inc, Santa Clara, CA) is a polyether ether ketone (peek) implant (PEEK-OPTIMA$^®$) which is advanced via a transpedicular approach through a Nitinol (nickel titanium) Kiva wire (Fig. 5). This device is currently being investigated in a multicenter trial, the KAST Study (Kiva^{TM} System as a Vertebral Augmentation Treatment—A Safety and Effectiveness Trial).

The StaXx FX Structural Kyphoplasty System$^®$ (Spine Wave, Shelton, CT) is another remodeling device which consists of wafers implanted in the fractured vertebra via a percutaneous peripedicular approach and a wide-based inserting needle. StaXx wafers are made from polyether ether ketone and are 1 mm thick each. Wafers are inserted one at a time, using a wedge action to create vertical lift and reduce the fractured vertebral body. The first wafer, or base wafer, acts as a foundation for subsequently inserted wafers. Once all wafers are inserted, bone cement is injected into the vertebral body for further fixation and stabilization. A small volume of cement is also specifically injected anteriorly at the base of the wafer stack, securing the anterior column.

The Optimesh$^®$ device (Spineology, Saint-Paul, MN) is a surgical mesh made of polyethylene terephthalate (PET). The mesh pouch, which contains impacted granular bone graft, is inserted in its empty state through a small cannula and then packed in situ with bone graft once in place. As more bone graft material is added to the mesh, the gradually increasing volume deploys the OptiMesh$^®$ implant in its final geometric state and generates significant distractive force. When completely filled, the OptiMesh$^®$ implant fibers become taut and granular mechanics transforms the contained graft into a custom-fit, rigid, load-bearing graft pack. The Optimesh$^®$ device is radiolucent and compatible with all imaging modalities.

The VerteLift^{TM} implant (SpineAlign Medical Inc, Pleasanton, CA) is a wire made of Nitinol alloy which comes in two basic shapes and a range of sizes. The device acts as an internal scaffold to engage the vertebral body endplates, while providing and maintaining lift until bone cement is injected. Prior to injection of bone cement, the VerteLift^{TM} implant is fully retrievable. The VerteLift^{TM} implant is currently approved in Europe, and undergoing investigational device exemption evaluation in the United States.

4 Indications and Contraindications

Currently accepted indications include painful vertebral compression fractures from (a) osteoporosis (primary or secondary), (b) neoplastic infiltration, (c) painful, "aggressive" vertebral hemangiomas, and (d) trauma when minimal displacement is present and surgery is contraindicated (Fig. 3).

There are no absolute contraindications to vertebroplasty or other vertebral augmentation procedures. There are relative contraindications to vertebral augmentation procedures that include (1) the presence of a systemic infection, and (2) lack of appropriate surgical backup, which could delay treatment. Bleeding conditions are not considered a contraindication, as they can be adequately controlled in the majority of patients prior to the procedure.

5 Complications

All complications of vertebral augmentation procedures are relatively uncommon, particularly severe ones. In the early 1990s, the United States FDA initiated the Manufacturer and User Facility Device Experience (MAUDE), a nationwide database which was designed to record the details of medical complications occurring from the use of medical devices associated with indexed procedures. Recorded data consists of user facility reports from 1991, distributor reports from 1993, voluntary reports from June 1993, and manufacturer reports from August 1996.

The earliest reports concerning vertebroplasty and kyphoplasty original clinical reports were filed in 1999. In November 2004, the first FDA MAUDE report on complications resulting from the use of medical devices associated with vertebroplasty and kyphoplasty was published.

A total of 43 adverse events were reported out of approximately 190,000 procedures (0.02 %). Reported complications included 4 deaths, 21 instances of neurologic deficits related to cement canal intrusion or epidural hematoma (6 of which were permanent), 3 episodes of blood pressure drop, 2 pulmonary embolisms, 2 infections (1 diskitis, 1 osteomyelitis), 1 pneumothorax, and 11 technical reports of inconsequential equipment breakage. Twenty-five of the 43 events were major, including 4 deaths and 21 cord compressions requiring surgery, with 6 permanent neurologic injuries (Nussbaum et al. 2004). These data, however, likely underrepresent the actual complication rate from these procedures which is better reflected in clinical studies. Deaths were presumed and reported to occur as a result of reactions to the acrylic bone cement, the free polymer portion of which has known cardiotoxicity and can cause cardiac arrhythmias and hemodynamic instability (Kaufmann et al. 2002). As the

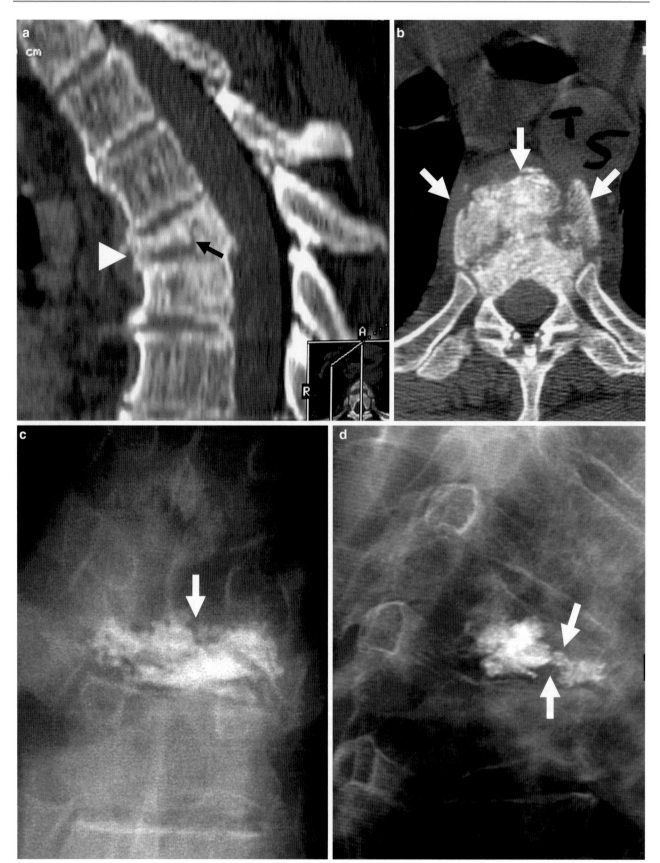

◀ **Fig. 3** Example of traumatic fracture in 66-year-old man treated with vertebroplasty with excellent pain relief. **a** Sagittal reconstruction of thoracic spine CT shows marked anterior wedging and height loss (*arrowhead*), and fracture line (*arrow*). **b** Axial imaging at T5 shows several fracture lines (*arrows*) in the vertebral body resulting in a "burst" pattern. **c** Anteroposterior view shows discontinuous cement deposition within the vertebral body (*arrow*). **d** Lateral view also shows irregular cement deposition in the vertebral body of T5, with apparent vertebral reconstruction and no posterior cement leakage (*arrows*)

risk is dose-dependent, this complication has only been reported when a large number of vertebrae were treated per session.

Neurologic compromise can occur from spinal cord compression because of leakage of large amounts of cement into the epidural venous plexus (Shapiro et al. 2003; Lee et al. 2002; Harrington 2001), requiring expedited surgical evacuation (Shapiro et al. 2003). Cement leakage may also cause direct nerve root compression which can cause new pain or exacerbation of pain (Lee et al. 2002).

Leaking cement in the paravertebral space surrounding the vertebral body usually does not lead to clinical complications, and may occur in as many as 10 % of procedures, (Coumans et al. 2003; Mathis et al. 2001) although transient dysphagia has been specifically reported at the cervical level from esophageal compression (Depriester et al. 1999). Leakage of cement into the intervertebral disk, especially in osteoporotic fractures with rupture of the inferior vertebral body endplate, may occur, without reported clinical consequences (Depriester et al. 1999). With vertebral puncture, there is also a risk of fracture, avoided by meticulous positioning with directed fluoroscopic technique (Pierot and Boulin 1999) or CT guidance in selected instances (Gangi et al. 1998).

With a posterolateral approach (Laredo et al. 1994), there is a risk of pneumothorax at the thoracic level, and of psoas hematoma at the lumbar level (Table 1).

6 Specific Issues with the Geriatric Population

In the elderly, a number of specific issues require special attention, including pre-treatment work-up, procedural technique, and follow-up.

6.1 Adequate Identification of Fractures

Compression fractures have been traditionally diagnosed on plain radiographs, which allow evaluation of bone structure, including the posterior vertebral body wall, and quantification of height loss when present. In the elderly population, several fractures of various ages may coexist, which can complicate identification of the symptomatic level on X-ray imaging alone, even if combined with fluoroscopic-guided provocative manual palpation and a reliable clinical examination. The age of a fracture is an important determinant of response to treatment, and plays an important role in treatment option selection, i.e. in considering the potential superiority of kyphoplasty or other augmentation procedures over vertebroplasty (Spiegl et al. 2009). Magnetic resonance imaging (MRI) is the mainstay of patient evaluation. It is very useful in dating a fracture, showing bone marrow edema in the early stages of a fracture that is not present in older fractures (Fig. 6) (Do 2000; Lindsay et al. 2001). In particular for patients with multiple myeloma, MRI has been shown to be superior to bone scintigraphy (Masala et al. 2005).

The work-up of metastatic spinal lesions also heavily relies on MRI which allows objective and reproducible quantitative assessment of the degree of compression, epidural extension, paraspinal extension, presence of other lesions, and the degree of vascularity (Georgy 2008).

A special mention must be made of SPECT/CT (single photon emission computed tomography/X-ray computed tomography), a relatively new hybrid application which combines metabolic information from SPECT images with accurate anatomical information from CT. This technique may be particularly useful in older patients with multiple fractures and severe claustrophobia, pacemaker, or other contraindication to MRI (Suárez et al 2009; Sudhakar et al. 2010) (Fig. 7).

6.2 Analgesia

Elderly patients who present for the evaluation and treatment of a vertebral compression fracture are often on narcotic pain medications for chronic pain from various causes, and their medication dependency may be exacerbated by the presence of a compression fracture. These patients commonly have a higher response threshold than average, for which higher doses of sedation are typically required during a procedure, and often they suffer from some degree of confusion. In anticipation of a procedure in such patients, it is helpful to reduce the oral intake of narcotics and attempt substituting anti-inflammatory drugs, i.e. ibuprofen or ketorolac (Toradol®), to better control intraprocedural sedation.

6.3 Patient Positioning

Elderly patients have a high incidence of spondylosis, arthritis, and advanced osteoporosis.

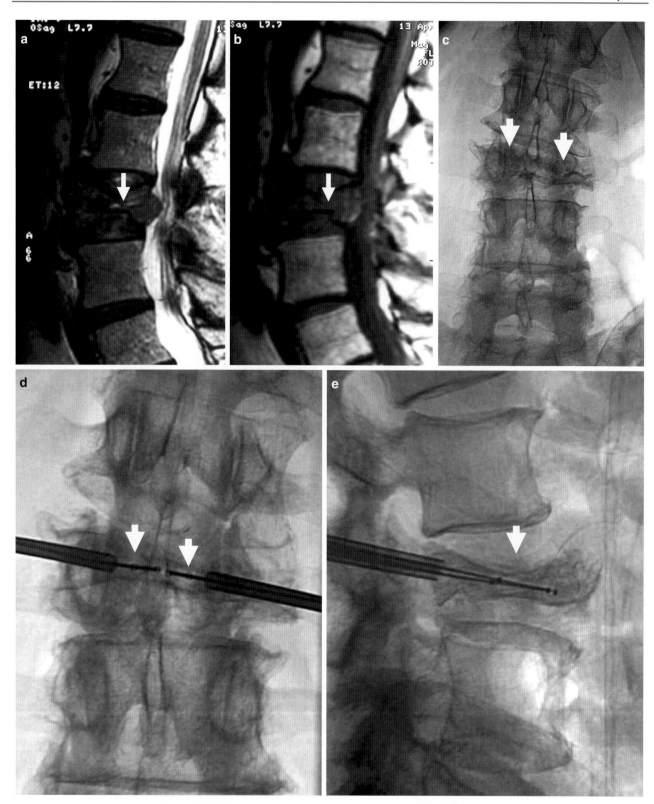

Fig. 4 Kyphoplasty using a bilateral transpedicular approach to treat an extremely painful fracture of L3 with significant retropulsion in a 75-year-old woman with scoliosis. **a** Sagittal T2 weighted MRI shows a hyperintense horizontal cleft in the superior aspect of the vertebral body of L3 (*arrow*). **b** Sagittal T1 weighted MRI shows hypointense signal within the cleft (*arrow*), confirming bone marrow edema. **c** X-ray of lumbar spine shows L3 fracture with 70 % height loss (*arrows*). **d, e**. Excellent placement of kyphoplasty balloons within L3 vertebral body (*arrows*). Note some degree of reduction of scoliosis. **f, g** Balloon inflation results in approximately 50 % height recovery (*arrows*). **h, i** After cement filling, there is approximately 30–40 % height recovery (*arrows*) with fracture reduction, and less pronounced scoliosis

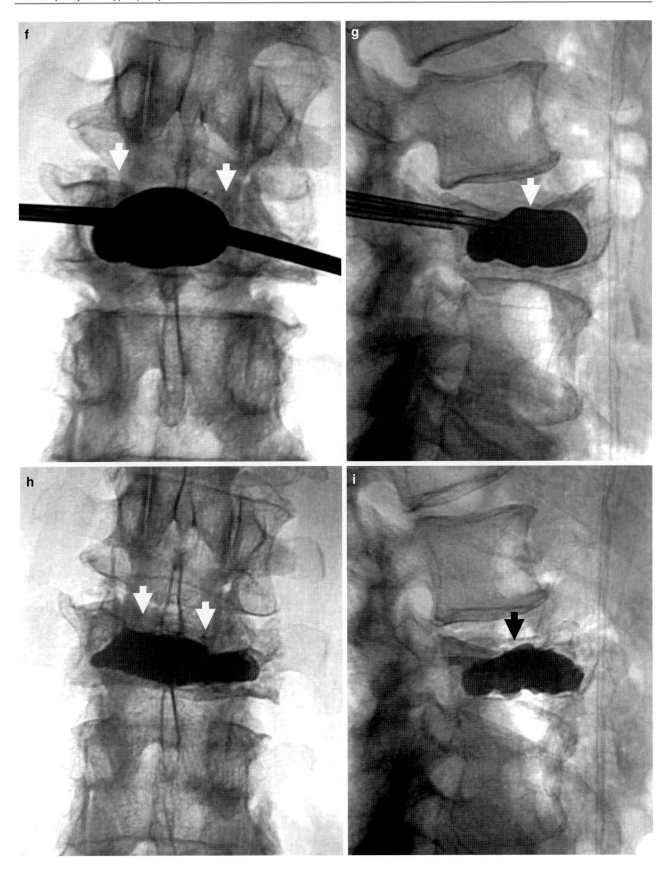

Fig. 4 (continued)

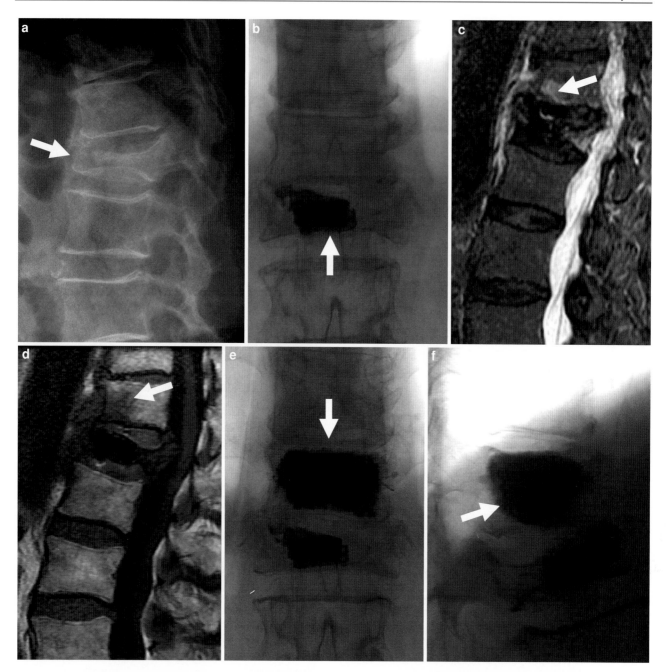

Fig. 5 72-year-old woman with painful L1 fracture treated with the Kiva™ device. Recurrent pain is caused by a fracture at T12, subsequently treated with vertebroplasty. **a** Thoraco-lumbar spine X-ray shows a fracture at L1 with 70 % height loss and moderate retropulsion (*arrow*). **b** Antero-posterior view of the lumbar spine shows the Kiva device and a small amount of bone cement within the vertebral body of L1 (*arrow*). T2-weighted (**c**) and T1-weighted (**d**) MRI shows bone marrow edema in fractured T12 vertebral body (*arrows*). Following vertebroplasty, AP (**e**) and lateral views (**f**) show diffuse and even filling of the T12 vertebral body (*arrows*). Pain relief was immediate

Careful and methodical positioning is particularly important in order to avoid causing new pathology, especially as osteoporosis results in challenging fluoroscopic visualization of bony structures. Rib fractures may occur relatively easily in these patients as a result of suboptimal positioning on the X-ray table, or from pressure on the ribcage from needle insertion through the pedicles. Particular attention should be directed to supplemental padding of contact points. Muscle spasms may also appear after such procedures and can be exacerbated by positioning maneuvers. Patients with a high level of confusion may be at risk for falling off the fluoroscopic table and therefore need to be closely monitored.

Table 1 Complications of vertebral augmentation procedures

Severe
Canal intrusion/epidural hematoma with permanent neurological damage
Infection (diskitis, osteomyelitis)
Pulmonary embolism
Myocardial infarction
Death
Moderate
Canal intrusion/epidural hematoma with transient neurological damage
Reactions to the acrylic (polymethylmethacrylate) bone cement -> cardiotoxicity, cardiac arrhythmias, and hemodynamic instability
Pneumothorax
Intraprocedural blood pressure drop
Minor
Uneventful equipment failure
Rib fractures
Transient post-kyphoplasty radicular pain

6.4 Procedural Sedation

Elderly patients may have significant age-related decreases in drug clearance, resulting in higher bioavailability of narcotic or other drugs taken at home prior to a procedure. In addition, renal and hepatic clearance of intravenous drugs may be significantly prolonged from age-related diminished enzyme activity, and in this patient population these complicating factors may not be accurately predicted from serum levels of creatinine and liver function tests. Particular care must be taken when midazolam is used for sedation, as a sudden drop in oxygenation may occur: severe drops in oxygen saturation levels may require emergent administration of a reversal agent. It is generally advisable to use as little sedation as possible in these patients, which emphasizes again the need for adequate patient preparation and education prior to the procedure (Luginbühl 2008).

6.5 Post-Procedural Care

Following procedures, elderly patients should be kept in observation for a reasonable and adequate amount of time which should cover a significant part of the half-life clearance of most drugs used. Even if spectacular pain relief results from the procedure, patients should be advised to be cautious when initially standing up and walking for a while following the procedure, as they remain at increased risk for falls. The effects of the procedure should be carefully monitored, as ancillary causes of pain may persist in these patients, i.e. facet disease, muscle spasm, undiagnosed, or new fractures, which may delay patient mobility, and may require intervention.

7 Effectiveness of Vertebral Augmentation Procedures

The first large-scale study to demonstrate the efficacy of pain relief with vertebroplasty in the United States is attributed to Jensen et al. (1997) who, in 1997, reported on 29 patients with painful osteoporotic vertebral fractures in whom a 90 % pain relief rate was obtained. This study played an important role in establishing vertebroplasty in the United States for the treatment of osteoporotic or neoplastic vertebral fractures. In 2000, a retrospective study by Barr et al. (2000) revealed that 95 % of 47 patients treated with vertebroplasty reported pain relief that was at least moderate.

Although an early metaanalysis of retrospective case series and uncontrolled studies reported rates of significant pain relief in the 70–80 % range in patients treated for a variety of osteolytic lesions including metastases, hemangiomas, multiple myeloma, and osteoporotic compression fractures, it was also noted that the durable positive response persisted for several months to several years after treatment (Levine et al. 2000). Later, larger scale meta analyses reported rates of pain relief for both vertebroplasty and kyphoplasty in the 90 % range (McGraw et al. 2002; Heini et al. 2000). McGraw et al. (2002) reported a series of 100 osteoporotic vertebral fractures treated with vertebroplasty, with a 97 % rate of significant pain relief at 24 h after treatment, and a 93 % rate of durable relief persisting at least 1 year (mean follow-up, 21.5 months). Similar data were demonstrated with kyphoplasty, with some authors reporting pain relief in 96.9 % of patients treated for osteoporotic fractures, mostly occurring within 24 h (Lane et al. 2000).

For neoplastic vertebral fractures, Weil et al. (1996) reported the first series of 37 patients with metastatic spinal fractures (20 men, 17 women; aged 33–86 years) treated successfully with vertebroplasty, and noted significant pain relief and increased stability in 73 %, with durable gains at 6 months. Later, Fourney et al. (2003) reported on 56 patients with cancer treated with vertebroplasty and kyphoplasty in whom complete pain relief was noted at a rate of 84 %, with persistent gains at 1 year.

A very interesting study is a retrospective evaluation of some of the earliest patients treated with vertebroplasty by the French group that described the original procedure (Deramond et al.) (Franc et al. 2010). Eighteen patients, treated between 1989 and 1998 for vertebral fractures due to osteoporosis ($n = 8$), hemangiomas ($n = 8$), and multiple myeloma ($n = 2$) were re-evaluated clinically and radiologically in 2007, nearly 20 years after their initial procedure. All patients experienced long-term pain relief and none demonstrated instability or disc degeneration disproportionate to that at adjacent vertebral levels (Franc et al. 2010). Similar pain relief rates are consistently reported for vertebroplasty

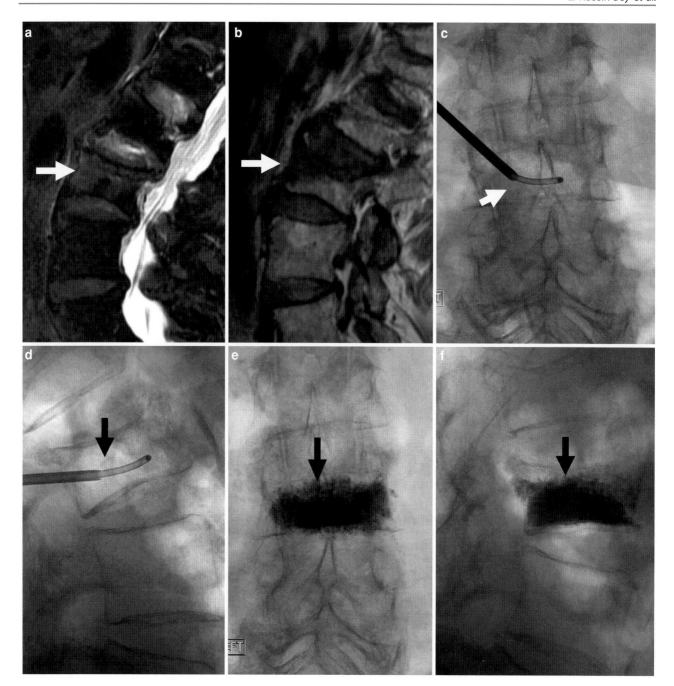

Fig. 6 86-year-old woman with very painful L3 fracture. Unilateral transpedicular vertebroplasty using an 11G curved needle. MRI, T2 (**a**), and T1 (**b**) weighted sagittal imaging shows diffused edema in the superior and anterior vertebral body of L3 (*arrows*). X-rays AP (**c**) and lateral (**d**) views show placement of the curved needle within the vertebral body (*arrows*). X-ray AP (**e**) and lateral (**f**) views show cement diffusely and evenly filling the L3 vertebral body (*arrows*), resulting in excellent pain relief

and kyphoplasty (Fourney et al. 2003; Wardlaw et al. 2009; Boonen et al. 2011; Lieberman and Reinhardt 2003; Ledlie and Renfro 2003; Lane et al. 2000).

Although kyphoplasty was initially marketed for the treatment of osteoporotic fractures as an improvement over vertebroplasty, by increasing vertebral height and reducing angular kyphosis, the overall comparative experience shows an average reduction of 4 mm for kyphoplasty versus 2.2 mm for vertebroplasty (Nussbaum et al. 2004). As yet, there is no indication as to whether the overall minimal difference in reduction is clinically significant. Another theoretical advantage of kyphoplasty is that "lower

Fig. 7 80-year-old woman with atrial fibrillation and a pacemaker. Severe back pain is evaluated by CT which shows a fracture of the T8 vertebral body. Severe residual pain is assessed with SPECT/CT which shows a fracture at T7. Repeat vertebroplasty at this level results in pain relief. **a** CT of the thoracic spine, sagittal reconstruction shows a fracture of T8 (*arrow*). Mild irregularity of T7 is also present (*arrowhead*). Note spinal cord stimulator (*thin long arrow*). **b** X-ray of the thoracic spine, AP view, shows cement in the T8 vertebral body. Note spinal cord stimulator (*thin long arrow*). **c** X-ray of the thoracic spine, AP view, shows cement in T7 and T8. Note spinal cord stimulator (*thin long arrow*). **d, e, f** SPECT/CT shows significant uptake of Tc-199 m not only in the vertebral body of recently treated T8 (*arrow*), but also in the T7 vertebral body (*arrowhead*)

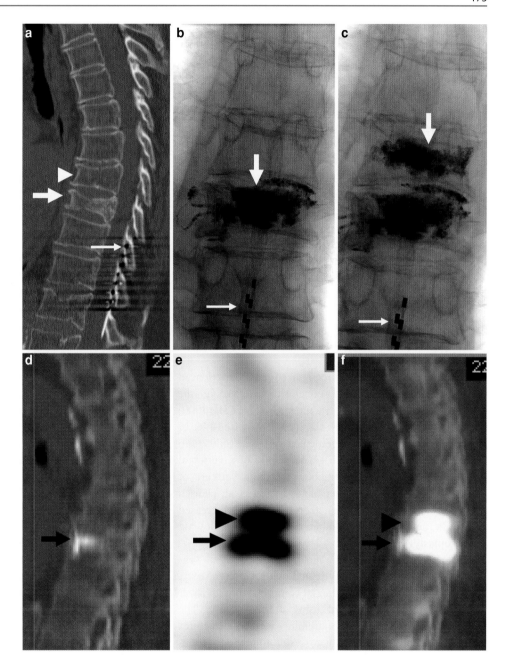

pressure" injections of cement are performed because a cavity is initially created in the vertebral body by the balloon tamp, rather than by injecting a "thinner" mixture as a forced intramedullary perfusate. Although one study found that there are more leaks with vertebroplasty than with kyphoplasty (Lieberman and Reinhardt 2003), another reported experimental evidence that higher pressures within voids created by bone tamps were noted with the use of larger systems (Agris et al. 2003).

With newer devices, pain relief rates seem to be consistent with the expected results from vertebroplasty and kyphoplasty. However, no large-scale data on outcomes are currently available.

8 Follow-Up and Risk of Subsequent Fractures

Patients should continue to be assessed after any vertebral augmentation procedure, particularly elderly patients. Some patients may have persistent pain despite adequate treatment. One reason for persistent pain may be incomplete treatment of the fractured vertebra, which might respond to a repeat procedure at the same level to obtain a more complete filling with cement (Kim et al. 2010). Another reason for persistent pain may be confounding facet joint pain: posterior facet instability and overload resulting from a wedge fracture has been identified as a significant cause of pain in as many as one-third of patients, particularly elderly patients (Wilson et al. 2011). Still, the most common reason for recurrent or persistent pain following vertebral augmentation procedures is the presence of another undiagnosed vertebral fracture, or a new fracture.

An increased risk of new fractures involving vertebrae adjacent to previously treated ones has been suggested (Uppin et al. 2003; Fribourg et al. 2004). It has been estimated that this risk is 12.4 % following vertebroplasty, and that 67 % of new fractures occur in vertebrae that are immediately adjacent to the treated vertebra (Uppin et al. 2003). Part of the concern is that reinforced vertebral bodies may alter the biomechanics of the spine and contribute to adjoining fractures. Following kyphoplasty, an early study of 40 patients reported that 26 % of those treated developed a new fracture within 8 months (Fribourg et al. 2004), while a larger, later study found an overall incidence of a new fracture of 22.6 % per patient and 15.1 % per kyphoplasty procedure (Harrop et al. 2004).

Two large studies from recognized and experienced groups provided conflicting conclusions regarding the effects on adjoining vertebral fractures. Grados et al. (2000) found a slight but statistically significant increased risk of vertebral fracture adjacent to cemented vertebrae (odds ratio 2.27, 95 % CI 1.1-4.56), with an odds ratio of a vertebral fracture adjacent to an uncemented fractured vertebra of 1.44 (0.82–2.55). On the other hand, Jensen et al. (Jensen and Dion 2000) suggested that there may be no increased risk of a new fracture in adjacent vertebrae following vertebroplasty.

A biomechanical study of a small number of spine segments, some healthy, some treated with vertebroplasty, aimed to assess unconstrained axial compression with shear forces and torque minimized using a robotic arm. The authors concluded that new adjoining vertebral fractures were significantly more likely to result following vertebroplasty, due to the mechanism of endplate deflection (Fahim et al. 2011). A recent study of 794 patients divided equally between those with prior vertebroplasty and those with no vertebral augmentation procedure found a similar incidence of new fractures in each group (Chosa et al. 2011).

It is conceptually possible that new fractures may be precipitated by a bone-strengthening, spine-straightening, vertebral augmentation procedure, but it is also clear that, because of the diffuse nature of osteoporosis and metastatic cancer, new fractures are to be expected as part of the natural course of the disease. This is particularly true in the elderly population. As a result, it is necessary and appropriate to carefully follow those patients, and to be prepared to offer treatment for new fractures.

9   Current Controversy

Recently, the efficacy of vertebroplasty in obtaining pain relief has been seriously challenged by two randomized controlled trials or critical reports, which were published in the same 2009 issue of the *New England Journal of Medicine* (*NEJM*) (Kallmes et al. 2009; Buchbinder et al. 2009) Although concerns were expressed about both the conduct and the conclusions of those two studies, these concerns did not receive the same degree of media attention as the studies themselves.

9.1   Concerns with the Critical Reports

One concern with the critical reports concerns offering sham or simulated procedures to patients in severe pain. In both *NEJM* studies (Kallmes et al. 2009; Buchbinder et al. 2009), patients with fractures were treated with either vertebroplasty or a simulated procedure, consisting of intravertebral placement of a needle alone. While in the study by Kallmes et al. (2009) the amount of cement injected into the vertebral bodies is not specified, it can be inferred that volumes similar to standard clinical practice were used. On the other hand, in the study by Buchbinder et al. (2009) only minimal amounts of cement (3 mls) were injected in the vertebrae of the 38/78 patients treated. Because this study does not specify which levels were treated, it has been rightly pointed out that the most commonly fractured vertebrae, i.e., T10 through L3, were most likely the treated ones (Noonan 2009). In these levels, such a small volume of cement is often considered a low volume, and may not be as effective at restoring vertebral body structure and axial integrity and providing pain relief as larger volumes (Noonan 2009).

In the study by Kallmes et al. (2009), 63 % of patients who received the sham procedure correctly guessed the type of procedure by 14 days, as opposed to 51 % in the treated group. In this study, patients were promised the right to have the other procedure if pain relief was not adequate, provided they wait at least 1 month after the initial intervention. Of the patients who had received the sham procedure, 43 % chose to "cross over" to a vertebroplasty procedure, while only 12 % of the vertebroplasty patients chose to cross over in the opposite direction (Kallmes et al. 2009). Such differences have been construed as indicating lack of confidence in the sham procedure on the part of patients (Noonan 2009).).

9.2   Concerns with the Timing of Treatment

Concern has been raised regarding the time window of patient enrollment in both studies, in which patients with back pain were treated within 12 months of their fracture. It is thought that patients with recent fractures of less than 8 weeks duration with unrelenting pain are most likely to benefit from vertebroplasty (Gangi and Clark 2010).).

9.3 Concerns with the Patient Population

In both critical reports the treated patients were outpatients. Prospective investigative evaluation of vertebroplasty may best be served by closely observing the pain syndrome in this patient population, rather than leaving such patients at home with potentially disabling pain which confines them to bed rest and narcotic analgesia. These patients are the most at risk for worsening of osteoporosis and other complications of bed rest and chronic narcotic intake. In the United States, by current Medicare standards, such patients would be considered candidates for vertebral augmentation on the basis of failure of conservative therapy. Of note, over half of the patients treated in the United States are admitted to hospitals for treatment of intractable pain, as indicated by the AMA resource-based data manager (2009 and 2010 data). This population is at high risk for hospital-associated morbidity (including nosocomial infections), additional bone loss, and increased costs for the hospital stay and pain control. Despite concerns regarding such a trial, it has been suggested that a randomized, prospective, double-blind study of hospital-bound patients with acute, painful osteoporotic vertebral fractures treated with vertebroplasty versus medical therapy would likely provide useful information regarding appropriately aggressive treatment (Wagner 2005)

9.4 Concerns with Evaluating the Effects of Treatment

In the study by Kallmes et al. (2009), a 30 % decrease in pain at 1 month was considered clinically meaningful pain relief. This study also reported a trend toward a higher rate of clinically meaningful improvement in pain in the vertebroplasty group when compared with controls (64 vs. 48 %), and concluded that vertebroplasty and simulated procedures produce "similar" effects. Similarly, in the study by Buchbinder et al. (2009) patient response was measured by using a 7-point ordinal scale, ranging from "a great deal worse" to "a great deal better." At 1 month, 34 % of the patients having undergone vertebroplasty classified their pain as "moderately better" or "a great deal better" versus 24 % of control patients, when compared with the stated conclusion that vertebroplasty and the sham procedure were essentially equivalent. An additional point for consideration is the expected statistical response to supposed minor differences between groups. The recommendation of the US FDA for

clinical trials that show small effect sizes is to examine the cumulative distribution function of responses between treatment groups to characterize the treatment effect (U.S. Department of Health and Human Services, Food and Drug Administration 2009). Therefore, reductions in pain of 30 % should be considered as clinically meaningful responses, having previously been shown to reflect improved pain by pooling of response data from many studies (Georgy 2011). For endpoints such as pain level, clinical trials typically seek to show not only a statistically significant improvement in the primary efficacy endpoint, but also that the magnitude of the effect is clinically relevant (Snapinn and Jiang 2007). The "responder analysis" statistical approach is particularly well suited for such purposes, as it allows clear separation of "responders" and "non-responders" to a continuous primary efficacy measure (Snapinn and Jiang 2007). It has been appropriately argued that, although both the studies by Kallmes and Buchbinder did conduct a "responder analysis", neither was powered to detect differences by using this approach (Georgy 2011).

A large responder analysis performed by the Initiative on Methods, Measurement, and Pain Assessment in Clinical Trials (IMMPACT) Group has shown that patients treated with vertebroplasty were overall 35 % more likely than control subjects to experience a clinically meaningful reduction in pain at 1 month (Dworkin et al. 2008).

The results of a large study, the Vertebroplasty versus Conservative Treatment in Acute Osteoporotic Vertebral Compression Fractures (VERTOS) II trial were published following the two *NEJM* studies (Klazen et al. 2010). VERTOS was a prospective randomized trial of vertebroplasty and conservative treatment for 202 patients and showed that vertebroplasty resulted in greater pain relief than conservative treatment with a significant difference in mean visual analog scale (VAS) score between baseline and 1 month. The study concluded that in a subgroup of patients with acute osteoporotic vertebral compression fractures and persistent pain, percutaneous vertebroplasty is both effective and safe, and provides pain relief which is immediate, sustained for at least 1 year, and significantly exceeds the relief achieved with conservative treatment at an acceptable cost. This study did not receive the same level of media and insurance carrier attention given to the *NEJM* articles (Klazen et al. 2010).

Not surprisingly, following the publication of the two critical *NEJM* reports, proposals to deny coverage decision and reimbursement of both percutaneous vertebroplasty and percutaneous vertebral augmentation for their previously approved indications have been advanced by large counseling and authoritative bodies, such as the Noridian Administrative Services, a Medicare intermediary for 11 United States Western states, and the Ontario Health Technology Advisory Committee in Ontario, Canada (Georgy 2011). Whether vertebroplasty and other augmentation procedures will continue to be covered remains to be seen.

10   Cost Considerations

Kyphoplasty and procedures that use remodeling devices cost more than vertebroplasty. For kyphoplasty, balloons and bone filler needles add expense to the procedure. In 2007, the cost of a KyphoPak kit (Kyphon) for a single-level vertebroplasty was $3423 as opposed to a few hundred dollars for vertebroplasty. Newer implantable devices will also incur costs that are higher than simple vertebroplasty. One study projects treatment costs at the current treatment rate of one in seven of the 700,000 fractures diagnosed each year in the United States. If kyphoplasty alone is used, treatment costs would add a global cost of $600 million (Nussbaum et al. 2004). In addition to the materials, fluoroscopy time and physician time are typically longer with newer, more complex procedures than vertebroplasty. It is likely that comparative effectiveness studies will be carried out to assess address and issues of cost.

11   Conclusion

Vertebroplasty has had a major impact on the management of vertebral compression fractures, by turning a potentially disabling and relatively common condition into an easily curable one. Whether technological improvements to the original procedure will translate into greater safety and effectiveness has yet to be established. Current concerns about the effectiveness of vertebral augmentation will need to be addressed as data continues to be collected. Improvements in technology may well include semi automated procedures using robotics and stereotactic guidance. Whether the cost and safety profile of the procedure and advances in our understanding of the epidemiology of osteoporosis and spine biomechanics will result in a potential prophylactic role for vertebral augmentation procedures in the future remains yet to be determined.

References

Agris JM, Zoarski GH, Stallmeyer MJB, Ortiz O (2003) Intravertebral pressure during vertebroplasty: a study comparing multiple delivery systems. Presented at the annual meeting of the American Society of Spine Radiology, Scottsdale, AZ, 19–23 Febr 2003

Barr JD, Barr MS, Lemley TJ, McCann RM (2000) Percutaneous vertebroplasty for pain relief and spinal stabilization. Spine 15(25):923–928

Boonen S, Van Meirhaeghe J, Bastian L, Cummings SR, Ranstam J, Tillman JB, Eastell R, Talmadge K, Wardlaw D (2011) Balloon

kyphoplasty for the treatment of acute vertebral compression fractures: 2-year results from a randomized trial. J Bone Miner Res 26(7):1627–1637

Buchbinder R, Osborne RH, Ebeling PR, Wark JD, Mitchell P, Wriedt C, Graves S, Staples MP, Murphy B (2009) A randomized trial of vertebroplasty for painful osteoporotic vertebral fractures. N Engl J Med 361:557–568

Chosa K, Naito A, Awai K (2011) Newly developed compression fractures after percutaneous vertebroplasty: comparison with conservative treatment. Jpn J Radiol 29(5):335–341. Epub 30 June 2011

Coumans JV, Reinhardt MK, Lieberman IH (2003) Kyphoplasty for vertebral compression fractures: 1-year clinical outcomes from a prospective study. J Neurosurg Spine 99:44–50

Depriester C, Deramond H, Toussaint P, Jhaveri HS, Galibert P (1999) Percutaneous vertebroplasty: indications, technique and complications. In: Connors JJ, III, Wojak JC (eds) Interventional neuroradiology, strategies and practical techniques. Saunders, Philadelphia, pp 346–357

Do HM (2000) Magnetic resonance imaging in the evaluation of patients for percutaneous vertebroplasty. Top Magn Reson Imaging 11:235–244

Dworkin RH, Turk DC, Wyrwich KW, Beaton D, Cleeland CS, Farrar JT, Haythornthwaite JA, Jensen MP, Kerns RD, Ader DN, Brandenburg N, Burke LB, Cella D, Chandler J, Cowan P, Dimitrova R, Dionne R, Hertz S, Jadad AR, Katz NP, Kehlet H, Kramer LD, Manning DC, McCormick C, McDermott MP, McQuay HJ, Patel S, Porter L, Quessy S, Rappaport BA, Rauschkolb C, Revicki DA, Rothman M, Schmader KE, Stacey BR, Stauffer JW, von Stein T, White RE, Witter J, Zavisic S (2008) Interpreting the clinical importance of treatment outcomes in chronic pain clinical trials: IMMPACT recommendations. J Pain 9:105–121

Fahim DK, Sun K, Tawackoli W, Mendel E, Rhines LD, Burton AW, Kim DH, Ehni BL, Liebschner MA (2011) Premature adjacent vertebral fracture after vertebroplasty: a biomechanical study. Neurosurgery 69(3):733–744

Fourney DR, Schomer DF, Nader R, Chlan-Fourney J, Suki D, Ahrar K, Rhines LD, Gokaslan ZL (2003) Percutaneous vertebroplasty and kyphoplasty for painful vertebral body fractures in cancer patients. J Neurosurg Spine 98:21–30

Franc J, Lehmann P, Saliou G, Monet P, Kocheida EM, Daguet E, Laurent A, Legars D, Deramond H (2010) Vertebroplasty: 10 years clinical and radiological follow-up. J Neuroradiol 37(4):211–2119. Epub 20 Mar 2010

Fribourg D, Tang C, Sra P, Delamarter R, Bae H (2004) Incidence of subsequent vertebral fracture after kyphoplasty. Spine 29:2270–2276

Galibert P, Deramond H, Rosat P, Le Gars D (1987) Preliminary note on the treatment of vertebral angioma by percutaneous acrylic vertebroplasty. Neurochirurgie 33:166–168

Gangi A, Clark WA (2010) Have recent vertebroplasty trials changed the indications for vertebroplasty? Cardiovasc Intervent Radiol 33(4):677–680

Gangi A, Dietemann JL, Mortazavi R, Pfleger D, Kauff C, Roy C (1998) CT-guided interventional procedures for pain management in the lumbosacral spine. Radiographics 18:621–633

Georgy BA (2008) Metastatic spinal lesions: state-of-the-art treatment options and future trends. AJNR Am J Neuroradiol 29(9):1605–1611

Georgy B (2011) Can meta-analysis save vertebroplasty? AJNR Am J Neuroradiol 32(4):614–616

Grados F, Depriester C, Cayrolle G, Hardy N, Deramond H, Fardellone P (2000a) Long-term observations of vertebral osteoporotic fractures treated by percutaneous vertebroplasty. Rheumatology (Oxf) 39(12):1410–1414

Grados F, Depriester C, Cayrolle G, Hardy N, Deramond H, Fardellone P (2000b) Long-term observations of vertebral osteoporotic fractures treated by percutaneous vertebroplasty. Rheumatology (Oxf) 39(12):1410–1414

Harrop JS, Prpa B, Reinhardt MK, Lieberman I (2004) Primary and secondary osteoporosis: incidence of subsequent vertebral compression fractures after kyphoplasty. Spine 29:2120–2125

Heini PF, Walchli B, Berlemann U (2000) Percutaneous transpedicular vertebroplasty with PMMA: operative technique and early results. A prospective study for the treatment of osteoporotic compression fractures. Eur Spine J 9:445–450

Harrington KD. Major neurological complications following percutaneous vertebroplasty with polymethylmethacrylate: A case report. *J Bone Joint Surg Am* 2001;83-A:1070–1073

Jensen ME, Dion JE (2000) Percutaneous vertebroplasty in the treatment of osteoporotic compression fractures. Neuroimaging Clin N Am 10(3):547–568

Jensen ME, Evans AJ, Mathis JM, Kallmes DF, Cloft HJ, Dion JE (1997a) Percutaneous polymethylmethacrylate vertebroplasty in the treatment of osteoporotic vertebral body compression fractures: technical aspects. AJNR Am J Neuroradiol 18:1897–1904

Jensen ME, Evans AJ, Mathis JM, Kallmes DF, Cloft HJ, Dion JE (1997b) Percutaneous polymethylmethacrylate vertebroplasty in the treatment of osteoporotic vertebral body compression fractures: technical aspects. AJNR Am J Neuroradiol 18:1897–1904

Kallmes DF, Comstock BA, Heagerty PJ, Turner JA, Wilson DJ, Diamond TH, Edwards R, Gray LA, Stout L, Owen S, Hollingworth W, Ghdoke B, Annesley-Williams DJ, Ralston SH, Jarvik JG (2009) A randomized trial of vertebroplasty for osteoporotic spinal fractures. N Engl J Med 361:569–579

Kaufmann TJ, Jensen ME, Ford G, Gill LL, Marx WF, Kallmes DF (2002) Cardiovascular effects of polymethylmethacrylate use in percutaneous vertebroplasty. AJNR Am J Neuroradiol 23:601–604

Kim HW, Kwon A, Lee MC, Song JW, Kim SK, Kim IH (2010) The retrial of percutaneous vertebroplasty for the treatment of vertebral compression fracture. J Kor Neurosurg Soc 47(4):278–281

Klazen CA, Lohle PN, de Vries J, Jansen FH, Tielbeek AV, Blonk MC, Venmans A, van Rooij WJ, Schoemaker MC, Juttmann JR, Lo TH, Verhaar HJ, van der Graaf Y, van Everdingen KJ, Muller AF, Elgersma OE, Halkema DR, Fransen H, Janssens X, Buskens E, Mali WP (2010) Vertebroplasty versus conservative treatment in acute osteoporotic vertebral compression fractures (VERTOS II): an open-label randomised trial. Lancet 376:1085–1092

Lane JM, Girardi F, Parvaianen H et al (2000a) Preliminary outcomes of the first 226 consecutive kyphoplasties for the fixation of painful osteoporotic vertebral compression fractures [abstract]. Osteoporosis Int 11(Suppl):S206

Lane JM, Girardi F, Parvaianen H et al (2000) Preliminary outcomes of the first 226 consecutive kyphoplasties for the fixation of painful osteoporotic vertebral compression fractures [abstract]. Osteoporosis Int 11(Suppl):S206

Laredo JD, Bellaiche L, Hamze B, Naouri JF, Bondeville JM, Tubiana JM (1994) Current status of musculoskeletal interventional radiology. Radiol Clin N Am 32:377–398

Ledlie JT, Renfro M (2003) Balloon kyphoplasty: one-year outcomes in vertebral body height restoration, chronic pain, and activity levels. J Neurosurg 98(Suppl 1):36–42

Lee BJ, Lee SR, Yoo TY (2002) Paraplegia as a complication of percutaneous vertebroplasty with polymethylmethacrylate: a case report. Spine 27:E419–E422

Levine SA, Perin LA, Hayes D, Hayes WS (2000) An evidence- based evaluation of percutaneous vertebroplasty. Manag Care 9:56–60

Lieberman I, Reinhardt MK (2003) Vertebroplasty and kyphoplasty for osteolytic vertebral collapse. Clin Orthop (Suppl 415):S176–S186

Lieberman IH, Dudeney S, Reinhardt MK, Bell G (2001) Initial outcome and efficacy of "kyphoplasty" in the treatment of painful osteoporotic vertebral compression fractures. Spine 26:1631–1638

Lindsay R, Silverman SL, Cooper C (2001) Risk of new vertebral fracture in the year following a fracture. JAMA 285:320–323

Luginbühl M (2008) Percutaneous vertebroplasty, kyphoplasty and lordoplasty: implications for the anesthesiologist. Curr Opin Anaesthesiol 21(4):504–513

Masala S, Tropepi D, Fiori R, Semprini R, Martorana A, Massari F, Bernardi G, Simonetti G (2004) Kyphoplasty: a new opportunity for rehabilitation of neurologic disabilities. Am J Phys Med Rehabil 83(10):810–812

Masala S, Schillaci O, Massari F, Danieli R, Ursone A, Fiori R, Simonetti G (2005) MRI and bone scan imaging in the preoperative evaluation of painful vertebral fractures treated with vertebroplasty and kyphoplasty. In Vivo (Athens, Greece) 19:1055–1060

Mathis JM, Barr JD, Belkoff SM, Barr MS, Jensen ME, Deramond H (2001) Percutaneous vertebroplasty: a developing standard of care for vertebral compression fractures. AJNR Am J Neuroradiol 22:373–381

McGraw JK, Lippert JA, Minkus KD, Rami PM, Davis TM, Budzik RF (2002) Prospective evaluation of pain relief in 100 patients undergoing percutaneous vertebroplasty: results and follow-up. J Vasc Interv Radiol 13(9 Pt 1):883–886

Noonan P (2009) Randomized vertebroplasty trials: bad news or sham news? AJNR Am J Neuroradiol 30(10):1808–1809

Nussbaum DA, Gailloud P, Murphy K (2004) A review of complications associated with vertebroplasty and kyphoplasty as reported to the food and drug administration medical device related web site. J Vasc Interv Radiol 15:1185–1192

Orler R, Frauchiger LH, Lange U, Heini PF (2006) Lordoplasty: report on early results with a new technique for the treatment of vertebral compression fractures to restore the lordosis. Eur Spine J 15(12):1769–1775

Ortiz O, Mathis JM (2010) Vertebral body reconstruction: techniques and tools. Neuroimaging Clin N Am 20(2):145–158

Pierot L, Boulin A (1999) Percutaneous biopsy of the thoracic and lumbar spine: transpedicular approach under fluoroscopic guidance. AJNR Am J Neuroradiol 20:23–25

Riggs BL, Melton LJ 3rd (1995) The worldwide problem of osteoporosis: insights afforded by epidemiology. Bone 17(Suppl 5):505S–511S

Shapiro S, Abel T, Purvines S (2003) Surgical removal of epidural and intradural polymethylmethacrylate extravasation complicating percutaneous vertebroplasty for an osteoporotic lumbar compression fracture. Case report. J Neurosurg 98(Suppl 1):90–92

Siminoski K, Jiang G, Adachi JD, Hanley DA, Cline G, Ioannidis G, Hodsman A, Josse RG, Kendler D, Olszynski WP, Ste Marie LG, Eastell R (2005) Accuracy of height loss during prospective monitoring for detection of incident vertebral fractures. Osteoporos Int 16(4):403–410

Snapinn SM, Jiang Q (2007) Responder analyses and the assessment of a clinically relevant treatment effect. Trials 25(8):31

Spiegl UJ, Beisse R, Hauck S, Grillhösl A, Bühren V (2009) Value of MRI imaging prior to a kyphoplasty for osteoporotic insufficiency fractures. Eur Spine J 18(9):1287–1292

Suárez MS, Andrés RP, de Pablo PP, Collsamata PC, Bota EC, Arroyo VV, López-Amor MF (2009) Utility of bone SPECT-CT in percutaneous vertebroplasty. Rev Esp Med Nucl 28(6):291–294. Epub 22 Oct 2009

Sudhakar P, Sharma AR, Bhushan SM, Ranadhir G, Narsimuhulu G, Rao VV (2010) Efficacy of SPECT over planar bone scan in the diagnosis of solitary vertebral lesions in patients with low back pain. Indian J Nucl Med 25(2):44–48

Uppin AA, Hirsch JA, Centenera LV, Pfiefer BA, Pazianos AG, Choi IS (2003) Occurrence of new vertebral body fracture after percutaneous vertebroplasty in patients with osteoporosis. Radiology 226:119–124

U.S. Department of Health and Human Services, Food and Drug Administration (2009) Guidance for industry: patient reported outcome measures—use in medical product development to support labeling claims. Dec 2009. http://www.fda.gov/ucm/groups/fdagov-public/@fdagov-drugs-gen/documents/document/ucm193282.pdf

Wagner AL (2005) Vertebroplasty and the randomized study: where science and ethics collide. AJNR Am J Neuroradiol 26(7):1610–1611

Wardlaw D, Cummings SR, Van Meirhaeghe J, Bastian L, Tillman JB, Ranstam J, Eastell R, Shabe P, Talmadge K, Boonen S (2009) Efficacy and safety of balloon kyphoplasty compared with non-surgical care for vertebral compression fracture (FREE): a randomised controlled trial. Lancet 373:1016–1024

Weill A, Chiras J, Simon JM, Rose M, Sola-Martinez T, Enkaoua E (1996) Spinal metastases: indications for and results of percutaneous injection of acrylic surgical cement. Radiology 199:241–247

Wilson DJ, Owen S, Corkill RA (2011) Facet joint injections as a means of reducing the need for vertebroplasty in insufficiency fractures of the spine. Eur Radiol 21(8):1772–1778. Epub 13 April 2011

Radiation Protection and Quality Assurance in Bone Densitometry

J. Damilakis and G. Solomou

Contents

J. Damilakis (✉)
Department of Medical Physics,
University of Crete, P.O. Box 2208,
71003 Heraklion, Crete, Greece
e-mail: john.damilakis@med.uoc.gr

G. Solomou
Department of Medical Physics,
University Hospital of Heraklion, P.O. Box 1352,
71110 Heraklion, Crete, Greece

Abstract

It is widely recognized that early diagnosis of osteoporosis is of paramount importance to prevent fractures. Several X-ray based imaging techniques capable of assessing bone quantity and quality have been developed. However, exposure to ionizing radiation carries a potential risk and, for this reason, it is necessary to ensure adequate radiation protection for patients and staff. This chapter provides (a) the general terminology used in quantifying radiation, (b) a brief review of the system of radiation protection, and (c) data on the levels of radiation exposure associated with methods used for diagnosis of osteoporosis. Moreover, the importance of quality assurance in bone densitometry is discussed and quality control tests are proposed to ensure that DXA devices are operating according to specifications.

1 Introduction

Evaluation of bone status is essential to clinicians for diagnosis of osteoporosis, osteoporosis treatment planning, and monitoring the effectiveness of treatment. Dual energy X-ray absorptiometry (DXA) is the most widely used method for measuring 'areal' bone mineral density (BMD_a; g/cm^2) at the lumbar spine and hip. Quantitative computed tomography (QCT) has the important advantage of separately measuring cortical and trabecular bone mineral density (BMD; mg/cm^3) and is less influenced by the presence of degenerative disease in the lumbar spine than DXA. A drawback of bone densitometry is that the bone density measurements provided are dependent on bone mass and not on trabecular architecture and bone tissue quality. For this reason, imaging techniques capable of providing structural information about bone, such as high resolution (HR) CT and micro CT (μCT) have been developed. Methods based on non-ionizing radiation such as quantitative ultrasound (QUS) and HR magnetic resonance imaging

G. Guglielmi (ed.), *Osteoporosis and Bone Densitometry Measurements*, Medical Radiology. Diagnostic Imaging,
DOI: 10.1007/174_2012_612, © Springer-Verlag Berlin Heidelberg 2013

(MRI) have also been proposed to examine bone status. However, QUS and MRI techniques for the diagnosis of osteoporosis currently are not well established and MRI remains a research tool. Despite considerable progress made recently, technical challenges have to be addressed before these methods have a true impact on daily clinical practice.

An integral part of bone densitometry methods used in daily clinical practice is exposure of patients and personnel to diagnostic X-rays. However, exposure to ionizing radiation carries a potential risk (Damilakis et al. 2010a, b). Therefore, the use of these methods must be responsible to ensure appropriate radiation protection. Furthermore, information produced by the bone densitometry devices should be accurate, reliable and reproducible. Facilities that operate bone densitometers have long recognized the value of quality assurance (QA) programs to ensure that services are of the highest quality and devices are operating according to specifications. This chapter aims to provide information related to the radiation protection of patients, health professionals, comforters, and research volunteers from radiation exposures resulting from the use of ionizing radiation in bone densitometry. An overview of a QA program needed to assure the quality of procedures performed in bone densitometry is also presented.

2 Radiation Protection in Bone Densitometry

2.1 The Quantities and Units of X-rays Used in Bone Densitometry

When ionizing radiation passes through a patient or a phantom, some of the energy of that radiation is absorbed. *Absorbed dose* is defined as the amount of energy per unit mass absorbed by the patient or phantom. For purposes of radiation protection the quantity normally calculated is the mean absorbed dose in an organ or tissue. Absorbed dose is measured in gray (Gy). *Entrance skin dose* is a measure of the radiation dose absorbed by the skin at the area where the X-ray beam enters the body and is typically measured in Gy. *Organ dose* refers to the absorbed dose delivered to the organs of an individual undergoing an X-ray examination. The unit used is Gy. The *conceptus absorbed dose* is the dose delivered to the unborn child of a pregnant individual. KERMA (Kinetic Energy Released per unit Mass) is the amount of energy extracted from the X-ray beam per unit mass of a specified material in a small irradiated volume of that material (for example air, soft tissue, fat, bone). Thus, air kerma is the energy extracted from an X-ray beam per unit mass of air in a small irradiated air volume. For diagnostic X-rays, kerma is equivalent to absorbed dose. Kerma is measured in Gy, which is the same as for absorbed dose.

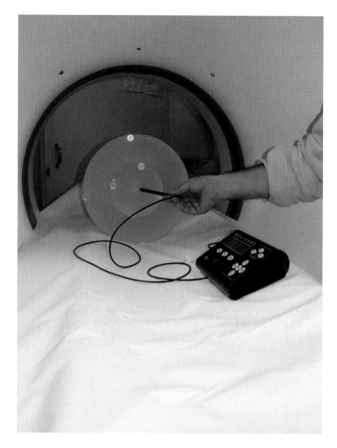

Fig. 1 Instrumentation used for CTDI determination: CTDI phantom, 10 cm long ionization chamber and electrometer

Air kerma–area product is the area integral of the air kerma over the area of the X-ray beam in a plane perpendicular to the beam axis. Kerma area product is measured in Gy·cm². The air kerma area product provides a good estimation of the total radiation energy delivered to a patient during an X-ray examination. The dosimetric quantity used in MDCT is the *Computed Tomography Dose Index* (CTDI). Medical physicists measure the quantity CTDI_{100}, which is given by

$$\text{CTDI}_{100} = \frac{1}{NT} \int\limits_{-50}^{+50} D(z)dz \qquad (1)$$

where, D(z) is the radiation dose profile along the axis of rotation, N the number of data channels used in a particular axial acquisition, and T is the slice width of one data channel. The value of NT represents the total z-axis width of the active detector i.e., the beam collimation. CTDI_{100} is measured using a calibrated pencil ionization chamber, 10 cm long, connected to a calibrated electrometer. The integration limits ($\pm$ 50 mm) correspond to the 100 mm length of the pencil ionization chamber. CTDI is expressed in Gy.

CTDI_{100} can be measured free-in-air or using cylindrical poly(methyl methacrylate) (PMMA) phantoms having one central and four peripheral holes for the placement of the pencil ionizing chamber (Fig. 1). Medical physicists use a 16 cm phantom to estimate the CTDI for head examinations and a 32 cm phantom to calculate the CTDI for body examinations. From $CTDI_{100}$ measurements at the center and at the periphery of a PMMA phantom, $CTDI_W$ is calculated as

$$CTDI_W = \frac{1}{3}\, CTDI_{100,\ center} + \frac{2}{3}\, CTDI_{100,\ periphery} \qquad (2)$$

CTDI volume ($CTDI_V$) is defined as

$$CTDI_V = \frac{CTDI_W}{pitch} \qquad (3)$$

The $CTDI_V$ is independent of patient size and acquisition length. To take into account the length of the acquisition, the *Dose Length Product* (DLP) has been introduced, which is defined as

$$DLP = CTDI_V \cdot SL \qquad (4)$$

where *SL* is the scanning length. The unit of DLP is mGy·cm. The $CTDI_V$ value and/or the DLP value of CT examinations are indicated on the scanner console. Although CTDI and DLP are useful tools for patient dose management, they do not quantify the amount of patient radiation dose.

All organs and tissues of the human body are not equally sensitive to the possible biological effects of radiation such as cancer induction. To account for the different radiosensitivity of body tissues and organs, organs and tissues have been assigned weighting factor values in a recent publication by the International Commission on Radiologic Protection (ICRP) (International Commission on Radiological Protection 2007). For example, lung, colon, breast, stomach, and red bone marrow have a tissue weighting factor of 0.12, whereas the corresponding value for bladder, liver, esophagus, and thyroid is 0.04. The sum of these factors is equal to 1.0. The *effective dose* is calculated using

$$E = \sum_T w_T D_T \qquad (5)$$

where w_T is the tissue T weighting factor and D_T is the absorbed dose to organ/tissue T. Effective dose is expressed in Sievert (Sv). If two or more areas have been exposed, the total body effective dose is the sum of the effective doses for each area. Therefore, the total body effective dose from a spine and a hip DXA acquisition is the sum of the effective doses from each acquisition. The effective dose is the most appropriate dose quantity to compare patient dose for different X-ray examinations, for example to compare the dose from a QCT and a DXA examination. Effective dose represent an estimate of risk from an X-ray examination.

A rough estimation of patient effective dose from CT examinations is possible using the equation

$$E = DLP \cdot k \qquad (6)$$

where k is the normalized effective dose expressed in $mSv\ mGy^{-1}cm^{-1}$. Sex- and age-specific normalized effective dose values can be found in the literature (Deak et al. 2010). Patient- and scanner-specific Monte Carlo simulation methods provide accurate estimation of patient dose (Damilakis et al. 2010a, b). The output of the simulation is a series of images that depict patient radiation dose. Figure 2 shows a CT image and corresponding dose image where each pixel represents a dose value.

2.2 Background Radiation Levels

Background radiation is a consistent source of low exposure natural and man-made ionizing radiation to all inhabitants of earth. Natural background radiation comes from cosmic radiation and terrestrial sources. The average effective dose from natural background radiation is 2.4 mSv per year. Man-made radiation comes from medical uses of radiation and nuclear industry. There is an increasing trend in medical radiation exposures due to the greater availability of medical radiation services. Figure 3 shows the percentage contribution of various radiation sources to the background radiation (World Nuclear Association 2011). It is evident that most radiation is from natural sources such as radon and cosmic radiation. Background radiation is sometimes used as a benchmark for judging radiation doses from medical exposures such as exposures from DXA or MDCT.

2.3 Low-Level Radiation Risks

Biological effects can be categorized as deterministic or stochastic. Deterministic effects such as cataract and erythema occur when radiation dose exceeds a dose threshold. Stochastic effects occur without a threshold, their probability increases with radiation dose and consist primarily of cancer and genetic effects. The response by human beings to low-level radiation doses has been the subject of many research studies. The health effect of concern at low doses of radiation is cancer. Risk estimates are based on the linear no-threshold model. This model assumes that there is a linear relationship between radiation dose and cancer risk at all dose levels. The risks of developing radiation-induced cancer at any time subsequent to the age at exposure can be estimated using age-, sex-, and organ-specific risk data provided by the National Research Council Committee on the Biological Effects of Ionizing Radiation reports or factors provided by ICRP (International Commission on

Radiological Protection 2007; National Research Council Committee on the Biological Effects of Ionizing Radiation 2006). Unborn children and children are much more radiosensitive than adults. There is evidence of cancer induction at effective doses above 5 mSv (Preston et al. 2003; Sont et al. 2001). Radiogenic risks at very low doses such as those measured during DXA examinations are uncertain. They may be zero, lower, or higher than those anticipated based on the linear no-threshold model.

2.4 The System of Radiation Protection

The radiation protection principles are justification, optimization, and dose limitation. Many X-ray examinations are unavoidable; however, it is a primary objective of medical radiation protection to keep unjustified exposures to a minimum. *Justification* is the process that ensures that no X-ray examination is performed unless the expected benefit to the exposed individual clearly outweighs the potential risks. Justification includes consideration of alternative examinations that use non-ionizing radiation. Exposures of pregnant patients to diagnostic X-rays as well as pediatric radiologic examinations require a higher level of justification. Screening programs for osteoporosis must be justified in terms of overall benefits and risks. Self-referral for a DXA or other bone densitometry examination should be discouraged. *Optimization* is the process to keep radiation exposures as low as reasonably achievable taking into account social and economic factors but still provide adequate diagnostic information. *Dose limitation* requires that radiation doses to the whole body or to specified organs should not exceed limits imposed by regulatory authorities. Dose limits do not apply for patient examinations, since the decision to perform an exposure is considered justified. Table 1 shows the annual limits as currently recommended by ICRP (International Commission on Radiological Protection 2007).

2.5 Patient Radiation Doses in Bone Densitometry

2.5.1 Assessment of Osteoporotic Fractures Using Radiography, DXA and MDCT

2.5.1.1 Assessment of Osteoporotic Fractures Using Radiography
Osteoporotic fractures occur in response to low-energy trauma at the wrist, spine, and proximal femur. Conventional radiography is the standard technique for the detection of vertebral and other fractures.

Patient dose from a radiograph depends on several parameters including exposure parameters (kV, mAs), filtration, grids, the speed of the detector system, and patient body size. Over the past years, many conventional screen-film systems have been replaced by digital radiography systems. The wide dynamic range of digital detectors in combination with the capabilities of post-processing allow digital radiography systems to obtain more diagnostic information with lower patient dose. Digital radiography has several advantages over conventional screen-film radiography including ease of use. However, attention is needed to the potential increase of radiation doses due to the tendency of acquiring more images than actually needed. Another point of concern is the possibility of patient overexposure for long periods because of selection of higher exposure parameters than actually needed. Overexposure is readily visible in radiographs produced with film-screen radiography because of film blackening. With digital radiography, high exposure parameters produce excellent image quality. For this reason, newly installed digital radiography systems should be optimized to achieve the best balance between image quality and patient radiation dose. After installation, continuous patient dose monitoring is needed to ensure patient radiation protection. Table 2 shows typical effective doses for an adult patient for various radiographic examinations (Damilakis et al. 2010a, b). The actual dose for an individual patient can be two or three times higher or smaller than estimates shown in Table 2.

2.5.1.2 Assessment of Osteoporotic Fractures Using DXA
Vertebral fractures may be identified by using images acquired with DXA. Morphometric X-ray absorptiometry is a widely used method for assessment of the patient's fracture status. The lateral projection covers the distance from T4 to L4 and the software provides information on the vertebral body heights and their ratios.

Morphometric X-ray absorptiometry is associated with a low radiation dose. Studies show that the patient effective dose ranges from 2 to 50 µSv (Vokes et al. 2006; Blake et al. 1997; Ferrar et al. 2005). The recent improvement in the image quality of DXA images in combination with low patient doses suggests that DXA is effective alternative to spine radiography for the identification of vertebral fractures.

2.5.1.3 Assessment of Osteoporotic Fractures Using MDCT
Vertebral fractures are being increasingly diagnosed fortuitously from midline sagittal reconstructions in patients having 3D multi-detector CT (MDCT) of the thorax and abdomen for other clinical reasons. In these cases, MDCT allows fracture assessment of the spine to be done without additional exposure to the patient. Bauer et al. have found that the thinnest available axial slice thickness with sagittal reconstructions of 0.6 mm performed best in fracture

Table 1 The radiation dose limits recommended by the international commission on radiological protection

Type of limit	Occupational	Public (mSv/year)
Effective dose		
	20 mSv/year	1
	100 mSv in 5 years with the further provision that the effective dose should not exceed 50 mSv in a single year	
Absorbed dose		
Eye lens	150 mSv/year	15
Skin	500 mSv/year	50
Hands and feet	500 mSv/year	–
Embryo/fetus	1 mGy once pregnancy has been declared	–

Table 2 Typical patient effective doses for radiographs acquired for assessment of osteoporotic fractures

Examination	Projection	Effective dose (mSv)
Thoracic spine	AP	0.4
Thoracic spine	LAT	0.3
Lumbar spine	AP	0.7
Lumbar spine	LAT	0.3
Pelvis	AP	0.6
Hand	AP	0.001

AP anteroposterior, *LAT* lateral

grading compared with conventional radiography (Bauer et al. 2006). Reconstructions based on 3 mm sections, however, also had good performance in identifying fractures. The improved spatial resolution in the longitudinal direction decreases partial volume artifacts and improves contrast depicting fine detail of the bone. When thin axial images are required, the patient dose need not be increased to obtain acceptable image noise. Thick images with good signal to noise ratios can be generated and displayed from the thinner image data.

2.5.2 Assessment of Trabecular Bone Structure Using Radiography and Texture Analysis

It is well-known that radiography is insensitive to the early and intermediate stages of osteoporosis. However, there are several features of osteoporosis that can be visualized and quantified with HR radiography and texture analysis. For this purpose, sophisticated image processing techniques such as fractal analysis or fast Fourier transforms have been used (Majumdar et al. 1999). The main limitation of these methods is that radiography records the mean absorption by all the tissues through which the X-ray beam has penetrated. Thus, cortical and trabecular bone are superimposed and the 3D bone architecture is not accurately displayed within the framework of a 2D radiograph. In vivo assessment of trabecular bone structure using radiographs is usually performed on calcaneus or distal radius images (Majumdar et al. 2000; Lespessailles et al. 2008). Lespessailles et al. have found that the combination of BMD and texture parameter values derived from calcaneus radiographs provided a better assessment of the fracture risk than obtainable only by BMD_a (Majumdar et al. 2000). Patient effective dose from a calcaneus or distal radius radiograph is about 1 μSv.

2.5.3 Dual Energy X-ray Absorptiometry

DXA is based on the measurement of the transmission of photons through the body at two different X-ray energies. DXA produces dual energy photons using either rapid switching of the X-ray tube potential from 70 kVp to 140 kVp or filters developed to produce dual energy peaks by selectively removing photons at the middle of the X-ray spectrum (Damilakis et al. 2007). The detector unit discriminates between high- and low-energy photons.

Studies have focused on patient radiation dose from pencil-beam and fan-beam DXA devices (Bezakova et al. 1997; Huda and Morin 1996; Steel et al. 1998; Lewis et al. 1994; Cawte et al. 1999; Njeh et al. 1997; Steel et al. 1998; Blake et al. 2006). Patient effective dose from pencil beam DXA is about 1 μSv. With the introduction of fan-beam technology, the performance capability of DXA devices has increased considerably. However, doses to patients have also been increased. Ranges of effective doses for DXA

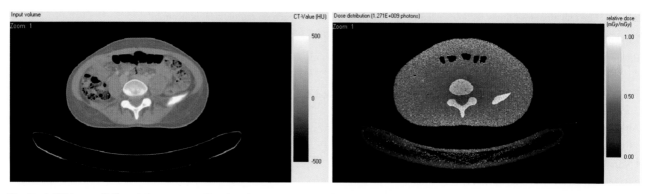

Fig. 2 A CT image (*left*) and the corresponding dose image generated using patient specific Monte Carlo simulation (*right*). Black corresponds to the lowest dose whereas white corresponds to the highest

acquisitions performed on fan-beam devices are presented in Fig. 4. The effective dose to 5-year-old children from spine or hip examinations can approach 50 μSv and 30 μSv, respectively using the default adult imaging protocol on Hologic scanners (Blake et al. 2006). However, using a pediatric protocol, pediatric doses similar to those for adult patients have been recorded. Forearm scans result in negligible dose i.e., about 1 μSv. Patient radiation doses from DXA are much lower than those from most radiologic examinations. Thus, the average effective dose from mammography is about 400 μSv, from an abdominal radiographic procedure is about 700 μSv and from head CT about 2000 μSv (Mettler et al. 2008).

In addition to effective dose, organ radiation doses are important, especially when organs are exposed primarily, partly included or marginally excluded from the direct X-ray beam. For these organs, radiation doses from a DXA acquisition have been estimated to be from about 0.001 mGy to about 0.01 mGy (Bezakova et al. 1997; Huda and Morin 1996; Steel et al. 1998; Lewis et al. 1994; Cawte et al. 1999; Njeh et al. 1997; Blake et al. 2006). Organs receiving the greatest amount of radiation from spine DXA are bone marrow, stomach, large intestine, and ovaries. Corresponding organs for hip DXA are large intestine and testes.

The patient dose from a DXA acquisition performed on a specific DXA device depends on the acquisition mode, the body region examined, and on the patient size. Patient doses vary considerably between DXA systems of different models and manufacturers depending on several parameters such as the acquisition technology (single-sweep wide-angle vs. multi-sweep narrow-angle fan-beam systems), detector efficiency and tools developed to reduce patient dose. Even for the same examination, when different DXA systems are compared, the effective dose may vary by a factor of five or more.

With the rapid increase in the use of DXA, women of childbearing age who are unaware of their pregnancy may accidentally expose their unborn child during a DXA examination. Referring clinicians should inform radiologists

Sources of Background Radiation

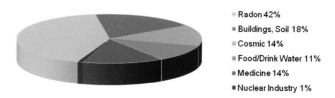

Fig. 3 The relative percentage of all sources of background radiation

before examination if their patient is pregnant. A sign that asks patients to inform staff about a possible pregnancy before the examination should be posted in the waiting area. Investigation of the reproductive status of patients of menstrual age (age range 12–50 years) is needed prior to examination. It is prudent to consider as pregnant any woman of menstrual age when a menstrual period is overdue, or missed, unless there is evidence that precludes a pregnancy (International Commission on Radiological Protection 2000). Conceptus doses from DXA performed on the mother are very low even when the unborn child is exposed primarily. Doses are lower than 5 μGy for a DXA acquisition performed using a pencil-beam device (Damilakis et al. 2002). Conceptus doses below 100 mGy should not be a reason for abortion (International Commission on Radiological Protection 2000). Therefore, termination of pregnancy due to conceptus radiation exposure during a DXA procedure is not justified. DXA examinations are rarely performed on patients known to be pregnant for the diagnosis or the differential diagnosis of pregnancy-associated osteoporosis. In these cases, the pregnant patient must understand the expected benefits and possible risks posed by the procedure. Informed consent should be obtained prior to examination.

Although radiation dose from bone densitometry techniques used in everyday clinical practice is very low, clinical justification is important for each imaging procedure and should be considered on an individual basis. A request form for a DXA examination should provide up-to-date

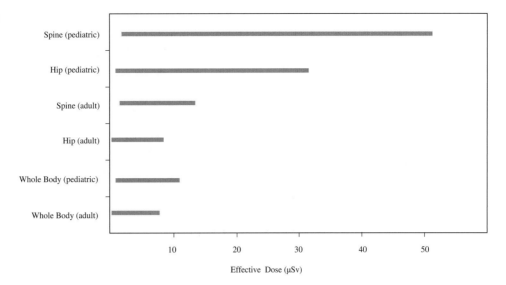

Fig. 4 Ranges of effective doses for acquisitions performed on fan-beam DXA devices

clinical information to demonstrate the necessity for the study. In most patients, the DXA examination includes acquisitions of the hip and lumbar spine. DXA is increasingly used to estimate BMD_a in children and adolescents. DXA examinations performed in children must be adjusted based on the size of the child's body. In children, a lumbar spine and/or total body imaging usually provide enough information to answer the specific medical question. Additional skeletal sites should be imaged only when the expected benefits clearly outweigh the potential risks. The necessity for follow-up studies should be carefully considered. Multiple imaging over the years performed on the same individual for follow-up evaluation may increase radiation risks. Follow-up imaging is sometimes performed too early, when according to the known biological data; measured differences in BMD_a are due solely to system variability and not to a true change in BMD_a.

2.5.4 Quantitative CT and HR MDCT Imaging

QCT examinations are performed using a dedicated software package and a calibration phantom (Fig. 5) imaged simultaneously with the patient to convert the CT numbers into volumetric density (BMD; mg/cm^3). In the 2D QCT protocol, three vertebral bodies (L1–L3) are measured using a single 10 mm slice through the center of each vertebra. The gantry is tilted appropriately so that the imaging plane is parallel to the vertebral endplates. The BMD measurements of the vertebrae are averaged and compared with data of a normal reference data population. Low exposure parameters (80 kVp tube potential and 120–140 mAs tube load) are used to reduce patient dose below standard CT examinations. Patient doses from 2D QCT examinations have been reported to be 60–300 µSv (Huda and Morin 1996; Kalender 1992). These dose levels, however, are above DXA dose levels.

Recently, multi-detector (MD) CT protocols have been proposed to make precise measurement of BMD and bone geometry (Engelke et al. 2008, 2009a, b; Genant et al. 2008). Typical parameter settings for acquiring MDQCT data are 120 kVp, 100–150 mAs, pitch 1. An anterior-posterior scout image from the iliac crest to mid-thigh is obtained and two vertebrae (L1-L2) are usually imaged. Also, MDQCT protocols have been developed to measure BMD of the hip. Studies show that 3D MDQCT protocols of the spine and hip provide an effective dose of 1500 µSv and 2900 µSv, respectively (Engelke et al. 2008, 2009a, b; Genant et al. 2008; Khoo et al. 2009). Patient doses from MDQCT are significantly higher than doses from other methods used for estimation of BMD. Studies are needed to investigate possibilities for dose reduction while maintaining diagnostic confidence. Modern MDCT have also allowed densitometric evaluation of distal radius with good accuracy and precision. Patient effective dose from this examination is lower than 10 µSv (Engelke et al. 2009a, b). QCT at the distal radius is associated with a low radiation dose because radiosensitive organs are distant from the area being exposed primarily. However, currently peripheral QCT is most commonly performed using dedicated small peripheral QCT.

Abdominal MDCT is a frequently performed diagnostic examination that includes information on lumbar vertebrae density. Recent studies have shown that routine abdominal MDCT images can be utilized to determine lumbar spine BMD and differentiate osteoporotic from healthy individuals. Link et al. showed that there is a significant correlation in the densitometric measurements between routine spiral CT and QCT (Link et al. 2004). Quantitative CT BMD values can be derived using BMD values from routine spiral CT multiplied by a conversion factor. In a recent study, Papadakis et al. have found that QCT data derived from

Fig. 5 The calibration phantom
used in QCT (*left*) and CT
measurement of bone mineral
density and the calibration
phantom positioned under the
patient (*right*). The phantom
consists of materials equivalent
to soft and bone tissue

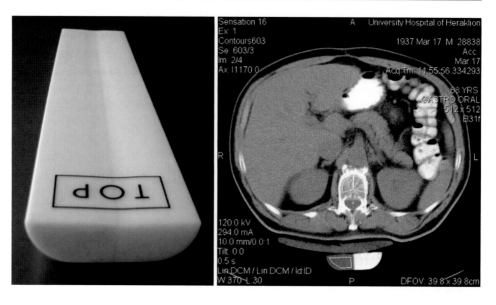

abdominal MDCT examinations can discriminate osteoporotic from healthy female subjects (Papadakis et al. 2009). These studies show that useful BMD information can be obtained of the lumbar spine without an additional radiation burden to the patient. However, more work is needed before routine abdominal MDCT can be considered as a method of diagnosing spinal osteoporosis.

Fast data acquisition and isotropic resolution achieved with the advent of MDCT systems has resulted in a significant increase in the use of CT in routine clinical practice over the recent years. Depending on technical parameters used, MDCT allows imaging with spatial resolution in the submillimeter range. The X-ray source-detector geometry, the field of view, the slice thickness, the reconstruction algorithms, and other factors are optimized for routine CT examinations. This limits the x-y resolution and the capability of standard MDCT to depict and quantify the 3D structure of trabecular bone. A spatial resolution better than 100 μm appears to be critical taking into account the typical dimension of trabeculae, which is 60–300 μm (Griffith and Genant 2008; Adams 2009). Although MDCT is not capable of depicting individual trabeculae, analysis of HR image provides important quantitative information regarding characteristics of the trabecular bone network (Issever et al. 2009; Krebs et al. 2009). HR MDCT is associated with patient effective doses of the order of 3000 μSv (Ito et al. 2005; Graeff et al. 2007).

During the past years, strategies have been developed for CT to deliver the lowest radiation dose to the patient necessary to obtain the information needed. Optimization of acquisition parameters (kVp, mAs, pitch, and beam collimation) may lead to a substantial decrease in patient dose from a CT examination. The use of 80 kVp for 2D QCT significantly decreases dose because of the quadratic

relationship between patient dose and tube potential. An increase in tube current will proportionally increase patient dose. MDCT scanners allow automatic exposure control as the tube rotates around the patient and along z-axis. Studies have shown that the use of these tools is associated with 10–53 % reduction in tube current for adult patients and 26–43 % for pediatric patients (Greess et al. 1999, 2000, 2004 Hundt et al. 2005; Tack et al. 2003; Das et al. 2005; Gies et al. 1999; Papadakis et al. 2008). A recent study has shown that the reduction in the modulation mA may be considered as a rough approximation of the patient effective dose reduction (Papadakis et al. 2011).

The length of the acquisition should be minimal. To reconstruct the first and last slice of imaged volume of a helical CT acquisition, reconstruction algorithms require a number of extra rotations. During these additional rotations patient tissues beyond the boundaries of the area to be imaged are exposed to radiation. This feature of helical scanners is known as z overscanning. The effect of z overscanning on patient effective dose is described in detail in recent publications (Tzedakis et al. 2005, 2007). Users should maximize the distance between the boundaries of the area to be imaged and radiosensitive organs. To avoid z overscanning, axial acquisition should be selected instead of helical acquisition. Manufacturers have developed recently adaptive dose shields to reduce the effect of z overscanning (Deak et al. 2009).

2.5.5 HR Peripheral QCT

HR peripheral QCT (HR p-QCT) is a new imaging technique that assesses BMD and trabecular and cortical structural bone parameters of the radius and tibia in vivo. To improve image quality an X-ray tube with 80 μm focal spot size is employed. The spatial resolution of this technique permits quantification of bone structure characteristics since the nominal isotropic pixel dimension is 82 μm (field-of-view 12.6 cm, matrix size 1536 × 1536). Typical exposure parameters for acquiring data are 60 kVp, 900 μA and the total acquisition time is 2.8 min. Several studies have focused on this method recently to investigate bone microstructure (Burrows et al. 2010; Bacchetta et al. 2010; Rizzoli et al. 2012). HR p-QCT is a low-dose method for evaluation of bone status. The effective dose from HR p-QCT examinations is lower than 10 μSv (Engelke et al. 2008; Burrows et al. 2010).

2.5.6 Micro CT

High resolution anatomical information can be obtained using μCT and synchrotron CT usually in vitro or for small animal studies. This technology is based on principles similar to CT used in everyday clinical practice. The most important advantage of μCT systems is that acquisition of CT slices with a nominal spatial resolution to the order of down to 1 μm can be obtained. To achieve this spatial resolution, the field of measurement is much smaller than that used by clinical CT systems. As a consequence, this technology is limited to in vitro and small animal imaging because of the small bore size. A very small X-ray tube focus size is also needed to improve image quality. HR images have been used to resolve individual trabeculae and examine properties of the trabecular bone network in a manner analogous to that of histomorphometry. Furthermore, μCT has served as a gold standard to validate results of other methods (Krebs et al. 2009).

In μCT, the small tube focus size results in significantly lower X-ray tube output power. This in turn leads to prolonged acquisition times. A moderate to high radiation dose is associated with each μCT. Repeated imaging may damage organs and tissues and may have effects on the skeletal growth of living animals. Examining doses and radiation effects in different species provides information about the number of examinations each animal can undergo during its experimental lifetime. Organ radiation doses range from several mGy to a few hundreds mGy, depending upon the device model, imaging geometry, imaging protocol and method of dose estimation (Klinck et al. 2008; Brouwers et al. 2007; Obenaus and Smith 2004). Boone et al. provided normalized data for dose estimation over a range of mouse imaging geometries (Boone et al. 2004).

2.6 Occupational Radiation Doses in Bone Densitometry

During a DXA examination the patient becomes a source of scattered radiation when the X-ray beam passes through body. Assuming a workload of 20 patients per day, the annual dose at 1 m from the central axis of the examination table ranges from about 100 μSv to 1500 μSv (Larkin et al. 2008; Sheahan et al. 2005). These dose levels are much lower than the annual dose limit for staff of 20 mSv/year (International Commission on Radiological Protection 2007). Methods used to reduce patient dose will also reduce occupational dose. Additional techniques can be used to reduce staff exposure. The most effective way for the staff to reduce occupational dose from DXA is to remain as far from the patient as possible during X-ray exposure. According to inverse square law, if distance is doubled, beam intensity will decrease by a factor of four. Manufacturers provide data about the intensity and distribution of scattered radiation around the examination table (isodose curves). The intensity and distribution of scattered radiation depend on many parameters including exposure parameters, patient size and the use of shielding. Isodose curves should be taken into account to limit the risk of radiation exposure in the workplace. Installation of a DXA device requires a room with adequate size (15–20 m^2) to ensure that the location of the operator is at least 2 m from the patient. In a confined space, protective shield for the operator's console may be required for fan-beam systems. Occasionally, wall shielding may be necessary for fan-beam devices to ensure that they operate within dose limits. Certified radiation experts should assess shielding requirements and local radiation protection requirements must be strictly followed. Parameters to be taken into account in the design of protective shielding include the model of DXA device, maximum workload, the distance of the wall from the patient, the material of the walls, and the occupancy of the adjoining areas.

The ICRP has recommended a dose limit of 1 mGy to the conceptus during the remainder of pregnancy of a declared pregnant worker (International Commission on Radiological Protection 2000). Conceptus dose is usually estimated using a personal radiation meter placed on the mother's abdomen.

2.7 Radiation Protection of Comforters

Staff should not hold a patient during an X-ray based imaging technique used in osteoporosis. Comforters and carers are persons assisting children or incapable adult patients during radiation exposure. In many cases comforters are friends or relatives of the patient. These individuals are willingly and voluntarily exposed to ionizing radiation to help and support the patient. Comforters and carers should be informed of the radiation risk involved. Radiation dose to a supporter from a DXA examination performed on a patient can be estimated, for the purposes of risk assessment, using isodose maps. Measures such as the use of protective clothing should be taken to reduce exposure of these individuals.

2.8 Radiation Protection in Bone Densitometry Research

Sometimes volunteers accept to undergo a bone densitometry examination which involves exposure to ionizing radiation during the course of medical research. In these cases, the risks and benefits from the procedure must be considered and the research study should be undertaken after approval by ethics committees and/or competent authority (European Commission 1998). The European Commission guidance on medical exposures in medical and biomedical research states that 'investigators should seek relevant information on previous radiation doses in order to identify individuals who repeatedly take part in research projects which expose them to risks including those of ionizing radiation exposures. The pre-existing and proposed risks should both be explained' (European Commission 1998).

Regarding pregnancy and biomedical research involving radiation exposure, ICRP discourages involvement of pregnant individuals in such research. In publication 84 ICRP states that 'Pregnant women should not be involved in biomedical research projects involving radiation exposure unless the pregnancy itself is central to the research and only if alternative techniques involving less risk cannot be used. Even in such a situation, there remains a very difficult ethical issue if a pregnant female receives radiation exposure while serving as a control subject in a research project' (International Commission on Radiological Protection 2000).

3 Quality Assurance in Bone Densitometry

QA in bone densitometry is 'all those organized actions necessary to (a) maintain adequate equipment performance with minimum exposure and (b) assure that adequate diagnostic information is provided at the lowest possible cost' (Damilakis and Guglielmi 2010). Quality control (QC) is a program that periodically tests the performance of bone densitometry devices to ensure they are operating at acceptable level. If the performance is suboptimal, steps must be taken to correct the problem. Therefore, QC focuses on bone densitometry equipment while QA is a wider term and includes all these activities needed to provide confidence that every aspect of work in a bone densitometry unit will fulfill requirements for quality. This part of the chapter focuses on the main aspects of QA in bone densitometry and describes QC tests that can be adapted to any DXA device.

3.1 Quality Assurance Program

A continuing QA program is of great importance for bone densitometry. QA program should include policies and guidelines, acceptance tests, QC tests, maintenance procedures, education, and training. The development of a series of policies and guidelines for QA in a bone densitometry facility is an important step toward implementation of an effective QA program. A QA manual should include staff responsibilities, policy for the purchase of new bone densitometry equipment, specifications of the examinations performed in adult and pediatric patients, QC and audit processes, strategies for minimizing exposure to patients and staff, policy for staff education, and policy for record keeping. The selection of proper bone densitometry equipment is very important to the production of a quality examination. Over the past decade, several noninvasive devices have been developed for the assessment of bone status. DXA measurement of the spine and femur is the gold standard for BMD measurement. For these measurements, central DXA devices are used. QCT packages are offered by manufacturers as CT scanner accessories for the measurement of spine and hip BMD. Peripheral DXA or QUS devices can be used to screen for low bone mass. The technical specifications of these devices or accessories should reflect the facility's clinical requirements. More information about specifications of bone densitometry equipment can be found in a previous publication (Damilakis and Guglielmi 2010).

3.2 Cross-Calibration

BMD measured on a DXA device cannot be compared with BMD measured on a different device due to differences in DXA geometry and design, differences in calibration standards, and differences in algorithms used for image processing and BMD calculation. BMD measurements from different manufacturers can differ by 15 % (Gundry et al. 1990; Pocock et al. 1992). Thus, standardization efforts are necessary to reduce differences between DXA devices.

In vivo cross-calibration is the best way to ensure that BMD measured on one DXA instrument is comparable with that from another. Alternatively, phantoms such as the European spine phantom or the GE-Lunar aluminum spinal phantom can be used for in vitro cross-calibration. Equations have been derived for the conversion of manufacturer-specific BMD to standardized BMD (Steiger 1995; Hanson 1997; International Committee for Standards in Bone Measurement 1997; Hui et al. 1997). Standardized values can reduce the differences between DXA devices made by different manufacturers to <6 %. Data provided to solve this comparability problem have been derived using pencil-bean DXA devices. A recent study examined whether the standardization equations derived from pencil beam DXA systems are still appropriate for modern DXA devices (Fan et al. 2010). This study found that standardized BMD values were equivalent within 1.0 % for hip but were statistically significantly different for spine on the Hologic Delphi and GE-Lunar Prodigy DXA systems. Therefore, there is a need to update standardization formulas with DXA technological advances. In general, use of different equipment to longitudinally monitor the BMD of a patient is not recommended.

Comparability of BMD values between different CT scanners is a concern related also to the interpretation of QCT results. The European spine phantom has been used as a tool for standardization in spinal BMD measurements by QCT (Kalender et al. 1995).

3.3 Accuracy and Precision

Accuracy is the difference between the true BMD value and the measured BMD value and is expressed in terms of accuracy error. Accuracy error (%) is given by

$$\%\text{Accuracy} = \frac{(\text{True BMD} - \text{Measured BMD})}{\text{True BMD}} \cdot 100 \quad (7)$$

Precision measures the reproducibility of a bone densitometry method and is usually expressed in terms of the coefficient of variation (%CV). The %CV is given by

$$\%CV_p = \frac{SD_p}{\overline{x_p}} \cdot 100 \quad (8)$$

where $\overline{x_p}$ is the mean BMD value and SD_p is the standard deviation of BMD measurements performed in a phantom or in a patient p

$$SD_p = \sqrt{\frac{\sum_{i=1}^{n_p} (x_{ip} - \overline{x_p})}{n_p - 1}} \quad (9)$$

where x_{ip} is the value of the ith BMD measurement, $\overline{x_p}$ is the mean BMD, and n_p is the number of BMD measurements.

The accuracy of a bone densitometry method is determined by measuring cadaveric bone specimens. DXA devices are calibrated so that the measured bone mineral content in bone specimens matches specimens' ash weight. The accuracy errors of DXA devices are mainly due to the inhomogeneous distribution of adipose tissue in the body. Accuracy of DXA devices is better than 10 % (Kanis et al. 1994). This level of accuracy is sufficient taking into account that for the distribution of bone density in healthy individuals of the same age and sex a standard deviation of about 30 % is typical (Kalender 2005). The accuracy errors

of QCT are due to the presence of marrow fat, partial volume, and beam hardening effects. Accuracy of QCT ranges between 5 and 15 % (Adams 2009).

The short-term in vivo precision of DXA measurements is 1–2.5 % (Adams 2008). A wide range of parameters influences precision including site of measurement, age, and clinical status of the patient, and skill and training of technical staff performing the DXA. Precision is better at the spine than the hip. Precision errors affect the use of DXA when measuring change in BMD$_a$ in longitudinal studies; the smallest change in BMD$_a$ that is statistically significant is known as least significant change (LSC) and is given by

$$\text{LSC} = 2.8 \cdot (\%CV) \quad (10)$$

Intervals of at least 18–24 months between DXA are required to measure significant changes.

For each DXA device, a precision study should be performed including estimation of in vitro and in vivo precision. To estimate in vitro short-term precision, the manufacturer's calibration phantom should be scanned several times without repositioning. From these measurements, precision is estimated in terms of SD or CV Eqs. (8) and (9). In routine QA, a phantom scan is performed daily and the in vitro long-term precision is estimated by the QA software of the DXA device. In vivo short-term precision includes errors due to patient repositioning and movement. Precision is dependent on population age and health status; therefore, it should be determined on a well-defined group of individuals, for example young healthy subjects or postmenopausal osteoporotic female patients. All individuals must give their voluntary informed consent for participation in the precision study. For a specific skeletal site, two or three BMD$_a$ measurements should be performed in 30 or 15 patients, respectively. For each individual, measurements should be performed within a short period of time, i.e., the same day or within a few days, to exclude the possibility of a true change in BMD$_a$. To obtain independent measurements, individuals should be repositioned between measurements. The combined precision is given by the root mean square (RMS) SD:

$$SD_{\text{RMS}} = \sqrt{\frac{\sum_{p=1}^{q} SD_p^2}{q}} \quad (11)$$

where q is the number of patients.
The RMS CV is given by

$$CV_{\text{RMS}} = \sqrt{\frac{\sum_{p=1}^{q} CV_p^2}{q}} \quad (12)$$

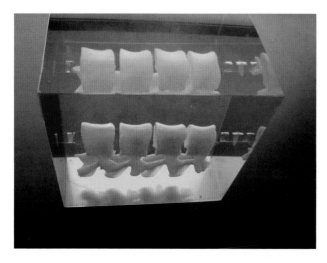

Fig. 6 A spine phantom used for routine DXA quality control tests, developed by Hologic

Long-term in vivo precision includes short-term in vivo precision errors and errors related to long-term densitometer stability. A study has shown that the long-term CVs were about twice the short CVs for two Hologic scanners i.e., the fan-beam QDR 4500 A and the pencil-beam QDR 1000 W (Tothill and Hannan 2007).

Precision of QCT depends upon many parameters such as beam hardening, patient position, and patient size. The precision of QCT in vivo is 2–4 %. A recent study showed that with 3D QCT in vivo precision errors of 1–1.5 % for trabecular and 2.5–3 % for cortical bone can be obtained in postmenopausal women (Engelke et al. 2009a, b). Boutroy et al. have evaluated the short-term precision of a HR pQCT system (Boutroy et al. 2005). They found that reproducibility of measurements was 0.7–1.5 % for total, trabecular, and cortical densities and 2.5–4.4 % for trabecular architecture. Several QUS devices have been developed for the assessment of bone status. The short-term in vivo precision of BUA ranges from about 2 % to about 3 % depending upon the QUS device and the site of measurement. This reproducibility is from six to nine times larger than the average annual loss rate in postmenopausal women. The corresponding precision for SOS is 0.3–1.5 %, which is about two to eight times larger than the average annual loss rate in postmenopausal individuals (Damilakis et al. 2007).

3.4 Quality Control Tests

A QC program is needed for CT systems to evaluate accuracy, reproducibility, patient safety, and personnel safety. This is important not only for routine examinations performed on these scanners but also for bone densitometry procedures. Routine monitoring of CT equipment parameters

is performed to achieve high quality images with as low a dose as reasonably practicable. QUS scanners require regular QC tests performed using tools and phantoms to ensure the reliability of results. Information about the testing procedures and the equipment required to develop a QC program for CT and QUS can be found in the literature (Seeran 2001; Fuerst et al. 1999). QC tests for DXA scanners are proposed in this section.

TEST 1. Calibration—In vitro reproducibility

Equipment. A phantom provided by the manufacturer of DXA device. These phantoms contain tissue equivalent materials. Figure 6 shows a spine phantom developed by Hologic and Fig. 7 shows a calibration phantom developed by GE-Lunar.

Measurement. The phantom is scanned at a position defined by the manufacturer. The user follows the manufacturer's instructions to measure BMD. Simultaneously with BMD measurements, additional tests are usually performed to test mechanical and electronic parts of the DXA system. The long-term precision in terms of SD or CV and a summary of test results is reported in the QC report. Figure 8 shows QC results from a GE Lunar DXA device.

Acceptance limits. The QC plot provides a pass/fail indication.

Frequency. Daily before patients' examinations.

TEST 2. Linearity

Equipment. A phantom provided by the manufacturer of DXA device. Figure 9 shows the aluminum spine phantom developed by GE Lunar. This phantom consists of four rectangular sections simulating vertebrae with a range of BMD values to test linearity.

Measurement. The phantom is placed in a water bath. An acquisition is performed using the spine protocol. The relationship between measured BMD and nominal BMD values is examined using linear regression analysis.

Acceptance limits. The measured BMD values are compared with the nominal values provided by the manufacturer. The percentage difference between each value and the corresponding nominal value should be <5 %.

Frequency. Weekly

TEST 3. X-ray tube output

Equipment. A radiation dosimeter with 180 cm^3 ionization chamber or an X-ray multimeter with a solid state detector designed for low-dose measurements.

Measurement. The detector is centered in the radiation field. An acquisition is performed using the spine protocol to measure the X-ray tube output. Five measurements should be performed to calculate reproducibility (%CV). This procedure is repeated to estimate reproducibility for all protocols.

Acceptance limits. The percentage difference between each value and the corresponding nominal value should be <15 %. The reproducibility should be better than 5 %.

Fig. 7 A calibration phantom used for daily quality control tests by GE Lunar (*left*) and a projection radiograph of the calibration phantom showing the internal structures (*right*)

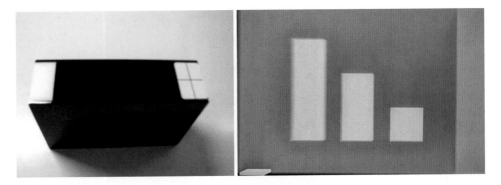

Frequency. Biannually and after maintenance

TEST 4. Half value layer

Equipment. A radiation dosimeter with 6 cm^3 ionization chamber or an X-ray multimeter with a solid state detector designed for low dose measurements and a set of aluminum filters.

Measurement. The X-ray tube output is measured with no attenuator in the beam. The measurement is repeated by adding increasing thicknesses of aluminum until the dose falls to below 50 % of the unattenuated value. The relationship between output and thickness of aluminum added is examined by plotting a graph.

Acceptance limits. The estimated HVL is compared with the value provided by the manufacturer. The HVL should be >2.5 mm Al. In practice, most models exceed 3.0 mm Al HVL.

Frequency. Annually or after maintenance

TEST 5. Kerma-Area Product

Equipment. A radiation dosimeter with 180 cm^3 ionization chamber or an X-ray multimeter with a solid state detector designed for low dose measurements and a 20 cm thick block of tissue equivalent material to provide backscattering radiation.

Measurement. An acquisition of the block is performed using the spine protocol. The detector is centered in the radiation field to measure the entrance dose. Kerma-area product is calculated by multiplying entrance dose with field size. This procedure is repeated to estimate kerma-area product for all protocols.

Acceptance limits. See acceptance limits for tests 3 and 6.

Frequency. Annually or after maintenance

TEST 6. Radiation Field Size

Equipment. An X-ray film cassette or CR plate

Measurement. An acquisition is performed using the spine protocol with the X-ray cassette (or CR plate) placed on the patient table. The radiation produces a dark area on the film that indicates where the radiation struck the film. The length and width values of exposed area are recorded. This procedure is repeated using other protocols to test different field sizes.

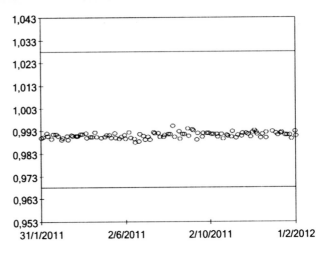

Fig. 8 Quality control daily results from a GE Lunar DXA device

Acceptance limits. The difference between each value and the corresponding nominal value should not be >1 cm.

Frequency. Annually and after maintenance

TEST 7. Fan Angle

Equipment. Two X-ray film cassettes or CR plates

Measurement. An acquisition is performed using the spine protocol with an X-ray cassette (or CR plate) placed on the patient table and another cassette at h cm (∼ 40 cm) above cassette A. An acquisition is performed so that radiation produces a narrow dark band on each film (Fig. 10). The width value of exposed areas is recorded. The fan angle φ is given by

$$\tan \varphi = \frac{\text{width difference}}{h} \qquad (13)$$

Acceptance limits. The difference between estimated angle and the corresponding nominal value should not be >10 %.

Frequency. Annually and after maintenance

TEST 8. Spatial resolution

Equipment. A resolution test pattern and a 20 cm thick block of tissue equivalent material.

Measurement. An acquisition is performed using the spine protocol with the test pattern placed on the patient

Fig. 9 A DXA acquisition of the aluminum spine phantom developed by GE Lunar (*left*) and the aluminum spine phantom (*right*)

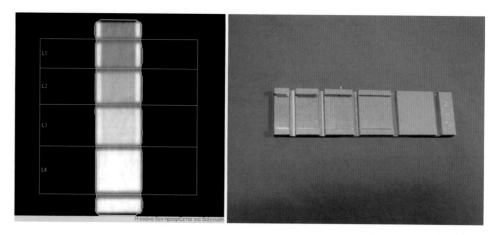

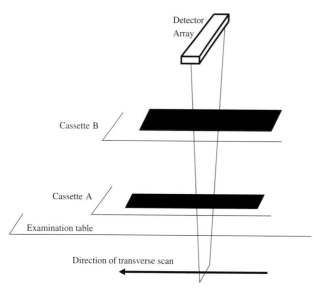

Fig. 10 Schematic diagram of the set up used for fan angle measurement in a GE Lunar Prodigy DXA device. The fan beam is oriented parallel to the long axis of the patient body. A narrow dark band is produced on films as the X-ray beam moves toward the transverse direction

Measurement. The phantom is placed on the patient table to provide radiation scatter and an acquisition is performed. The exposure rate is measured at several locations, paying particular attention to control panel, and to locations where personnel might stand during an examination. Measurements are repeated for different acquisition modes.

Acceptance limits. Measurements should be compared with data specified by the manufacturer. The difference between measured values and corresponding values provided by the manufacturer should not be >10 %.

Frequency. Annually and after maintenance

3.5 Education and Training of Health Professionals in Bone Densitometry

Each bone densitometry unit should have a team made-up of qualified health care professionals who have undergone specialized training in bone densitometry. High standard training programs are the key prerequisites to ensure excellence in diagnosis of osteoporosis. Diagnostic radiologists, radiologic technologists, maintenance engineers, nurses, medical physicists, and referring physicians should participate in continuing education programs adapted to their specialty to maintain and expand their knowledge in osteoporosis. Scientific societies and international organizations have an important role in the promotion, organization, and implementation of training activities in bone densitometry. The International Society for Clinical Densitometry provides educational courses in bone densitometry and vertebral fracture assessment and allows the certification of the training for the attendants (International Society for Clinical Densitometry 2012). The International Osteoporosis Foundation organizes educational and training courses on osteoporosis for physicians and other health professionals (International Osteoporosis Foundation 2012). The American College of Radiology (ACR) has developed practice guidelines and technical standards including

table. The number of resolvable groups of lines is scored from the display. The measurement is repeated with the resolution test object placed at 15 cm above patient table surface. This procedure is repeated using other protocols to test image quality using different tube current load. Images should be printed for future reference.

Acceptance limits. Baseline measurements should be established during acceptance testing. Subsequent tests should be compared with this baseline.

Frequency. Biannually and after maintenance

TEST 9. Room safety

Equipment. A survey meter with a large volume ion chamber designed to be used in diagnostic X-ray suites for low-level radiation monitoring and an anthropomorphic phantom or 20 cm thick water phantom or 20 cm block of tissue equivalent material.

qualifications and responsibilities of professionals in bone densitometry devices (American College of Radiology 2008). Additionally, ACR has recently published guidelines for the development of the science of radiology and encourages continuing education for radiologists and medical physicists (ACR 2011). The European Commission program SENTINEL has developed training syllabi in radiation protection and QA for DXA (O'Connor et al. 2008). The American Society of Radiologic Technologists has released the Bone Densitometry Curriculum, which provides essential components of a bone densitometry educational program designed for technologists involved in bone densitometry units (American Society of Radiologic Technologists 2009).

4 Conclusion

The patient effective dose from DXA examinations of the spine or hip performed on adults using fan-beam devices is up to 15 µSv. DXA examinations performed in children and adolescents must be adjusted based on the body size of the patient. The dose from bone densitometry techniques performed at peripheral sites (forearm DXA, pQCT and QCT at the forearm using whole-body MDCT) is negligible (i.e. <10 µSv). This dose level is comparable to daily natural background radiation. Patient dose from 2D spine QCT ranges from 60 to 300 µSv. The dose from a lateral radiograph of the thoracic and lumbar spine is about 300 µSv. Morphometric X-ray absorptiometry is associated with considerably lower effective dose to the patient i.e., from 2 to 50 µSv. Spine MDQCT, hip MDQCT and HR MDCT for evaluation of bone microstructure is associated with doses of 1000–3000 µSv. The necessity for justification of each bone densitometry examination and the optimal use of equipment and techniques is a critical issue that deserves attention. The establishment of a QA program is of great importance for all bone densitometry facilities.

5 Key Points

- The effective dose associated with DXA examinations of the spine or hip performed on adult patients using fan-beam devices is up to 15 µSv. The actual dose depends on several parameters including the model of the DXA equipment and the acquisition protocol used during the examination.
- DXA examinations performed in children must be adjusted based on the size of the child's body. Pediatric DXA protocols and dose-saving tools must be used during pediatric DXA examinations to reduce patient dose.

- Patient doses from 2D QCT examinations have been reported to be 60–300 µSv. The 3D MDQCT protocols of spine and hip provide an effective dose of 1500 µSv and 2900 µSv, respectively.
- The effective dose from HR p-QCT examinations is lower than 10 µSv.
- Patient dose associated with morphometric X-ray absorptiometry ranges from 2 to 50 µSv.
- The effective dose from a radiograph performed for assessment of osteoporotic fractures is considerably higher than morphometric X-ray absorptiometry.
- Manufacturers provide data about the intensity and distribution of scattered radiation around the examination table (isodose curves). This information can be used for anticipation of occupational exposure.
- Quality assurance in bone densitometry ensures that adequate diagnostic information is provided with the least possible radiation exposure of the patient and staff at the lowest possible cost.
- Quality control tests for DXA and other bone densitometry equipment should be performed to ensure that devices are operating according to specifications.

References

Adams JE (2008) Dual-energy X-ray absorptiometry. In: Grampp S (ed) Radiology of osteoporosis, 2nd edn. Springer, New York, pp 105–124

Adams JE (2009) Quantitative computed tomography. Eur J Radiol 71:415–424

American College of Radiology (2008) Practice guidelines for the performance of dual-energy X-ray absorptiometry (DXA). In: Practice guidelines and technical standards, pp 1–10. Available via http://www.acr.org/SecondaryMainMenuCategories/quality_safety/guidelines/dx.asp. Accessed 26 March 2012

American College of Radiology (2011) ACR practice guideline for continuing medical education (CME), pp. 1–3. Available via http://www.acr.org/SecondaryMainMenuCategories/quality_safety/guidelines/cme/cme.aspx. Accessed 23 March 2012

American Society of Radiologic Technologists (2009) Bone densitometry curriculum Albuquerque (NM). Am Soc Radiol Technol 1–70

Bacchetta J, Boutroy S, Vilayphiou N et al (2010) Early impairment of trabecular microarchitecture assessed with HR-pQCT in patients with stage II–IV chronic kidney disease. J Bone Miner Res 25:849–857

Bauer JS, Muller D, Ambekar A et al (2006) Detection of osteoporotic vertebral fractures using multidetector CT. Osteoporos Int 17:608–615

Bezakova E, Collins PJ, Beddoe AH (1997) Absorbed dose measurements in dual energy X-ray absorptiometry (DXA). Br J Radiol 70:172–179

Blake GM, Rea JA, Fogelman I (1997) Vertebral morphometry studies using dual-energy X-ray absorptiometry. Semin Nucl Med 27:276–290

Blake G, Naeem M, Boutros M (2006) Comparison of effective dose to children and adults from dual X-ray absorptiometry examinations. Bone 38:935–942

Boone JM, Velazquez O, Cherry SR (2004) Small-animal X-ray dose from micro-CT. Mol Imaging 3:149–158

Boutroy S, Bouxsein ML, Munoz F, Delmas PD (2005) In vivo assessment of trabecular bone microarchitecture by high-resolution peripheral quantitative computed tomography. J Clin Endocrinol Metab 90:6508–6515

Brouwers JE, van Rietbergen B, Huiskes R (2007) No effects of in vivo micro-CT radiation on structural parameters and bone marrow cells in proximal tibia of Wistar rats detected after eight weekly scans. J Orthop Res 25:1325–1332

Burrows M, Liu D, McKay H (2010) High resolution peripheral QCT imaging of bone micro-structure in adolescents. Osteoporos Int 21:515–520

Cawte SA, Pearson D, Green DJ, Maslanka WB, Miller CG, Rogers AT (1999) Cross-calibration, precision and patient dose measurements in preparation for clinical trials using dual energy X-ray absorptiometry of the lumbar spine. Br J Radiol 72:354–362

Damilakis J, Guglielmi G (2010) Quality assurance and dosimetry in bone densitometry. Radiol Clin N Am 48:629–640

Damilakis J, Perisinakis K, Vrahoriti H, Kontakis G, Varveris H, Gourtsoyiannis N (2002) Embryo/fetus radiation dose and risk from dual X-ray absorptiometry examinations. Osteoporos Int 13:716–722

Damilakis J, Maris T, Karantanas A (2007) An update on the assessment of osteoporosis using radiologic techniques. Eur Radiol 17:1591–1602

Damilakis J, Adams J, Guglielmi G, Link T (2010a) Radiation exposure in X-ray-based imaging techniques in osteoporosis. Eur Radiol 20:2707–2714

Damilakis J, Perisinakis K, Tzedakis A, Papadakis A, Karantanas A (2010b) Radiation dose to the conceptus from multidetector CT during early gestation: a method that allows for variations in maternal body size and conceptus position. Radiology 257:483–489

Das M, Mahnken AH, Muhlenbruch G et al (2005) Individually adapted examination protocols for reduction of radiation exposure for 16-MDCT chest examinations. Am J Roentgenol 184:1437–1443

Deak PD, Langner O, Lell M, Kalender WA (2009) Effects of adaptive section collimation on patient radiation dose in multisection spiral CT. Radiology 252:140–147

Deak PD, Smal Y, Kalender WA (2010) Multisection CT protocols: sex- and age-specific conversion factors used to determine effective dose from dose-length product. Radiology 257:158–166

Engelke K, Adams JE, Armbrecht G et al (2008) Clinical use of quantitative computed tomography and peripheral quantitative computed tomography in the management of osteoporosis in adults: the 2007 ISCD official positions. J Clin Densitom 11:123–162

Engelke K, Libanati C, Liu Y et al (2009a) Quantitative computed tomography (QCT) of the forearm using general purpose spiral whole-body CT scanners: Accuracy, precision and comparison with dual-energy X-ray absorptiometry (DXA). Bone 45:110–118

Engelke K, Mastmeyer A, Bousson V, Fuerst T, Laredo J, Kalender W (2009b) Reanalysis precision of 3D quantitative computed tomography (QCT) of the spine. Bone 44:566–572

European Commission, Radiation Protection 99 (1998) Guidance on medical exposures in medical and biomedical research, Directorate-General Environment. Nuclear Safety and Civil Protection

Fan B, Lu Y, Genant H, Fuerst T, Shepherd J (2010) Does standardized BMD still remove differences between Hologic and GE-Lunar state-of-the-art DXA systems? Osteoporos Int 21:1227–1236

Ferrar L, Jiang G, Adams J, Eastell R (2005) Identification of vertebral fractures: an update. Osteoporos Int 16:717–728

Fuerst T, Njeh C, Hans D (1999) Quality assurance and quality control in quantitative ultrasound. In: Njeh CF, Hans D, Fuerst T, Gluer CC, Genant H (eds) Quantitative ultrasound. Assessment of osteoporosis and bone status, 1st edn. Martin Dunitz, London, pp 163–175

Genant HK, Engelke K, Prevrhal S (2008) Advanced CT bone imaging in osteoporosis. Rheumatology 47:iv9–iv16

Gies M, Kalender WA, Wolf H et al (1999) Dose reduction in CT by anatomically adapted tube current modulation. I. Simulation studies. Med Phys 26:2235–2247

Graeff C, Timm W, Nickelsen TN, Farrerons J et al (2007) Monitoring teriparatide-associated changes in vertebral microstructure by high-resolution CT in vivo: results from the EUROFORS study. J Bone Miner Res 22:1426–1433

Greess H, Wolf H, Baum U et al (1999) Dosage reduction in computed tomography by anatomy-oriented attenuation-based tube-current modulation: the first clinical results. Rofo 170:246–250

Greess H, Wolf H, Baum U et al (2000) Dose reduction in computed tomography by attenuation-based on-line modulation of tube current: evaluation of six anatomical regions. Eur Radiol 10:391–394

Greess H, Lutze J, Nomayr A et al (2004) Dose reduction in subsecond multislice spiral CT examination of children by on-line tube current modulation. Eur Radiol 14:995–999

Griffith J, Genant H (2008) Bone mass and architecture determination: state of the art. Best Pract Res Clin Endocrinol Metab 22:737–764

Gundry CR, Miller CW, Ramos E et al (1990) Dual-energy radiographic absorptiometry of the lumbar spine: clinical experience with two different systems. Radiology 174:539–541

Hanson J (1997) Standardization of femur BMD (letter to the editor). J Bone Miner Res 12:1316–1317

Huda W, Morin RL (1996) Patient doses in bone mineral densitometry. Br J Radiol 69:422–425

Hui SL, Gao S, Zhou XH et al (1997) Universal standardization of bone density measurements: a method with optimal properties for calibration among several instruments. J Bone Miner Res 12:1463–1470

Hundt W, Rust F, Stabler A et al (2005) Dose reduction in multislice computed tomography. J Comput Assist Tomogr 29:140–147

International Commission on Radiological Protection [ICRP publication 103] (2007) Recommendations of the international commission on radiological protection. Ann ICRP 37:1–332

International Commission on Radiological Protection [ICRP publication 84] (2000) Pregnancy and medical radiation. Ann ICRP 30:1–43

International Committee for Standards in Bone Measurement (1997) Standardization of proximal femur bone mineral density (BMD) measurements by DXA. Bone 21:369–370

International Osteoporosis Foundation (2012) Training and education courses. Available via http://www.iofbonehealth.org/bonehealth/training-and-education-courses. Accessed 29 March 2012

International Society for Clinical Densitometry (2012) Education. Available via http://www.iscd.org/Visitors/education/. Accessed 29 March 2012

Issever A, Link T, Kentenich M et al (2009) Assessment of trabecular bone structure using MDCT: comparison of 64- and 320-slice CT using HR-pQCT as the reference standard. Eur Radiol 20:458–468

Ito M, Ikeda K, Nishiguchi M et al (2005) Multidetector row CT imaging of vertebral microstructure for evaluation of fracture risk. J Bone Miner Res 20:1828–1836

Kalender WA (1992) Effective dose values in bone mineral measurements by photon absorptiometry and computed tomography. Osteoporos Int 2:82–87

Kalender W (2005) Computed tomography, fundamentals, system technology, image quality, applications. Publicis Corporate Publishing, Erlangen, pp 209–230

Kalender WA, Felsenberg D, Genant HK et al (1995) The European Spine Phantom—a tool for standardization and quality control in spinal bone mineral measurements by DXA and QCT. Eur J Radiol 20:83–92

Kanis JA, Melton LJ III, Christiansen C et al (1994) The diagnosis of osteoporosis. J Bone Miner Res 9:1137–1141

Khoo BC, Brown K, Cann C et al (2009) Comparison of QCT-derived and DXA-derived areal bone mineral density and T scores. Osteoporos Int 20:1539–1545

Klinck R, Campbell G, Boyd S (2008) Radiation effects on bone architecture in mice and rats resulting from in vivo micro-computed tomography scanning. Med Eng Phys 30:888–895

Krebs A, Graeff C, Frieling I et al (2009) High resolution computed tomography of the vertebrae yields accurate information on trabecular distances if processed by 3D fuzzy segmentation approaches. Bone 44:145–152

Larkin A, Sheahan N, O'Connor U et al (2008) QA/Acceptance testing of DEXA X-ray systems used in bone mineral densitometry. Radiat Prot Dosim 129:279–283

Lespessailles E, Gadois C, Kousiqnian I et al (2008) Clinical interest of bone texture analysis in osteoporosis: a case control multicenter study. Osteoporos Int 19:1019–1028

Lewis MK, Blake GM, Fogelman I (1994) Patient dose in dual X-ray absorptiometry. Osteoporosis Int 4:11–15

Link TM, Koppers BB, Licht T et al (2004) In vitro and in vivo spiral CT to determine bone mineral density: initial experience in patients at risk for osteoporosis. Radiology 231:805–811

Majumdar S, Lin J, Link T et al (1999) Fractal analysis of radiographs: assessment of trabecular bone structure and prediction of elastic modulus and strength. Med Phys 26:1330–1340

Majumdar S, Link TM, Millard J et al (2000) In vivo assessment of trabecular bone structure using fractal analysis of distal radius radiographs. Med Phys 27:2594–2599

Mettler F, Huda W, Yoshizumi T, Mahesh M (2008) Effective doses in radiology and diagnostic nuclear medicine: A catalog. Radiology 248:254–263

National Research Council Committee on the Biological Effects of Ionizing Radiation, Committee to Assess Health Risks from Exposure to Low levels of Ionizing Radiation; Nuclear and Radiation Studies Board, Division on Earth and Life Studies, National Research Council of the National Academies (2006) Health Risks from Exposure to low Levels of Ionizing Radiation: BEIR VII Phase 2. The National Academy Press, Washington

Njeh CF, Samat SB, Nightingale A, McNeil EA, Boivin CM (1997) Radiation dose and in vitro precision in bone mineral density measurement using dual X-ray absorptiometry. Br J Radiol 70:719–727

O'Connor U, Dowling A, Larkin A et al (2008) Development of training syllabi for radiation protection and quality assurance of dual-energy X-ray absorptiometry (DXA) systems. Radiat Prot Dosim 129:211–213

Obenaus A, Smith A (2004) Radiation dose in rodent tissues during micro-CT imaging. J X-ray Sci Tech 12:241–249

Papadakis AE, Perisinakis K, Damilakis J (2008) Automatic exposure control in pediatric and adult multidetector CT examinations: a phantom study on dose reduction and image quality. Med Phys 35:4567–4576

Papadakis AE, Karantanas AH, Papadokostakis G, Petinellis E, Damilakis J (2009) Can abdominal multi-detector CT diagnose spinal osteoporosis? Eur Radiol 19:172–176

Papadakis A, Perisinakis K, Oikonomou I, Damilakis J (2011) Automatic exposure control in pediatric and adult computed tomography examinations. Invest Radiol 46:654–662

Pocock NA, Sambrook PN, Nguyen T et al (1992) Assessment of spinal and femoral bone density by dual X-ray absorptiometry: comparison of Lunar and Hologic instruments. J Bone Miner Res 7:1081–1084

Preston DL, Shimizu Y, Pierce DA, Suyama A, Mabuchi K (2003) Studies of mortality of atomic bomb survivors: report 13—solid cancer and noncancer disease mortality, 1950–1997. Radiat Res 160:381–407

Rizzoli R, Chapurlat R, Laroche J et al (2012) Effects of strontium ranelate and alendronate on bone microstructure in women with osteoporosis. Results of a 2-year study. Osteoporos Int 23:305–315

Seeram E (2001) Computed tomography. physical principles, clinical applications and quality control, 2nd edn. W. B. Saunders, Philadelphia

Sheahan NF, Dowling A, O'Reilly G et al (2005) Commissioning and quality assurance protocol for dual energy X-ray absorptiometry (DEXA) systems. Radiat Prot Dosimetry 117:288–290

Sont WN, Zielinski, Ashmore JM, Jiang H, Krewski D, Fair ME, Band PR, Letourneau EG (2001) First analysis of cancer incidence and occupational radiation exposure based on the national dose registry of Canada. Am J Epidemiol 153:309–318

Steel SA, Baker AJ, Saunderson JR (1998) An assessment of the radiation dose to patients and staff from a lunar expert-xl fan beam densitometer. Physiol Meas 19:17–26

Steiger P (1995) Standardization of measurements for assessing BMD by DXA (letter to the editor). Calcif Tissue Int 57:469

Tack D, De Maertelaer V, Gevenois PA (2003) Dose reduction in multidetector CT using attenuation-based online tube current modulation. Am J Roentgenol 181:331–334

Tothill P, Hannan W (2007) Precision and accuracy of measuring changes in bone mineral density by dual-energy X-ray absorptiometry. Osteoporos Int 18:1515–1523

Tzedakis A, Damilakis J, Perisinakis K, Stratakis J, Gourtsoyiannis N (2005) The effect of z overscanning on patient effective dose from multidetector helical computed tomography examinations. Med Phys 32:1621–1629

Tzedakis A, Perisinakis K, Raissaki M, Damilakis J (2007) The effect of z overscanning on radiation burden of pediatric patients undergoing head CT with multidetector scanners: a Monte Carlo study. Med Phys 33:2472–2478

Vokes T, Bachman D, Baim S et al (2006) Vertebral fracture assessment: the 2005 ISCD official positions. J Clin Densitom 9:37–46

World Nuclear Association. Nuclear Radiation and Health Effects (updated November 2011). Available via http://www.world-nuclear.org/info/inf05.html. Accessed 27 March 2012

Index

Printing: Ten Brink, Meppel, The Netherlands
Binding: Stürtz, Würzburg, Germany